Surgical Critical Care

Editor

JOHN A. WEIGELT

SURGICAL CLINICS
OF NORTH AMERICA

www.surgical.theclinics.com

Consulting Editor
RONALD F. MARTIN

December 2012 • Volume 92 • Number 6

ELSEVIER

1600 John F. Kennedy Blvd., Suite 1800, Philadelphia, PA 19103-2899

http://www.surgical.theclinics.com

SURGICAL CLINICS OF NORTH AMERICA Volume 92, Number 6
December 2012 ISSN 0039–6109, ISBN-13: 978-1-4557-4966-9

Editor: John Vassallo, j.vassallo@elsevier.com

Developmental Editor: Teia Stone

Surgical Clinics of North America (ISSN 0039–6109) is published bimonthly by Elsevier Inc., 360 Park Avenue South, New York, NY 10010-1710. Months of publication are February, April, June, August, October, and December. Business and Editorial Offices: 1600 John F. Kennedy Blvd., Suite 1800, Philadelphia, PA 19103-2899. Periodicals postage paid at New York, NY and additional mailing offices. Subscription prices are $339.00 per year for US individuals, $575.00 per year for US institutions, $166.00 per year for US students and residents, $415.00 per year for Canadian individuals, $714.00 per year for Canadian institutions, $468.00 for international individuals, $714.00 per year for international institutions and $229.00 per year for Canadian and foreign students/residents. To receive student/resident rate, orders must be accompanied by name of affiliated institution, date of term, and the *signature* of program/residency coordinator on institution letterhead. Orders will be billed at individual rate until proof of status is received. Foreign air speed delivery is included in all *Clinics* subscription prices. All prices are subject to change without notice. POSTMASTER: Send address changes to *Surgical Clinics*, Elsevier Health Sciences Division, Subscription Customer Service, 3251 Riverport Lane, Maryland Heights, MO 63043. **Customer Service (orders, claims, online, change of address): Telephone: 1-800-654-2452 (U.S. and Canada); 314-447-8871 (outside U.S. and Canada). Fax: 314-447-8029. E-mail: journalscustomerservice-usa@elsevier.com (for print support); journalsonline support-usa@elsevier.com (for online support).**

Reprints. For copies of 100 or more, of articles in this publication, please contact the Commercial Reprints Department, Elsevier Inc., 360 Park Avenue South, New York, New York 10010-1710. Tel. (212) 633-3812, Fax: (212) 462-1935, e-mail: reprints@elsevier.com.

The Surgical Clinics of North America is also published in Spanish by McGraw-Hill Interamericana Editores S.A., P.O. Box 5-237 06500 Mexico D.F. Mexico; and in Portuguese by Interlivros Edicoes Ltda., Rua Comandante Coelho 1085, CEP 21250, Rio de Janeiro, Brazil; and in Greek by Paschalidis Medical Publications, Athens Greece.

The Surgical Clinics of North America is covered in *MEDLINE/PubMed (Index Medicus), EMBASE/Excerpta Medica, Current Contents/Clinical Medicine, Current Contents/Life Sciences, Science Citation Index*, and *ISI/BIOMED.*

Printed and bound by CPI Group (UK) Ltd, Croydon, CR0 4YY

Transferred to digital print 2012

Contributors

CONSULTING EDITOR

RONALD F. MARTIN, MD
Staff Surgeon, Department of Surgery, Marshfield Clinic, Marshfield, Wisconsin; Clinical
Associate Professor, University of Wisconsin School of Medicine and Public Health,
Madison, Wisconsin; Colonel, Medical Corps, United States Army Reserve

GUEST EDITOR

JOHN A. WEIGELT, MD, DVM, MMA
Milt and Lidy Lunda Aprahamian Professor of Surgery, Department of Surgery; Professor
and Chief, Division of Trauma and Critical Care, Medical College of Wisconsin, Milwaukee,
Wisconsin

AUTHORS

PHILIP S. BARIE, MD, MBA, FIDSA, FCCM, FACS
Professor, Department of Surgery and Public Health, Joan and Sanford I. Weill Medical
College of Cornell University, New York, New York

GREG J. BEILMAN, MD, FACS
Chief, Division of Critical Care and Acute Care Surgery, Professor and Vice-Chair,
Department of Surgery, University of Minnesota, Minneapolis, Minnesota

CIARÁN T. BRADLEY, MD
Department of Surgery, Memorial Sloan-Kettering Cancer Center, New York, New York

KAREN J. BRASEL, MD, MPH
Departments of Surgery, Bioethics and Medical Humanities, Medical College of
Wisconsin, Milwaukee, Wisconsin

PANNA A. CODNER, MD, FACS
Assistant Professor, Division of Trauma and Critical Care, Department of Surgery, Medical
College of Wisconsin, Milwaukee, Wisconsin

RAUL COIMBRA, MD, PhD, FACS
The Monroe E. Trout Professor of Surgery, Executive Vice-Chairman, Chief, Division of
Trauma, Surgical Critical Care, and Burns, Department of Surgery, University of California
San Diego School of Medicine, San Diego, California

TODD W. COSTANTINI, MD
Assistant Professor of Surgery, Division of Trauma, Surgical Critical Care, and Burns,
Department of Surgery, University of California San Diego School of Medicine, San Diego,
California

CHARLES E. EDMISTON Jr, PhD, CIC
Professor of Surgery, Division of Vascular Surgery; Director, Surgical Microbiology Research Laboratory, Department of Surgery, Medical College of Wisconsin; Hospital Epidemiologist, Froedtert Hospital, Milwaukee, Wisconsin

VANESSA P. HO, MD, MPH
Fellow in Surgical Critical Care, Department of Surgery, New Jersey Medical School, University of Medicine and Dentistry of New Jersey, Newark, New Jersey

GALEN HOLMES, MD
Department of Surgery, Ventura County Health Care Agency, Ventura, California

MOLLIE M. JAMES, DO, MPH, FACOS
Assistant Professor, Division of Critical Care and Acute Care Surgery, Department of Surgery, University of Minnesota, Minneapolis, Minnesota

JEREMY S. JUERN, MD
Assistant Professor, Division of Trauma and Critical Care, Department of Surgery, Medical College of Wisconsin, Milwaukee, Wisconsin

LESLIE KOBAYASHI, MD, FACS
Assistant Professor of Surgery, Division of Trauma, Surgical Critical Care, and Burns, Department of Surgery, University of California San Diego School of Medicine, San Diego, California

STEPHEN LANZAROTTI, MD, FACS
Evansville Surgical Associates, Trauma Medical Director, St. Mary's Hospital, Evansville, Indiana

LARRY LINDENBAUM, MD
Assistant Professor, Department of Anesthesiology, Medical College of Wisconsin, Milwaukee, Wisconsin

DAVID J. MILIA, MD
Assistant Professor, Division of Surgery and Trauma Critical Care, Medical College of Wisconsin, Milwaukee, Wisconsin

FREDERICK A. MOORE, MD, FACS, FCCM
Professor and Chief of Acute Care Surgery, Department of Surgery, The University of Florida, Gainesville, Florida

LAURA J. MOORE, MD, FACS
Assistant Professor, Department of Surgery, The University of Texas Health Science Center, Houston, Texas

LENA M. NAPOLITANO, MD, FACS, FCCP, FCCM
Professor of Surgery, Division Chief, Division of Acute Care Surgery [Trauma, Burns, Surgical Critical Care, Emergency Surgery], Director, Trauma and Surgical Critical Care, Associate Chair, Department of Surgery, University of Michigan Health System, Ann Arbor, Michigan

TODD NEIDEEN, MD, MS
Assistant Professor in General Surgery, Division of Trauma and Critical Care Surgery, Medical College of Wisconsin, Milwaukee, Wisconsin

RAM NIRULA, MD
Division of General Surgery, University of Utah School of Medicine, Salt Lake City, Utah

JASMEET S. PAUL, MD
Assistant Professor, Division of Trauma and Critical Care, Department of Surgery, Medical College of Wisconsin, Milwaukee, Wisconsin

SARAH R. PEPPARD, PharmD, BCPS
Assistant Professor of Pharmacy Practice, Concordia University Wisconsin School of Pharmacy, Mequon, Wisconsin

WILLIAM J. PEPPARD, PharmD, BCPS
Surgical Critical Care Pharmacist, Director, Critical Care Residency Program, Department of Pharmacy, Froedtert Hospital, Milwaukee, Wisconsin

TIMOTHY J. RIDOLFI, MD
Department of Surgery, Medical College of Wisconsin, Milwaukee, Wisconsin

JENNIFER ROBERTS, MD
Department of Surgery, Division of Trauma and Surgical Critical Care, Medical College of Wisconsin, Milwaukee, Wisconsin

PETER J. ROSSI, MD, FACS
Assistant Professor of Surgery and Radiology, Division of Vascular Surgery, Department of Surgery, Medical College of Wisconsin, Milwaukee, Wisconsin

LEWIS SOMBERG, MD, FACS
Associate Professor, Division of Trauma Surgery, Medical College of Wisconsin, Milwaukee, Wisconsin

KATHLEEN B. TO, MD
Assistant Professor of Surgery, Division of Acute Care Surgery [Trauma, Burns, Surgical Critical Care, Emergency Surgery], Department of Surgery, University of Michigan Health System, Ann Arbor, Michigan

KENNETH S. WAXMAN, MD
Medical Director of Quality, Ventura County Health Care Agency, Ventura, California

JESSICA L. WEAVER, MD
Department of Surgery, School of Medicine, University of Louisville, Louisville, Kentucky

JOHN A. WEIGELT, MD, DVM, MMA
Milt and Lidy Lunda Aprahamian Professor of Surgery, Department of Surgery; Professor and Chief, Division of Trauma and Critical Care, Medical College of Wisconsin, Milwaukee, Wisconsin

Contents

Improving the quality and safety of intensive care unit (ICU) care in the United States is a significant challenge for the future. Obtaining improvement in systems of care is difficult given the reactionary mode physicians tend to enter when dealing with moment-to-moment crises. It will be important to implement quality and safety measures that are already supported by evidence. Improvement of device safety will be critical to reducing the large number of device-related complications that occur in US ICUs. Prospective collection of adverse events with rigorous analysis will be important to allow systematic errors to be exposed and corrected.

Monitors in the intensive care unit are imperative to taking adequate care of these critically ill patients. Cardiovascular, pulmonary, and neurologic monitors are key to performing these tasks. This article gives an overview of the most common monitors that are used in the intensive care unit.

Several changes in the way patients with hemorrhagic shock are resuscitated have occurred over the past decades, including permissive hypotension, minimal crystalloid resuscitation, earlier blood transfusion, and higher plasma and platelet-to-red cell ratios. Hemostatic adjuncts, such as tranexamic acid and prothrombin complex, and the use of new methods of assessing coagulopathy are also being incorporated into resuscitation of the bleeding patient. These ideas have been incorporated by many trauma centers into institutional massive transfusion protocols, and adoption of these protocols has resulted in improvements in mortality and morbidity. This article discusses each of these new resuscitation strategies and the evidence supporting their use.

Sepsis in the surgical patient continues to be a common and potentially lethal problem. Early identification of patients and timely implementation of evidence-based therapies continue to represent significant clinical challenges for care providers. The implementation of a sepsis screening program in conjunction with protocol for the delivery of evidence-based care and rapid source control can improve patient outcomes. The article provides definitions and guidelines for the screening and management of sepsis and septic shock.

The primary focus of this review is on the cost-effectiveness of critical care. The rapid growth in health care expenditures has engendered careful scrutiny of the practice of medicine with regard not only to effectiveness but also to efficiency. This shift necessitates that physicians understand the effectiveness of their interventions and the cost at which this effectiveness is obtained. Cost-effectiveness and cost-utility analyses have become crucial evaluative tools in medicine. Explicit articulation of comparative cost-effectiveness facilitates the allocation of limited resources. Physicians and policy-makers must evaluate such studies with caution, skepticism, and attention to the methods used.

The treatment of respiratory failure requiring mechanical ventilation has advanced significantly over the last 20 years. The goal of therapy in patients with acute respiratory distress syndrome should be to optimize oxygenation while minimizing the risk of ventilator-induced lung injury and providing adequate ventilation. Appropriate use of ventilation modes and strategies, positive-end expiratory pressure levels, and recruitment maneuvers can improve oxygen delivery. Salvage therapies, such as prone positioning, inhaled epoprostenol and nitric oxide, and high-frequency oscillatory ventilation, have a well-established role in supportive management and are associated with improved oxygenation but not survival.

Weaning from mechanical ventilation is usually straightforward but is occasionally challenging. Sedation must be used at the appropriate times and with appropriate dosing. A protocol that calls for a daily sedation holiday with a spontaneous breathing trial decreases time on the ventilator. Early tracheostomy is beneficial in traumatic brain injury patients. Noninvasive ventilation is most useful in patients with baseline obstructive sleep apnea and chronic obstructive pulmonary disease.

Timing and route of nutrition provided to critically ill patients can affect their outcome. Early enteral nutrition has been shown to decrease specifically infectious morbidity in the critically ill patient. There is a small group of patients who are malnourished on arrival to the intensive care unit and in these patients parenteral nutrition is beneficial.

it even more critical for the ICU practitioner to understand the typical causes of pain in this setting and the applicability of many pain management regimens.

The Institute of Medicine strongly recommends a health care system that supports family members. Nowhere is the need for family-centered care greater than with critically ill patients. Simplistically, family-centered care is primarily about communication. Unfortunately, family perception of communication in the intensive care unit (ICU) is quite poor. This article reviews some strategies to improve communication, including family meetings and family presence at resuscitation. It also highlights some of the areas within the realm of ICU care in which family engagement is particularly important, including advance directives, end-of-life care, brain death, and organ donation.

Initial evaluation of severely injured patients requires an organized, rapid, and thorough evaluation of the patient where life-threatening injuries are identified and treated simultaneously. A case study provides the basis for discussion of the management of the multiply injured trauma patient. The ultimate goal in rehabilitation of a multiply injured patient is to return each patient to as much independent function and ability to contribute to society as possible.

Intra-abdominal infections are a common problem for the general surgeon and major sources of morbidity and mortality in the intensive care unit. Some of these patients present with peritonitis that can rapidly progress to septic shock. The basic principles of care include prompt resuscitation, antibiotics, and source control. This article will use a detailed case study to outline the management of a patient with severe intra-abdominal infection from diverticulitis from initial resuscitation to reconstruction. Components of the Surviving Sepsis Campaign as they pertain to surgical patients are discussed and updated, and the concept of damage control general surgery is applied.

Intra-abdominal hypertension falsely elevates the pulmonary artery pressure. Volumetric pulmonary artery catheter monitoring is an option-for estimating preload in this condition. Treatment of intra-abdominal hypertension begins with medical therapy but once abdominal compartment syndrome develops it requires decompressive laparotomy for definitive management. Pulmonary hypertension reduces cardiac function which may be improved with inotropes that simultaneously reduce pulmonary artery pressure. Oxygenation may be improved with elevated PEEP and FiO_2.

SURGICAL CLINICS OF NORTH AMERICA

**DOWNLOAD
Free App!**

Review Articles
THE CLINICS

NOW AVAILABLE FOR YOUR iPhone and iPad

Foreword
Surgical Critical Care

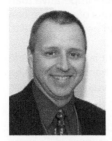

Ronald F. Martin, MD
Consulting Editor

At the time of completion of this issue of the *Surgical Clinics of North America*, we are in series of transitions. I suppose one could always say we are in a series of transitions and be right, but now we seem to be at the confluence of some of the bigger ones. The general election for President and the Congress has not yet been decided but will be by the time you read this. We have not yet gone over the fiscal cliff nor have we avoided it. We really don't know how many Accountable Care Organization applications have or will be approved nor do we know how that will affect our delivery of health care.

On a lesser scale, the *Surgical Clinics of North America* is undergoing a transition; we are changing our cover and over time we will continue to modify our format. The primary reason for these changes is to align our print products and our electronic products better. I would like to assure all that we remain absolutely committed to bringing the best content and best context to the readership as we possibly can in *any* format. The reality of modern information sharing, though, remains that cross-platform capability is critical to serving the needs of the totality of our readership—and that is my primary objective: getting the reader what he or she needs to do the job better. As always, we will want your feedback and observations about how these changes work for you.

For this specific issue, which has been wonderfully orchestrated by Dr Weigelt and his colleagues, we also deal with transitions. One could argue that the 2 areas of greatest change in the near future will be those at each end of the spectrum: primary care and critical care. Primary care changes will affect very large groups of people and will involve large amounts of money based just on the sheer volume of business. The critical care environment will also change as we wrestle with how to manage the sometimes fine lines between doing things to people and doing things for people. The number of patients in the critical care settings are minuscule compared to the general population but the cost per patient is sometimes astronomical. Assuring that we are utilizing resources to good advantage will be necessary for us and scrutinized by others.

Surg Clin N Am 92 (2012) xiii–xiv
http://dx.doi.org/10.1016/j.suc.2012.09.013
0039-6109/12/$ – see front matter © 2012 Elsevier Inc. All rights reserved.

surgical.theclinics.com

As the shift in health cares slowly but inexorably moves away a bit from focusing on just the individual patient and more toward the health of populations, the tensions of how much we expend on care and how effective that care is will increase. The critical care setting is perhaps the ultimate challenge for balancing the needs of the many and the needs of the individual. Under such circumstances, it will be more imperative than ever to have the best understanding of the capabilities and limitations of what we can do for people. Dr Weigelt's format of content plus scenarios should be very helpful to readers of all levels of sophistication for many of these topics.

While it has been said that the only thing that remains constant is change, some changes are good and others, well, perhaps not so much. Yet all change is a learning opportunity. Please let us know how our changes are affecting you. Your input is valued and needed.

Ronald F. Martin, MD
Department of Surgery
Marshfield Clinic
1000 North Oak Avenue
Marshfield, WI 54449, USA

E-mail address:
martin.ronald@marshfieldclinic.org

Preface

Surgical Critical Care

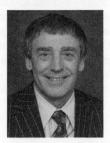

John A. Weigelt, MD, DVM
Guest Editor

The last time I wrote a preface for a book on surgical critical care it was 1996.[1] Our focus stressed areas of the discipline important to surgeons. My goal for this issue of *Surgical Clinics* was similar. I chose topics that surgical patients and their caregivers face everyday. Providing a clinical perspective about critical care topics was my objective as I asked practicing surgical intensivists from around the country to contribute. We added some case studies in critical care that emphasize how many of the principles discussed in various articles are used. I thank all of my authors for providing an up-to-date review of their topic.

An area that is not covered in this treatise is the organizational structure of surgical critical care. I originally thought, as others did, that this was an important topic that needed attention.[2-4] I even thought we could define a best practice to emulate. Alas, I believe there are many ways to provide safe, high-quality, and cost-effective critical care. Additionally, we are in the dawn of a new way to organize medicine as the Patient Protection and Affordable Care Act (ACA) moves forward. The American Association for the Surgery of Trauma has produced a position paper about surgical critical care in the world of ACA.[5] It emphasizes that critically ill surgical patients have better outcomes when cared for by surgeons with critical care training. This report challenges a small workforce of surgeons to embrace their role in improving the quality of care and controlling costs that are increasing despite other hospital costs decreasing. It represents a true challenge!

So what is the future of critical care, especially for surgical patients? It is clear to everyone that the emphasis for the next few years will be on the value of our health care. Value is defined as quality/cost.[6] Cost-effective care will be sought in all areas of medicine, including critical care. Since we are a high cost center, our practices are bound to be scrutinized. We must learn to be more efficient with our resources. How we will accomplish this is unclear, although some suggestions are gaining ground.

Surg Clin N Am 92 (2012) xv–xvii
http://dx.doi.org/10.1016/j.suc.2012.08.020
0039-6109/12/$ – see front matter © 2012 Published by Elsevier Inc.

surgical.theclinics.com

Better admission and discharge criteria will avoid misuse of the critical care resources. Team care will be predominant and will need a crisp definition. Care by a committee of physicians caring for individual organs is not team care and will need to be curtailed if we are to maximize cost effectiveness. Introducing advanced practitioners to the care team is beginning to occur and will probably increase.[7] Use of remote electronic monitoring still remains questionable, but will improve and eventually be accepted.[8,9] Patient-centered care will truly achieve center stage with better engagement of families and patients.[10] Part of this engagement will be better discussions and application of palliative care.[5] Critical care specialists must assist in technology assessment and use. We must demand proper evaluation and proof of benefit before newer devices are introduced into our care plans. Finally, our care environment is extremely complex; maybe we need help in redesigning it to be more efficient and cost effective. Systems modeling and simulation using the domains of ecology, social sciences, economics, engineering, and medicine just might help us achieve a better intensive care unit.[11]

I still believe critical care is a great way to practice medicine. It allows us to assess and treat critically ill patients. Our knowledge focuses on derangements in a patient's normal healthy state. Our interventions correct the derangements, allowing the patient to recover and return to a functional position in society. This sequence is what the discipline of critical care is all about and when done correctly it is always fulfilling. While we have our successes and failures, we continue to bring our knowledge to the bedside to advocate for what is best for our patients.

John A. Weigelt, MD, DVM
Department of Surgery
Medical College of Wisconsin
9200 W. Wisconsin Avenue
Milwaukee, WI 53226, USA

E-mail address:
jweigelt@mcw.edu

REFERENCES

1. Weigelt JA. Definition of surgical critical care. In: Weigelt JA, Lewis FR, editors. Surgical Critical Care. 1st ed. Philadelphia, PA: W.B. Saunders Company; 1996. p. 3–6.
2. Pronovost PJ, Thompson DA, Holzmueller CG, et al. The organization of intensive care unit physician services. Crit Care Med 2007;10(35):E1–17.
3. Napolitano LM, Fulda GJ, Davis KA, et al. Challenging issues in surgical critical care, trauma, and acute care surgery: A report from the Critical Care Committee of the American Association for the Surgery of Trauma. J Trauma 2010;69(6):1619–33.
4. Brilli RJ, Spevetz A, Branson RD, et al. Critical care delivery in the intensive care unit: defining clinical roles and the best practice model. Crit Care Med 2001; 29(10):2007–19.
5. Frankel HL, Butler KL, Cuschieri J, et al. The role and value of surgical critical care, an essential component of acute care surgery, in the Affordable Care Act: a report from the Critical Care Committee and Board of Managers of the American Association for the Surgery of Trauma. J Trauma Acute Care Surg 2012;73(1):20–6.
6. Kaplan RS, Porter ME. How to solve the cost crisis in health care. Harv Bus Rev 2011;89(9):46–64.

7. Boyle WA, Beyatte MB, Grabent R. Non physician providers in critical care. http://www.sccm.org/Publications/Critical_Connections/Archives/August2009/Pages/CodingCorner.aspx. Accessed August 21, 2012.
8. Berenson RA, Grossman JM, November EA. Does telemonitoring of patients—the eICU—improve intensive care? Health Affairs 2009;28(5):w937–47.
9. Willmitch B, Golembeski S, Kim SS, et al. Clinical outcomes after telemedicine intensive care unit implementation. Crit Care Med 2012;40(2):450.
10. McCauley K, Irwin RS. Changing the work environment in ICUs to achieve patient-focused care. Chest 2006;130(5):1571–8.
11. Dong Y, Chbat NW, Gupta A, et al. Systems modeling and simulation applications for critical care medicine. Ann Intensive Care 2012;2(18):1–10.

Patient Safety in the Critical Care Environment

Peter J. Rossi, MD[a],*, Charles E. Edmiston Jr, PhD[a,b,c]

KEYWORDS

- Infection control • Isolation • Hand hygiene • Care-bundles • Medical device safety
- Imaging safety • Intensive care

KEY POINTS

- In the United States, more than 5 million patients per year are admitted to the intensive care unit (ICU), composing 30% of the acute care cost or approximately $160 billion per annum nationwide.
- Errors in patient care at some level cause up to 10% of patient fatalities in trauma ICUs in patients with otherwise survivable injuries; estimates are that critically ill patients may suffer up to 1.7 medical errors a day, mostly from medication administration errors.
- It will be of utmost importance to implement quality and safety measures that are already supported by evidence, such as hand hygiene, implementation of evidenced-based care bundles, adequate identification and treatment of health care–acquired infections, and increasing the percentage of patients in ICU settings that are cared for by dedicated intensivists.

INTRODUCTION: CREATING A CULTURE OF SAFETY

In the United States, more than 5 million patients per year are admitted to the intensive care unit (ICU), composing 30% of the acute care cost or approximately $160 billion per annum nationwide.[1] The ICU would intuitively be one of the safest places within the hospital environment; however, the reverse is often true. A recent multinational study found that, on average, 38.8 sentinel events occur per 100 patient ICU days.[2] The genesis for these sentinel events revolves around 2 separate but intertwined factors: the complex interactions between medical/nursing/technician health care professionals and therapeutic intervention per disease entity.[3] The complexity of care within the ICU requires that health care professionals exhibit a transdisciplinary level of competency. This circumstance has lead critical care teams to embrace

The authors have nothing to disclose.
[a] Division of Vascular Surgery, Medical College of Wisconsin, 9200 West Wisconsin Avenue, Milwaukee, WI 53226, USA; [b] Froedtert Hospital, Milwaukee, WI 53226, USA; [c] Surgical Microbiology Research Laboratory, Department of Surgery, Medical College of Wisconsin, Milwaukee, WI 53226, USA
* Corresponding author.
E-mail address: prossi@mcw.edu

evidence-based guidelines that encourage the use of standardized process measures for managing ICU patient populations. For example, the concept of the *care bundle* (aggregated evidence-based interventional practices) has reduced the risk of central line–associated blood stream infections (CLABSIs), ventilator-associated pneumonia (VAP), deep vein thrombosis, and stress ulcers, which are frequent hospital-acquired conditions.[3,4]

In the past decade, creating a safe patient-care environment has placed a spotlight on preventable medical errors within health care organizations. This emphasis, which encompasses a broad spectrum of care, is focused on improving patient outcomes. This commitment to improving the quality of care and creating a safe patient-care environment does not come without a significant investment in both infrastructure and resources. A recent study demonstrated that the implementation of a hospital-wide culture of safety required a significant fiscal investment, suggesting that hospitals with greater financial and institutional resources are more effective at promoting patient safety through effective infection control interventions.[5,6] A pivotal component of effective quality improvement is leadership, that is, a leader who cannot only implement change but who can also anticipate the need for change.[7] Finally, the relationship between leadership, culture of safety, and outcome cannot be dismissed. In a recent study by Huang and colleagues,[8] a lowered perception of management or lowered institutional commitment to safety was independently associated with an increase in both length of stay (LOS) and mortality. Perceptions of management and a safe patient environment for ICUs in the United States were moderately linked to patient outcomes. The concept of a *safety climate* refers to a tangible perception of a strong and proactive organizational commitment to safety, which exists not just for the benefit of patients but also for the staff. The present article reviews several selective patient-care practices that are vulnerable to errors, placing patients at an increased risk for morbidity and death but amendable to selective interventional practices leading to enhanced patient outcomes.

HEALTH CARE–ASSOCIATED INFECTIONS IN THE ICU: EPIDEMIOLOGY OF A PATIENT SAFETY ISSUE

Health care–associated infections (HAIs) adversely impact approximately 5% of hospitalized patients, leading to increased morbidity and death. HAIs are, in fact, the fifth leading cause of death in acute care hospitals.[9] The total economic burden for all HAIs in the acute care environment approaches $20 billion per year. A large number of these events are associated with temporarily placed biomedical devices, such as endotracheal tubes, indwelling urinary catheter, and central venous access devices. The personal and fiscal morbidity associated with these HAIs is significant; a CLABSI is estimated to increase mortality by 18%, increasing ICU LOS on average by 13 days while adding $10 531 to $56 167 to the total hospital cost.[10–12] The risk for infection is actually greater within the ICU patient population. A multi-institutional study revealed that 19% of ICU patients develop an infection sometime during their ICU stay.[13] The microbial pathogens and the percent occurrence of selective HAIs have been documented by the Centers for Disease Control and Prevention's (CDC) National Healthcare Safety Network (**Table 1**).[14] Many of these infections occurring within the ICU pose a significant safety burden to this high-risk patient population. The implementation of evidence-based interventions directed against specific mechanistic components of selective HAIs offers the best opportunity for reducing risk and creating a safe and effective health care environment.

Table 1
Microbial pathogens associated with HAIs in critical care patients

Pathogen	Overall Percentage (%)	CLABSI (%)	CAUTI (%)	VAP (%)	SSI (%)
CNS	15.3	34.1	2.5	1.3	13.7
Staphylococcus aureus	14.5	9.9	2.2	24.4	30.0
Enterococcus faecalis	3.5	5.5	3.6	0.4	2.8
Enterococcus faecium	5.6	8.2	6.0	0.6	4.9
Candida albicans	6.8	5.9	14.5	2.4	1.6
Candida spp	3.9	5.9	6.5	0.3	0.4
Escherichia coli	9.6	2.7	21.4	4.6	9.6
Pseudomonas aeruginosa	7.9	3.1	10.0	16.3	5.6
Klebsiella Pneumonia	5.8	4.9	7.7	7.5	3.0
Enterobacter spp	4.8	3.9	4.1	8.4	4.2
Acinetobacter baumannii	2.7	2.2	1.2	8.4	0.6
Klebsiella oxytoca	1.1	0.9	0.9	2.2	0.7
Other	15.6	10.5	14.1	23.1	19.4

Abbreviations: CAUTI, catheter-associated urinary tract infection; CNS, coagulase negative staphylococci; SSI, surgical site infection.

Adapted from Hidron AL, Edward JR, Patel J, et al. National Healthcare Safety Network team; participating healthcare network facilities. NHSN annual update: antimicrobial-resistant pathogens associated with healthcare-associated infection: annual summary of data reported to the National Healthcare Safety Network at the Centers for Disease Control and Prevention, 2006–2007. Infect Control Hosp Epidemiol 2008;29:996–1011.

IMPLEMENTING EVIDENCE-BASED PROCESS MEASURES: PROMOTING EFFECTIVE INFECTION CONTROL INITIATIVES
Care Bundles

The concept of the care bundle has become central to mitigating the risk of HAIs within the ICU environment. The care bundle was developed in an effort to move away from dependency on individual knowledge, motivation, and skills and focusing instead on a systematic approach for delivering structured care. The care bundle is comprised of a series of separate but interrelated elements that flow in a cohesive manner and have evidence-based validation for improving patient outcomes.[15] An interesting observation in the development of an early care bundle to reduce the risk of VAP found that the process as designed did not immediately result in a decreased risk of VAP in a trauma unit. It was only after a process tool was put into place that measured the daily compliance to the bundle that the rate of VAP actually declined in the trauma ICU.[16]

Although evidence-based medicine has been a guiding factor in the development of care bundles in the ICU, it should be recognized that evidence-based practice is a moving target and these interventions must evolve over time. Although stress ulcer prophylaxis was a prominent component of the bundle package in the original Institute for Healthcare Improvement (IHI) VAP bundle, subsequent iterations have omitted this element of the package and are instead substituting subglottic suctioning as new evidence emerges validating efficacy.[17,18] As these processes become standardized in the ICU, compliance rates should be in the 90% to 100% range. A high level of compliance with process measures, such as the ventilator bundle or central line bundle, is documented to improve patient outcomes by reducing morbidity and mortality.[10,15–17] Unfortunately, this has not been the case with all recent process initiatives. A case in point is the Surgical Care Improvement Project (SCIP).[19] High compliance with the SCIP core process measures has resulted in mixed reviews, with some reports documenting little to no decrease in the rate of surgical site infections (SSI), whereas others have observed an increased SSI in the presence of high compliance.[20] The complexities of surgical interventions, patient morbidities, and variations in surgical technique all challenge the concept of process standardization, especially in postoperative patients who end up in the ICU. However, the convergence of scientific inquiry, public perception, and legislative initiatives has targeted HAIs as a patient safety issue thereby creating the national momentum necessary for improving patient outcomes within a culture of safety.[21]

Hand Hygiene

Although hand washing is considered the cornerstone for disrupting the transmission of health care–associated pathogens, the strength of its scientific efficacy has produced mixed results. There is no argument that the hands of all health care workers become contaminated during the execution of their duties and that this contamination can be transferred to inert surfaces or other patients and/or staff members. Unfortunately, the current educational efforts aimed at improving hand hygiene tend to focus on personal consequences rather than patient consequences, which is a classic disconnect. Failure to practice appropriate hand hygiene creates an endangerment not necessarily to self but to that "next individual who you will be caring for."[22] The number of hand hygiene opportunities (HHOs) can vary greatly from one health care facility to another and are also influenced by the metrics used to document compliance. McArdle and colleagues[23] reported a total of 350 individual HHOs over a 24-hour period in an ICU; however, several HHOs (~190) did not fall within the World Health Organization's (WHO) 5 indications (HHOs) for hand hygiene (**Box 1**).[23,24]

Box 1
WHO 5 moments for hand hygiene

1. Before patient contact

    When: clean hands before touching patients

    Why: prevent transmission of organisms from hands to patients

2. Before performing any aseptic tasks

    When: clean hands immediately after aseptic technique

    Why: prevent transmission of intrinsic and extrinsic contamination

3. After exposure to blood or body fluids

    When: after removing gloves, cleans hands immediately after blood and body fluid exposure

    Why: protect yourself and health care environment from contamination

4. After patient contact

    When: clean hands after touching patients and/or the immediate patient-care environment before leaving the room

    Why: protect yourself and health care environment from contamination

5. After contact with patient environment

    When: clean hands after touching any object or furniture in patients' immediate environment, even if patients were not touched

    Why: protect yourself and health care environment from contamination

Adapted from World Health Organization. WHO guidelines for hand hygiene in health care. Geneva (Switzerland): World Health Organization; 2006.

Compliance rates measured in selected ICUs following patient contact reported in the literature were reported as 59% (surgical ICU [SICU]), 77% (medical ICU [MICU]), and 88% (neonatal ICU [NICU]), whereas hand hygiene compliance rates following contact with potentially infectious body fluids were reported as 49% (SICU), 76% (MICU), and 74% (NICU).[25] Although these rates are shockingly low, they agree with other published observational studies.[23,26,27]

Some investigators have reported a direct linkage between increased hand hygiene compliance and a reduction in infection.[28,29] Unfortunately, these studies have not been confirmed by recent observations that question the singular role of appropriate hand hygiene as a sentinel interventional strategy for reducing the risk of selective HAIs.[30,31] An interesting observation was recently published by a collaborative group in Australia. They found that multidrug-resistant (methicillin-resistant Staphylococcus aureus [MRSA] and vancomycin-resistant enterococci [VRE]) biofilm-forming microorganisms (MDROs) actually persisted on inert surfaces within the ICU following routine terminal cleaning. The investigators hypothesized that the relative humidity within the ICU was sufficient to produce surface condensation, allowing biofilms to develop with the resultant exopolysaccharide matrix-shielding microorganism from the biocidal cleansing activity of disinfectants or desiccation.[32] Mechanistically, these inert contaminated surfaces would be an excellent reservoir for subsequent transmission of MDROs via the hands of contaminated health care workers, supporting the rationale behind moment 5 of the WHO hand hygiene guidelines (see **Box 1**).[24] Finally, hand hygiene compliance is multifactorial and highly variable from unit to unit within a hospital. A recent study conducted among surgical services in 9 different countries found that staff workload was an important determinant of compliance; although educational campaigns had an effective short-term impact, the effect was not long lasting among clinical practitioners.[33] There is no debate that appropriate hand hygiene reduces the transmission of nosocomial pathogens; however, the disconnect between recognition and practice continues to be problematic.

Isolation Practices: Improving Outcome or Restricting Quality of Care?

Patients are placed in isolation as an intervention to prevent the spread of infectious agents among other patients or, in some cases, to protect the health care worker (tuberculosis [TB]). Airborne precautions (suspected patients with TB) require patients to be placed within a negative pressure room and all doors kept closed during the period of isolation. Health care professionals caring for known or suspected patients with TB must wear an N95 respirator mask and be fit tested at least once a year in areas where the burden of TB is considered high.[34] If patients are to be transported outside of the unit, they must wear a surgical mask. Removal from airborne isolation requires the following conditions: (1) patients are receiving effective therapy (TB) and are no longer considered infectious and/or (2) have had 3 consecutive negative sputum smears collected on different days ruling out pulmonary disease. Droplet precautions (influenza, meningococcal disease, and so forth) require that patients be placed in a private room or in cohort isolation. All health care workers are required to wear a surgical mask when working or coming within 3 ft of a patient. Protective eyewear and other personal protective equipment (PPE) may be appropriate depending upon the circumstances. Patients must wear a surgical mask when being transported outside of the unit, and patients must remain in droplet precautions for the duration of illness or following effective antibiotic therapy. Appropriate hand hygiene must be practiced when entering or leaving the patients' room (see **Box 1**).

Contact precautions (ie, MDRO gram-negatives, MRSA, VRE, and Clostridium difficile) dictates that patients be placed in private or cohort isolation. All personnel or visitors must wear gloves when entering the room and remove gloves on leaving the patients' room. Hands must be washed with an antimicrobial soap immediately on removal of the gloves. Gowns are to be worn if it is anticipated that clothing will have substantial contact with patients' blood or body fluids, environmental surfaces, if patients are incontinent, have diarrhea, an ileostomy, colostomy, or excessive wound drainage. Gowns are removed before leaving the patients' environment. Efforts should be made to insure that dedicated patient care equipment (blood pressure cuffs, stethoscopes, and so forth) not be shared with other patients. If not disposable, these items must be thoroughly cleaned and disinfected before used on other patients. Contact precautions cannot be discontinued unless a negative culture is obtained 48 hours after stopping antibiotics. Historically, patients with diarrhea from C difficile must be symptom free or have a negative stool toxin assay before discontinuation of contact isolation; however, these patients often shed the organism into the environment for several weeks after resolution of symptoms.[35] This circumstance has resulted in some institutions implementing policies that require patients to remain in isolation until discharged. Following discharge, the patients' room undergoes a thorough terminal cleaning, which includes disposal of all patient items, including privacy drapes, in an effort to reduce the risk of disseminating C difficile spores to the next patient occupying that room.

Isolation precautions should be based on current epidemiologic information that identifies transmission patterns of infectious agents within the hospital environment. The current guidelines from the CDC are intended to recognize the importance of body fluids in the transmission of HAIs while addressing adequate precautions for traditional routes of transmission (ie, droplet, airborne, and contact).[36] Isolation policies should always be viewed in an evidence-based-practices context, subject to review and updated as further data are available on acquisition and transmission of infectious agents within the hospital environment. Contact isolation has long been viewed as restrictive to patient care, especially within the ICU, potentially limiting physician and nursing encounters.[37–39] A recent report has suggested that patients in contact isolation were independently associated with lower compliance of selective hospital process-of-care measures for pneumonia and smoking cessation. Any barrier to the vaccination process-of-care measure for Pneumococcus and influenza can have a potential adverse clinical impact in this high-risk patient population.[40] Over the past 10 years, selective hospital process-of-care measures have increased significantly, with some evidence correlating compliance with lower mortality.[41,42] Infection control interventions, which include contact isolation, have contributed to decreased morbidity and mortality.[43] So although the implementation of some hospital care processes and infection interventions, such as contact isolation, would seem at times to be in conflict, they are both in essence part of the same culture-of-safety initiative. The intrinsic conflict between these two processes would suggest that further studies are warranted to investigate the unintended consequences that arise when one sentinel intervention practice directly conflicts with another.

MRSA Carriage, Surveillance, and Decolonization

The mean prevalence of nasal carriage of S aureus in the United States has been reported to be 32.4%, suggesting that a third of the US population is colonized with S aureus. Although asymptomatic colonization with MRSA has been described previously as a risk factor for subsequent MRSA infection, the use of nasal cultures as a screening tool is viewed as a controversial strategy for reducing the risk (incidence) of MRSA acquisition and dissemination within the hospitalized patient population.[44,45] Published studies clearly reveal that an active MRSA surveillance program will uncover previously occult patients colonized with MRSA, leading to an increase in the rate of contact isolation.[46] In light of numerous reports that point to an increased risk for infection associated with patients colonized with MRSA admitted to the ICU, several investigators have suggested that screening patients for MRSA colonization before ICU admission may be a prudent risk-reduction strategy in those high-risk individuals undergoing invasive medical or surgical procedures.[47,48] The CDC is currently revising the SSI prevention guidelines and, in all likelihood, active MRSA surveillance will be listed as a strong evidence-based practice for preoperative surgical patients. At present, the CDC has no recommendation for MRSA surveillance in either MICUs or SICUs.

Although many acute care facilities have active surveillance programs in the ICU, the question of whether or not to decolonize patients who are MRSA positive remains an open question. A recent study from Singapore where active MRSA surveillance was applied to all ICU admissions over a 12-month period found no significant difference in mean MRSA infection rate when compared with the previous 12-month baseline period.[49] Other recent studies in ICU patients have suggested that coupling active surveillance with topical decolonization (mupirocin or chlorhexidine gluconate) was beneficial in reducing MRSA transmission and selective HAIs.[50–52] It would seem that mupirocin is effective in eradicating nasal carriage and reducing the risk of infection over the short term; however, the longer-term benefits are presently unknown.[53] There is sufficient data to suggest that inappropriate use of mupirocin is associated with the emergence (rapid) of resistance, which is highly problematic because mupirocin is the primary agent for MRSA nares decolonization.[54,55] In addition to using mupirocin for nares decontamination, several evidence-based clinical studies have documented the benefits of daily patient skin cleansing with 2% chlorhexidine gluconate (CHG) on a polyester cloth to reduce the risk of selected HAIs in the critical care patient population.[56–58] An interesting study conducted by Peterson and colleagues[59] at 3 suburban hospitals outside of Chicago found that limiting MRSA surveillance to the critical care population did not achieve a significant reduction in MRSA disease. It was only after the adoption of a universal (hospital-wide) MRSA surveillance program in combination with decolonization did a significant reduction occur. The initial capital expense to establish this program was substantial (approximately $600 000) and the universal screening increased the overall burden of isolation by approximately 20%. However, the eventual fiscal savings associated with preventing MRSA-associated HAIs (50 less infections per year) approached $1 200 000 per year. The evidence-based benefits observed in each of these clinical studies required a uniform standard of practice, which was then applied to all eligible patients.

As the US population ages, so will the ICU patient population; many of these patients will express variable levels of immunosuppression, placing them squarely at risk for HAIs. Several well-designed and executed clinical studies have documented that the incidence of HAIs can be significantly reduced within the critical care environment through focused initiatives that embraced bundled interventional risk-reduction strategies. Although many of these processes have originated from the infection control literature and not the surgical literature, successful implementation of these evidence-based interventions requires the commitment of all members of the critical care team, surgeons, nursing, and ancillary health care professionals.

Imaging Safety and Intrahospital Transportation

Radiologic imaging of patients in the ICU is a universal event; although several studies can be performed at the bedside, transport to another department for routine imaging and image-guided procedures may be required for a large number of patients. Mazza and colleagues[60] documented a 32.4% complication rate in patients transported out of the ICU for imaging studies, although most of the imaging studies obtained were for follow-up of a previously documented abnormality. Complications included agitation, hypotension, hypoxemia, and hypertension with no patient deaths. Other investigators have documented multiple complications caused by transport for imaging studies and other procedures, including death directly attributed to this practice. One study demonstrated a 75% complication rate (hypotension and hypercarbia) in patients being transported for radiologic studies using a manual ventilation system compared with a 44% rate of the same complications in patients transported with a transport ventilator.[61] Another published series of patients being transported for imaging revealed deaths and severe morbidity related to transport and documented other significant complications, such as a drain being removed after being caught in a doorway.[62] In 1990, Smith and colleagues[63] demonstrated a 60% complication rate for patient transport out of the ICU for elective procedures compared with 40% for patients being transported for emergency procedures. An informative retrospective analysis in 1988 demonstrated a 68% rate of complications directly related to the transport of trauma patients out of the ICU for imaging studies and surprisingly revealed that 76% of all studies obtained had no influence on patient management.[64] Similar results are reported by other investigators.[65] A multidisciplinary transport team can reduce the risks associated with these "road trips."[60,66] The decision to undertake a 'road trip' for necessary diagnostic testing or operative intervention requires an analysis of the risk of transport, such as that reported in the present study. This is a quote from the article, next-to-last paragraph of "Discussion" section. Given the volume of literature documenting a large number of complications related to intrahospital transport of critically ill patients, substantial consideration of the potential for a study to alter patient management should be undertaken before sending patients out of the tightly controlled ICU environment for imaging. Bedside imaging and image-guided procedures provide an alternative to transport for radiologic studies in critically ill patients. Examples include portable chest radiography, lung ultrasound, renal ultrasound, and bedside placement of central venous access catheters and inferior vena cava filters.

The portable chest X ray (pCXR) is a mainstay of critical care. As with any other bedside procedure, pCXR entails some amount of risk for dislodging monitoring devices, endotracheal tubes, and invasive monitoring devices, along with the ergonomic risk to nursing and technical staff that have to reposition the patients. Recently, the utility of performing this study on a daily basis has been called into question. This debate is not new. In 1982, Greenbaum and Marschall[67] evaluated 200 routine morning pCXR studies and found that 54 revealed new or worsening findings when compared with previous films. This was confirmed in a study from the University of Chicago in 1992 whereby new abnormalities were detected in 17.6% of routine studies.[68] A randomized controlled trial from France demonstrated that a restrictive policy for pCXR in the ICU was associated with lower costs and no change in outcomes.[69] These results were replicated in a multicenter trial in 2009.[70] Given the risks associated with the procedure, the exposure of patients and staff to ionizing radiation, and the lack of a proven benefit of daily pCXR, a selective approach to these studies is preferred. Although lung ultrasound is being promulgated currently as an alternative to pCXR in critically ill patients,[71] its relative lack of sensitivity to pneumothorax[72] makes the utility of this technique in the SICU questionable at this time.

The cumulative effect of radiation exposure from routine radiologic studies should not be discounted for either patients or providers. The average effective radiation dose to patients from a single pCXR is 0.02 (mSv), whereas the annual average background radiation exposure to an adult in the United States is 3 mSv.[73] Short-term exposure to radiation doses between 10 to 50 mSv has been associated with the development of malignancies. A review of the National Dose Registry of Canada revealed that the excess relative risk (ERR) of developing any leukemia except chronic lymphocytic leukemia in health care workers was 2.7 per millisievert of occupational radiation exposure, and the ERR for developing any cancer except leukemia was 2.3 per millisievert. These relative risks were very similar to the relative malignancy risks observed in survivors of atomic bomb blasts.[74] Additionally, as imaging technology has improved, the effective radiation dose from traditionally obtained studies has increased. Katz and colleagues[75] demonstrated an increase in radiation exposure during CT urogram from 6.5mSv with single-detector computed tomography (CT) scan to 8.5 mSv with multi-detector row CT scan. Obviously, critically ill patients undergoing multiple imaging studies are at high risk of rapidly accumulating ionizing radiation doses, with the highest risk likely being to patients suffering from cardiac complications that undergo coronary catheterization. Limiting the exposure of health care workers and patients to unnecessary ionizing radiation is of significant importance.

Device Safety

The use of medical devices for monitoring, whether invasive or noninvasive, is ubiquitous in the ICU setting. Errors in the use of these devices can range from improperly set alarms leading to detrimental outcomes from unrecognized complications[76] to accidental removal of life-sustaining devices, such as endotracheal tubes and intra-aortic balloon pumps.[77] Although the exact incidence of device-related complications is unknown, errors can occur at 1 of 4 interactions (**Table 2**). Currently, at least 500 000 medical devices are available on the market in the United States.[76,78] Devices can range in complexity from a cotton-tipped applicator to a left ventricular support device. In the United States, these devices are classified as types I through III.

1. I: Noninvasive devices
2. II: Most diagnostic and treatment equipment, such as x-ray machines
3. III: Implantable and life-support devices, such as pacemakers and implantable defibrillators

These classifications are specified for each of 16 medical specialties. Clearly, not every provider is going to understand the technical nuances of every available device, and even familiar devices can malfunction and cause patient harm if improperly used. It has been reported that most reported critical incidents in the ICU are device-related and often caused by either inadequate training or faulty equipment.[79]

Few objective data exist regarding the incidence of patient-initiated device removal in the ICU. In a 2007 study of 49 adult ICUs, the overall incidence of removal of any

Table 2
Types and examples of medical device errors

Type of Interaction	Example
Patient-device	Self-extubation
Provider-device	Improperly set IV pump or PCA
Device-device	Interaction between device and plugged-in module (ie, brick for multiple wires and ICU physiologic monitor)
Device-environment	Device not plugged in for use or not charged, device malfunction caused by temperature extremes

Abbreviations: IV, intravenous; PCA, patient-controlled analgesia.

therapeutic device was 22.1 per 1000 patient-days, with most commonly removed devices being nasogastric tubes (28.9%), supplemental oxygen (23.5%), and peripheral intravenous (IV) catheters (20.8%). However, more serious issues were observed, including the accidental removal of external ventricular drains, endotracheal tubes, and surgical drains. Of interest, only 48.9% of patients that removed their own endotracheal tubes had to be reintubated, highlighting the supposition that perhaps these devices that are being removed are being left in place too long in the first place.[77]

The US Food and Drug Administration maintains a medical device safety database referred to as MAUDE (Manufacturer and User Facility Device Experience). A common device used in surgical patients, the patient-controlled analgesia (PCA) pump, was evaluated for all errors reported to the MAUDE database from January 1, 2002 to December 31, 2003.[80] This analysis disclosed that 2009 individual PCA-related events were reported during the data collection period. Of these events, 1590 (79.1%) were device safety-related issues, most often related to switch, motor, battery, display board, or software. Eight events (0.5%) resulted in patient harm, including one incident whereby a battery fell on a patient. A large number of operator errors were likewise identified (131), with the most common error being at the provider-device level with problems programming the pump. Three deaths were reported to directly result from programming errors.

As device criticality increases, so often does the complexity of use. Unfortunately, devices that are more complex and more critical to sustaining life are often used rarely, with a corresponding increase in possibility for errors.[81] In addition, the overall level of congestion of instruments, wires, IV lines, and monitors around ICU patients contributes to the number of errors in their care, with up to 30% of errors considered severe enough to potentially cause harm or death.[82] Clearly, improvement of the ergonomic environment of the ICU, along with improvement of device interfaces at all levels, is critical to the improvement of patient safety in the future and a necessary direction of future research.

ICU Staffing Models and Outcomes

From 1985 to 2000, the number of ICU beds in the United States increased by 26.2%. However, dedicated intensivists provide care to a minority of ICU patients in the United States. In fact, only 10% of ICUs have in-house physician staffing on weekend evenings, which compares poorly with staffing models in other countries.[83] There are currently more than 6000 ICUs in the United States, which provide care to more than 2.4 million patients per year.[84] Given that 1% of the US gross domestic product is spent on intensive care services, defining the optimal physician staffing model to deliver that care is of paramount importance.

Physician staffing models continue to be debated with regard to their roles in enhancing the safety of critically ill patients. Dedicated intensivist staffing in ICUs is thought to improve patient outcomes, but this conclusion remains controversial. A 2006 meta-analysis examined 26 studies of low-intensity (no or elective intensivist consultation) versus high-intensity (mandatory consultation or closed ICU) staffing patterns. This study ultimately included 14 356 patients in the high-intensity group and 13 117 patients in the low-intensity group. In 16 out of 17 studies reviewed, high-intensity staffing was associated with lower mortality (relative risk, 0.71).[85] Unfortunately, the opposite outcome has been observed in a large study of more than 101 000 patients by Levy and colleagues.[86] Their study showed that dedicated staffing by intensivists (95% of patients cared for by an intensivist for their ICU stay) was associated with an increased severity-adjusted mortality compared with low-intensity staffing. This study has been subjected to a significant amount of criticism,[83] but it remains a very large patient sample compared with all other studies.

The Leapfrog group has promulgated a set of guidelines related to critical care, and the Safe Practice Survey (SPS) is used to determine quality of care in the intensive care setting. A recent study examined the SPS related to the care of critically ill trauma patients. The 2006 Nationwide Inpatient Sample database was queried for all patients admitted to the ICU with a primary diagnosis of trauma (*International Classification of Diseases, Ninth Revision, Clinical Modification* codes 800.0–959.9, excluding burns, late effects of trauma, superficial trauma, and foreign bodies). HAIs and mortality were the defined end points because previous studies examining only mortality were criticized for exclusion of HAIs. The SPS score had no effect on mortality or HAIs. High-intensity staffing and low-intensity physician staffing models were not correlated with outcomes, and in fact the only outcome related to use of the SPS was that disclosure of medical errors to patient families was correlated with lower mortality.[87] Although this study has several limitations, including selection bias and the possibility of underreporting of HAIs in administrative databases, their analysis certainly suggests that we are missing opportunities to improve patient safety in the critical care environment.

As has been widely reported and discussed, up to 98 000 patients may die of human error in US hospitals every year.[88] Although the veracity of this number can be debated, the fact that a large number of human errors occur in critical care units cannot be denied. Up to 45.8% of ICU admissions are reported to involve an adverse event, with 17.7% of patients experiencing an adverse event that could be considered serious.[89] The Centers for Medicare and Medicaid Services now do not reimburse hospitals for treatment of certain adverse events, highlighting the necessity of preventing these events before they occur.

ICUs are complex environments with multiple interactions occurring between providers, patients, ancillary staff, and medical devices with increasingly complex interfaces. Errors in medical care can occur during any of these interactions and are divided into several broad categories. A 90-month study of a 13-bed ICU found that in 1127 documented critical incidents, hazards included errors in equipment use (30.0%), clinical practice (22.8%), pharmaceuticals (21.1%), administration (18.9%), and health and safety hazards (7.2%). Errors were reported by nursing and physician staff through an on-line data collection system and compared with regional hospitals. The two most common errors reported were "faulty equipment" (113 critical incidents) and "unfamiliarity or incorrect use of equipment" (72 critical incidents). The investigators determined that most of the incidents were related to a lack of training with specific pieces of equipment and addressed this by introducing a practice educator, which allowed for continuous performance improvement and education in the use of all equipment available in the ICU.[79]

Patient handoffs are another area where potentially serious errors in care can occur. The transfer of care between providers is a phenomenon that occurs on a daily basis in hospital settings and is a very common practice in the ICU. The transfer of patients between house staff (sign out) is extensively encouraged, but few rigorous studies are available to document its efficacy.[90] The transfer of patients from the ICU to the ward can result in a lack of transfer of crucial information. A recent study from the University of Calgary revealed that in 112 patient transfers from ICU care to ward care, 13 medical errors were identified as the result of transfer, with 2 patients being transiently "lost to care." Challenges to effective transfer of information include different focuses between disparate specialties and different workloads. Only 26% of accepting ward physicians received communication directly from the ICU physician at the time the patients were transferred. Additionally, only 32% of patients received communication from their ICU physicians regarding their transfer and ongoing medical care.[91]

ENHANCING PATIENT SAFETY: RISK REDUCTION, ERROR REPORTING, AND FUTURE DIRECTIONS

Errors in patient care at some level cause up to 10% of patient fatalities in trauma ICUs in patients with otherwise survivable injuries[92]; estimates are that critically ill patients may experience up to 1.7 medical errors a day, mostly from medication administration errors.[93,94] Risk reduction is the holy grail of the performance improvement arena.

Computerized physician order entry (CPOE) is proposed as a solution to medication errors, which are ultimately caused by errors in either communication or judgment. The expanded use of health information technology (HIT) is promulgated by the federal government as a way to improve health care quality and reduce risk. The Leapfrog group and the Institute of Medicine have endorsed the expanded use of HIT, and financial incentives are available to health care institutions that demonstrate its "meaningful use."[94] CPOE has not been clearly demonstrated to reduce medication errors in the ICU, and its initiation can in fact cause significant problems. An often-cited study from Pittsburgh[95] showed an increase in unadjusted mortality in a pediatric ICU after the start of CPOE, with CPOE being independently associated with increased mortality. A subsequent study from Seattle refuted this idea.[96] The available data illustrate a significant learning curve to CPOE; although this technology has the potential to reduce errors, there is currently no proof that this has occurred.

Reporting of errors is another area that can potentially lead to risk reduction and performance improvement by allowing rigorous study of modes of failure. It is widely perceived that critical incidents and errors in ICU care are underreported, and consistent error reporting is recommended by the Institute of Medicine as a key error reduction strategy.[97] Two studies show that paper-based reporting systems enhanced overall error reporting, with one study involving card-based replacement of a previously used Web-site–based program.[97,98] Physicians were more likely to report incidents if they caused harm to patients, and the rate of error reporting improved when switching from a computer-based system to a card-based system.[97] These reports suggest that simplicity in a reporting system increases its use and enhances the volume of data available for analysis regarding patterns of errors.

Improving the quality and safety of ICU care in the United States is a significant challenge for the future. Obtaining lasting improvement in our systems of care is difficult given the reactionary mode physicians tend to enter when dealing with moment-to-moment crises.[99] It will be of utmost importance to implement quality and safety measures that are already supported by evidence, such as hand hygiene, implementation of evidenced-based care bundles, adequate identification and treatment of HAIs, and increasing the percentage of patients in ICU settings that are cared for by dedicated intensivists. Improvement of device safety, especially at the device-provider level, will be critical to reducing the large number of device-related complications that occur on a yearly basis in US ICUs. Prospective collection of adverse events with rigorous analysis will be important to allow systematic errors to be exposed and corrected.

REFERENCES

1. Cornell-Vigorito M, McNicoll L, Adams L, et al. Improving safety culture in Rhode Island ICUs: lessons learned from development of action-oriented plans. Jt Comm J Qual Patient Saf 2011;37:509–14.
2. Valentin A, Capuzzo M, Guidet B, et al. Patient safety in intensive care: results from the multinational Sentinel Events Evaluation (SEE) study. Intensive Care Med 2006;32:1591–8.

3. Valentin A, Bion J. How safe is my intensive care unit? - An overview of error causation and prevention. Curr Opin Crit care 2007;13:697–702.

4. Krimsky WS, Mroz IB, McIlwaine JK, et al. A model for increasing patient safety in the intensive care unit: increasing the rate of proven safety measures. Qual Saf Health Care 2009;18:74–80.

5. Fukuda H, Imanaka Y, Hirose M, et al. Factors associated with system-level activities for patient safety and infection control. Health Policy 2009;89:26–36.

6. Yokoe DS, Classen D. Improving public safety through infection control: a new healthcare imperative. Infect Control Hosp Epidemiol 2008;29:S3–11.

7. Nelson S, Stone PW, Jordan S, et al. Patient safety climate: variation in perception by infection preventionist and quality directors [online]. Interdiscip Perspect Infect Dis 2011;2011:357121.

8. Huang DT, Clermont G, Kong LA, et al. Intensive care unit safety culture and outcomes: a US multicenter study. Int J Qual Health Care 2010;22:151–61.

9. Kleven RM, Edwards JR, Richards CL, et al. Estimating healthcare-associated infections and death in US hospitals, 2002. Public Health Rep 2007;122:160–6.

10. Waters HR, Korn R, Colantuoni E, et al. The business case for quality: economic analysis of the Michigan Keystone Patient Safety Program in ICU. Am J Med Qual 2011;26:333–9.

11. Dimick JB, Pronovost PJ, Heitmiller RF, et al. Intensive care unit physician staffing is associated with decreased length of stay, hospital cost and complication after esophageal resection. Crit Care Med 2001;29:753–8.

12. Halton K, Graves N. Economic evaluation and catheter-related bloodstream infections. Emerg Infect Dis 2007;13(6):815–23.

13. Alberti C, Brun-Buisson C, Burchardi H, et al. Epidemiology of sepsis and infection in ICU patients from an international multicenter cohort study. Intensive Care Med 2002;28:108–21.

14. Hidron AL, Edward JR, Patel J, et al. National Healthcare Safety Network Team; participating healthcare network facilities. NHSN annual update: antimicrobial-resistant pathogens associated with healthcare-associated infection: annual summary of data reported to the national healthcare safety network at the centers for disease control and prevention, 2006-2007. Infect Control Hosp Epidemiol 2008;29:996–1011.

15. Marwick C, Davey P. Care bundles: the holy grail of infectious risk management in hospitals? Curr Opin Infect Dis 2009;22:364–9.

16. Cocanour CS, Peninger M, Domonoske BD, et al. Decreasing ventilator-associated pneumonia in a trauma ICU. J Trauma 2006;61:122–9.

17. Resar R, Pronovost P, Haraden C, et al. Using a bundle approach to improve ventilator care processes and reduce ventilator-associated pneumonia. Jt Comm Qual Patient Saf 2005;31:243–8.

18. Krein SL, Kowalski CP, Damschroder L, et al. Preventing ventilator-associated pneumonia in the United States: a multicenter mixed-methods study. Infect Control Hosp Epidemiol 2008;29:933–40.

19. Hawn MT, Vick CC, Richman J, et al. Surgical site infection prevention: time to move beyond the surgical care improvement program. Ann Surg 2011;254:494–9.

20. Edmiston CE, Spencor M, Lewis BD, et al. Reducing the risk of surgical site infections: did we really think that SCIP was going to lead us to the promised land? Surg Infect (Larchmt) 2011;12:169–77.

21. The research Committee of the Society of Healthcare Epidemiology of America. Enhancing patient safety by reducing healthcare-associated infection: the role of discovery and dissemination. Infect Control Hosp Epidemiol 2010;31:118–23.

22. Grant AM, Hofman DA. It's not all about me: motivating hand hygiene among healthcare professionals by focusing on patients. Psychol Sci 2011;22:1494–9.
23. McArdle FL, Lee RJ, Gibb AP, et al. How much time is needed for hand hygiene in intensive care? A prospective trained observer study of rates of contact between healthcare workers and intensive care patients. J Hosp Infect 2006;62:304–10.
24. World Health Organization. WHO guidelines for hand hygiene in healthcare. Geneva (Switzerland): World Health Organization; 2006.
25. Scheithauer S, Haefner H, Schwanz T, et al. Compliance with hand hygiene on surgical, medical, and neurologic intensive care units: direct observation versus calculated disinfectant usage. Am J Infect Control 2009;37:835–41.
26. Boyce JM, Pittet D. Centers for Disease Control and Prevention (CDC) guidelines for hand hygiene in healthcare settings: recommendations of the healthcare infection control practice advisory committee and the HIPAC/SHEA/APIC/IDSA hand hygiene task force. MMWR Morb Mortal Wkly Rep 2002;52:1–16.
27. Larsen EL, Albrecht S, O'Keefe M. Hand hygiene behavior in a pediatric emergency department and a pediatric intensive care unit: comparison of use of 2 dispenser systems. Am J Crit Care 2005;14:304–11.
28. Pittet D, Sax H, Hugonnet S, et al. Cost implications of successful hand hygiene promotion. Infect Control Hosp Epidemiol 2004;25:264–6.
29. Trick WE, Vernon MO, Welbel SF, et al. Chicago Antimicrobial Resistance Project. Multicenter intervention program to increase adherence to hand hygiene recommendations and glove use and to reduce the incidence of antimicrobial resistance. Infect Control Hosp Epidemiol 2007;28:42–9.
30. Rupp ME, Fitzgerald T, Puumala S, et al. Prospective, controlled, cross-over trial of alcohol-based hand gel in critical care units. Infect Control Hosp Epidemiol 2008;29:8–15.
31. Mertz D, Dafoe N, Walter SD, et al. Effect of a multifaceted intervention on adherence to hand hygiene among healthcare workers: a cluster-randomized trial. Infect Control Hosp Epidemiol 2010;31:1170–6.
32. Vickery K, Deva A, Jacomb A, et al. Presence of biofilm containing viable multi-resistant organisms despite terminal cleaning on clinical surfaces ion an intensive care unit. J Hosp Infect 2012;80:52–5.
33. Lee A, Chalfine A, Daikos GL, et al. Hand hygiene practices and adherence determinants in surgical wards across Europe and Israel: a multicenter observational study. Am J Infect Control 2011;39:517–20.
34. Jensen P, Lambert LA, Iademarco MF, et al. Guidelines for preventing the transmission of mycobacterium tuberculosis in healthcare setting, 2005. MMWR Morb Mortal Wkly Rep 2005;54:1–147.
35. Owen RC. Clostridium difficile-associated disease: an emerging threat to patient safety. Pharmacotherapy 2006;26:299–311.
36. Siegel JD, Rhinehart E, Jackson M, et al. 2007 guidelines for isolation precautions: preventing transmission of infectious agents in healthcare settings. Infect Control Hosp Epidemiol 2007;25:S65–164.
37. Evans HL, Shaffer MM, Hughes MG, et al. Contact isolation in surgical patients: a barrier to care? Surgery 2003;134:180–8.
38. Kirkland KB, Weinstein JM. Adverse effect of contact isolation. Lancet 1999;354: 1177–8.
39. Saint S, Higgins IA, Nallamothu BK, et al. Do physicians examine patients in contact isolation less frequently? A brief report. Am J Infect Control 2003;31:354–6.
40. Morgan DJ, Day HR, Harris AD, et al. The impact of contact isolation on the quality of inpatient hospital care. PLoS One 2011;6:e22190.

41. Fiore AE, Shay DK, Broder K, et al. Prevention and control of seasonal influenza with vaccines: recommendation of the advisory committee on immunization practices (ACIP). MMWR Recomm Rep 2009;58:1–52.
42. Werner RM, Bradlow ET. Relationship between Medicare's hospital compare performance measure and mortality rates. JAMA 2006;296:2694–702.
43. Edmond MB, Ober JF, Bearman G. Active surveillance cultures are not required to control MRSA infections in the critical care setting. Am J Infect Control 2008;36: 461–3.
44. Harbarth S, Frankhauser C, Schrenzel L, et al. Universal screening for methicillin-resistant *Staphylococcus aureus* at hospital admission and nosocomial infection in surgical patients. JAMA 2008;299:1149–57.
45. Davis KA, Stewart JJ, Crouch HK, et al. Methicillin-resistant *Staphylococcus aureus* (MRSA) nares colonization at hospital admission and its effect on subsequent MRSA infection. Clin Infect Dis 2004;39:776–82.
46. Mangini E, Segal-Maurer S, Burns J, et al. Impact of contact and droplet precautions on the incidence of hospital-acquired methicillin-resistant *Staphylococcus aureus*. Infect Control Hosp Epidemiol 2007;28:1261–6.
47. Shorr AF, Combes A, Kollef MH. Methicillin-resistant *Staphylococcus aureus* prolongs intensive care unit stay in ventilator-associated pneumonia, despite initially appropriate antibiotic therap. Crit Care Med 2006;34:700–6.
48. Warren DK, Guth RM, Coopersmith CM, et al. Impact of a methicillin-resistant *Staphylococcus aureus* active surveillance program on contact precaution utilization in a surgical intensive care unit. Crit Care Med 2007;35:430–4.
49. Chlebicka KA, Tan KY, Chen EX, et al. Active surveillance testing and decontamination strategies in intensive care units to reduce methicillin-resistant *Staphylococcus aureus* infections. Am J Infect Control 2010;38:361–7.
50. Muller A, Talon D, Potier A, et al. Use of intranasal mupirocin to prevent methicillin-resistant *Staphylococcus aureus* infection in intensive care units. Crit Care 2005;9:R246–50.
51. Holmes JW, Williams MD. Methicillin-resistant *Staphylococcus aureus* screening and eradication in the surgical intensive care unit: is it worth it? Am J Surg 2010;200:827–30.
52. Edgeworth JD. Has decolonization played an central role in the decline of UK methicillin-resistant *Staphylococcus aureus* transmission: a focus on evidence from intensive care. J Antimicrob Chemother 2011;66:S41–7.
53. Laupland KB, Conly JM. Treatment of *Staphylococcus aureus* colonization and prophylaxis for infection with topical intranasal mupirocin: an evidence-based review. Clin Infect Dis 2003;37:933–8.
54. Hurdle JG, O'Neill AJ, Mody L, et al. In vivo transfer of high level mupirocin resistance from *Staphylococcus epidermidis* to methicillin-resistant *Staphylococcus aureus* associated with failure of mupirocin prophylaxis. J Antimicrob Chemother 2005;56:1166–8.
55. Cavdar C, Atay T, Zeybel M, et al. Emergence of resistance in staphylococci after long-term mupirocin application in patient on continuous ambulatory dialysis. Adv Perit Dial 2004;20:67–70.
56. Bleasdale SC, Trick W, Gonzalez IM, et al. Effectiveness of chlorhexidine bathing to reduce catheter-associated bloodstream infections in medical intensive care unit patients. Arch Intern Med 2007;167:2073–9.
57. Popovich KJ, Hota B, Hayes R, et al. Effectiveness of routine patient cleansing with chlorhexidine gluconate for infection prevention in the medical intensive care unit. Infect Control Hosp Epidemiol 2009;30:959–63.

58. Holder C, Zellinger M. Daily bathing with chlorhexidine in the ICU to prevent central line-associated infections. J Clin Outcomes Manag 2009;16:509–13.
59. Peterson LR, Hacek DM, Robicsek A. Case study: an MRSA intervention at Evanston Northwestern Healthcare. Jt Comm J Qual Patient Saf 2007;33: 732–8.
60. Mazza FB, Gomes do Amaral JL, Rosseti H, et al. Safety of intrahospital transportation: evaluation of respiratory and hemodynamic parameters. A prospective cohort study. Sao Paulo Med J 2008;126:319–22.
61. Braman SS, Dunn SM, Amico CA, et al. Complications of intrahospital transportation in critically ill patients. Ann Intern Med 1987;107:469–73.
62. Waddell G. Movement of critically ill patients within the hospital. BMJ 1975;2: 417–9.
63. Smith I, Fleming S, Cernaianu A. Mishaps during transport from the intensive care unit. Crit Care Med 1990;18:278–81.
64. Indeck M, Peterson S, Smith J, et al. Risk, cost and benefit of transporting ICU patients for special studies. J Trauma 1988;28:1020–5.
65. Hurst JM, Davis K Jr, Johnson DJ, et al. Cost and complications during in-hospital transport of critically ill patients: a prospective cohort study. J Trauma 1992;33: 582–5.
66. Szem JW, Hydo LJ, Fischer E, et al. High-risk intrahospital transport of critically ill patients: safety and outcome of the necessary "road trip". Crit Care Med 1995;23: 1660–6.
67. Greenbaum DM, Marschall KE. The value of routine daily chest x-rays in intubated patients in the medical intensive care unit. Crit Care Med 1982;10:29–30.
68. Hall JB, White SR, Karrison T. Efficacy of daily routine chest radiographs in intubated, mechanically ventilated patients. Crit Care Med 1991;19:689–93.
69. Clec'h C, Simon P, Hamdi L, et al. Are daily routine chest radiographs useful in critically ill, mechanically ventilated patients? A randomized study. Intensive Care Med 2008;34:264–70.
70. Hejblum G, Chalumeau-Lemoine L, Ioos V, et al. Comparison of routine and on-demand prescription of chest radiographs in mechanically ventilated adults: a multicentre, cluster-randomized, two-period crossover study. Lancet 2009; 374:1687–93.
71. Bouhemad B, Zhang M, Lu Q, et al. Clinical review: bedside lung ultrasound in critical care practice. Crit Care 2007;11:205–13.
72. Xirouchaki N, Magkanas E, Vaporidi K, et al. Lung ultrasound in critically ill patients: comparison with bedside chest radiography. Intensive Care Med 2011;37:1488–93.
73. Kaul P, Medvedev S, Hohmann S, et al. Ionizing radiation exposure to patients admitted with acute myocardial infarction in the United States. Circulation 2010;122:2160–9.
74. Gilbert ES. Invited commentary: studies of workers exposed to low doses of radiation. Am J Epidemiol 2001;153:319–22.
75. Katz SI, Saluja S, Brink JA, et al. Radiation dose associated with unenhanced CT for suspected renal colic: impact of repetitive studies. AJR Am J Roentgenol 2006;186:1120–4.
76. Balka E, Doyle-Walters M, Lecznarowicz D, et al. Technology, governance and patient safety: systems issues in technology and patient safety. Int J Med Inform 2007;76(Suppl 1):s35–47.
77. Mion LC, Minnick AF, Leipzig RM, et al. Patient-initiated device removal in intensive care units: a national prevalence study. Crit Care Med 2007;35:2714–20.

78. O'Shea JC, Kramer JM, Califf RM, et al. Sharing a commitment to improve cardio-vascular devices, part I: identifying holes in the safety net. Am Heart J 2004;147: 977–84.
79. Welters ID, Gibson J, Mogk M, et al. Major sources of critical incidents in intensive care. Crit Care 2011;15:R232 [epub ahead of print].
80. Hankin CS, Schein J, Clark JA, et al. Adverse events involving intravenous patient-controlled analgesia. Am J Health Syst Pharm 2007;64:1492–9.
81. Drews FA, Musters A, Samore MH. Error producing conditions in the intensive care unit. In: Henriksen K, Battles JB, Keyes MA, et al, editors. Advances in patient safety: new directions and alternative approaches (vol. 3: performance and tools). Rockville (MD): Agency for Healthcare Research and Quality; 2008. Available at: http://www.ncbi.nlm.nih.gov/books/NBK43691/.
82. Donchin Y, Gopher D, Olin M, et al. A look into the nature and causes of human errors in the intensive care unit. Crit Care Med 1995;23:294–300.
83. Gajic O, Afessa B. Physician staffing models and patient safety in the ICU. Chest 2009;135:1038–44.
84. Sawyer RG, Tache Leon CA. Common complications in the surgical intensive care unit. Crit Care Med 2010;38(9 Suppl):s483–93.
85. Pronovost PJ, Angus DC, Dorman T, et al. Physician staffing patterns and clinical outcomes in critically ill patients: a systematic review. JAMA 2002;288:2151–62.
86. Levy MM, Rapoport J, Lemeshow S, et al. Association between critical care physician management and patient mortality in the intensive care unit. Ann Intern Med 2008;148:801–9.
87. Glance LG, Dick AW, Osler TM, et al. Relationship between leapfrog safe prac-tices survey and outcomes in trauma. Arch Surg 2011;146:1170–7.
88. Kohn LT, Corrigan JM, Donaldson MS, editors. To err is human: building a safer health system. Washington, DC: National Academy Press; 2000. p. 1–16.
89. Andrews LB, Stocking C, Krizek T, et al. An alternative method to studying adverse events in medical care. Lancet 1997;349:309–13.
90. Horwitz LI, Krumholz HM, Green ML, et al. Transfer of patient care between house staff on medical wards: a national survey. Arch Intern Med 2006;166:1173–7.
91. Li P, Stelfox HT, Ghali WA. A prospective observational study of physician handoff for intensive-care-unit-to-ward patient transfers. Am J Med 2011;124:860–7.
92. Stahl K, Palileo A, Schulman CI, et al. Enhancing patient safety in the trauma/surgical intensive care unit. J Trauma 2009;67:430–5.
93. Rothschild JM, Landrigan CP, Cronin JW, et al. The critical care safety study: the incidence and nature of adverse events and serious medical errors in intensive care. Crit Care Med 2005;33:1694–700.
94. Maslove DM, Rizk N, Lowe HJ. Computerized order entry in the critical care envi-ronment: a review of current literature. J Intensive Care Med 2011;26:165–71.
95. Han YY, Carcillo JA, Venkataraman ST, et al. Unexpected increase in mortality after implementation of a commercially sold computerized physician order entry system. Pediatrics 2005;116:1506–12.
96. DeBeccaro MA, Jeffries HE, Eisenberg MA, et al. Computerized order entry im-plementation: no association with increased mortality rates in an intensive care unit. Pediatrics 2006;118:290–5.
97. Harris CB, Krauss MJ, Coopersmith CM, et al. Patient safety event reporting in critical care: a study of three intensive care units. Crit Care Med 2007;35: 1068–75.
98. Ilan R, Squires M, Panopoulos C, et al. Increasing patient safety event reporting in two intensive care units: a prospective interventional study. J Crit Care 2011;26:431e11–8.

99. Henriksen K, Oppenheimer C, Leape LL, et al. Envisioning patient safety in the year 2025: eight perspectives. In: Henriksen K, Battles JB, Keyes MA, et al, editors. Advances in patient safety: new directions and alternative approaches (vol. 1: assessment). Rockville (MD): Agency for Healthcare Research and Quality; 2008. Available at: http://www.ncbi.nlm.nih.gov/books/NBK43618/.

Monitoring Devices in the Intensive Care Unit

Todd Neideen, MD, MS

KEYWORDS

- Monitors • Pulmonary artery catheter • Central venous pressure • Pulse oximetry
- Capnography • Intracranial pressure

KEY POINTS

- Cardiovascular monitors help determine if patients' tissues are getting enough blood supply.
- The pulmonary monitors monitor the pulmonary mechanics of the patients' respiratory system.
- Neurologic monitors are used to maintain adequate blood flow to the brain.

MONITORING IN THE INTENSIVE CARE UNIT

Monitoring devices are the corner stone of the modern intensive care unit. Without these revolutionary devices, clinicians would not have the requisite information to care for the critically ill especially if patient status changes acutely. Monitors in the intensive care unit (ICU) are key to delivering treatment in the ICU. Current devices emphasize assessing cardiovascular (CV), pulmonary, and neurologic function. This article deals mostly with CV monitoring.

CV MONITORS

There are many different types of CV monitors. They can be broadly categorized into 2 types: those intrinsic to heart function and those that monitor blood or, more importantly, oxygen delivery to tissues.

TELEMETRY

Telemetry monitoring is the most common type of CV monitor in the ICU. It monitors the intrinsic electrical function of the heart. Every patient in the ICU has a telemetry monitor attached to them. Telemetry is a 2-lead continuous electrocardiogram. The leads II and

The author has nothing to disclose.
Division of Trauma and Critical Care Surgery, Medical College of Wisconsin, 9200 West Wisconsin Avenue, Milwaukee, WI 53226, USA
E-mail address: tneideen@mcw.edu

Surg Clin N Am 92 (2012) 1387–1402
http://dx.doi.org/10.1016/j.suc.2012.08.010
0039-6109/12/$ – see front matter © 2012 Published by Elsevier Inc.
surgical.theclinics.com

V1 are commonly used because the QRS complex in these leads is usually the largest of all leads and they have prominent P waves. Telemetry allows any arrhythmia to be detected immediately. Any new arrhythmia diagnosed gives a clue to many physiologic derangements of the patient. Electrolyte abnormalities, fluid shifts, and cardiac ischemia are the most common reasons for acute cardiac arrhythmias.[1]

Sinus tachycardia is the most common abnormality seen on telemetry and is usually a sign of cardiac excitability from many sources, including pain, hypoxia, sepsis, increased inflammation, increased adrenal output from trauma or other sources, or beta blocker withdrawal. Tachycardia may or may not need to be treated. Bradycardia is usually caused by medications but has many other causes. Bradycardia can be the first sign of severe hypoxia. Atrial arrhythmias are also common. Atrial fibrillation can be seen in surgical patients as they start mobilizing resuscitative fluids between 48 to 72 hours after resuscitation.[2] Atrial flutter is less common. Ventricular arrhythmias are worse. Early diagnosis and treatment are critical. Subtle changes in the telemetry strip, in conjunction with information received from other monitors, can give clues to bigger problems. T waves are the most labile individual wave on a telemetry strip. As a result, when a T-wave abnormality occurs, the differential diagnosis is long. The most common T-wave abnormality is an inversion of the wave.[3,4] As with any subtle telemetry change after assessing patients, the next step is a 12-lead electrocardiogram.

PULSE OXIMETER

The pulse oximeter is a useful tool in the ICU. It measures the percent saturation of oxygen on hemoglobin molecules in arterial blood. Without a pulse oximeter, a blood gas would be needed every time a physician wanted to know how well patients were being oxygenated. The development of the pulse oximeter took approximately 50 years. Starting in the 1930s, theory and crude instruments were developed, with the first commercially available device being used in hospitals starting in 1981.[5] The machine displays the percent saturation of hemoglobin molecules in arterial blood with oxygen. It does this by taking advantage of the fact that the hemoglobin molecule that has oxygen attached to it absorbs and reflects a different wavelength of light than a hemoglobin molecule without an oxygen molecule attached to it. The percentage of oxygen is calculated only from the reflected light that has a pulsatile nature, which corresponds to the pulsatile blood in the artery. Carbon monoxide will falsely elevate the pulse oximeter reading because it reflects the same wavelength of light that oxyhemoglobin reflects. For a pulse oximeter to work well, the probe must be attached to skin that is well perfused.

The ICU monitor will display the pulse oximeter information as a number but also as a waveform. The wave is a display of the pulsing blood that the sensor is reading. It looks like a blood pressure tracing on the monitor. The characteristic of this waveform corresponds to how accurate the reading is. A dampened waveform indicates poor tissue perfusion and cannot be accepted as an accurate reading.

The transducer probe that emits and measures the pulse can be placed almost anywhere on the body, but the areas with thinner skin are better. The most common places are the fingers, toes, ears, nose, and forehead. Unfortunately, the perfusion of too many of these body locations is compromised in low-flow states or when vasopressors are being used.

A normal pulse oximeter reading for someone without lung disease on room air should be between 94% and 100%. Patients with chronic lung problems can have a pulse oximetry reading of greater than 86%, but it is usually less than 92% on room air. Most pulse oximeters are accurate down to a reading of 70%. When pulse oximeters are providing consistent readings in the 70% range, it is recommended that an arterial blood gas be obtained to check the validity of the pulse oximeter.[6]

Tissue Hemoglobin Oxygen Saturation

The tissue hemoglobin oxygen saturation (StO2) monitor is a device that allows us to determine how much hemoglobin is saturated with oxygen in tissues deeper than the skin by using near-infrared spectroscopy technology. Usually it is set up to determine the StO2 in skeletal muscle but the monitor can be set up to determine StO2 in organs that are close to the body's surface, like a child's kidney. The StO2 can be followed to determine if fluid resuscitation is successful by increasing oxygen delivery to tissue. Increasing StO2 correlates with improved outcome, and an acute decrease in StO2 can be a harbinger of poor outcome; but having an StO2 monitor set up does not seem to change outcomes any better than following base deficit, lactate levels, or oxygen delivery calculations.[7]

Arterial Lines

Arterial lines give us access to arterial blood for sampling, measures blood pressure, and can help us determine if someone requires volume resuscitation or not. For patients who have CV instability requiring continuous blood pressure monitoring, an arterial line is indispensable. Continuous blood pressure measurement with an arterial line determines how effective our treatments are without continually recycling the blood pressure cuff, which can cause damage to the muscle and skin in patients.[8,9] Blood draws are frequently obtained from the arterial lines when in place. An arterial line does increase the number of blood draws and the volume of blood that is drawn when compared with patients without arterial lines. This increase in blood loss occurs without any measurable outcome benefit.[10]

Correct calibration of an arterial line is key to successful readings. The first step is to zero the pressure in the transducer. This action is done with the transducer at the level of the heart. Once the arterial line tubing is attached to the transducer, a waveform should be displayed on the monitor. The appearance of the waveform will help the physician interpret the recorded pressure. An inaccurate waveform can be described as overdamped or underdamped. Overdamping will appear as a narrowed and flattened tracing. This appearance implies that the pressure is being dulled or artificially lowered and the most common cause is air in the system. Most of the time, this is an air bubble next to the transducer. The air needs to be bled out of the system and the system recalibrated to obtain an accurate tracing and blood pressure reading. An underdamped arterial line tracing will appear as very sharp changes (sawtooth appearance). If this tracing appears, a kink in the tubing or obstruction in the system will be giving this elevated abnormal reading. Flushing the tubing or removing the kink will improve this waveform.

To test if an arterial line is overdamped or underdamped, one should flush the arterial line rapidly with pressurized saline and then abruptly stop flushing the line while watching the monitor. An underdamped waveform will display greater than 4 narrow waves before returning to a more natural-appearing wave. An overdamped waveform will go right back to a more natural-appearing wave after this rapid flush without any narrow waves. If 2 narrow waves appear after this rapid flush followed by the normal blood pressure tracing, it is perfect. **Figs. 1–3** show what the tracings should look like for these various scenarios.

Using the arterial line tracing to determine if patients will be fluid responsive is a nice technique. Patients' blood pressure changes depending on what part of the respiratory cycle they are in. It has to do with the fact that intrathoracic pressure changes

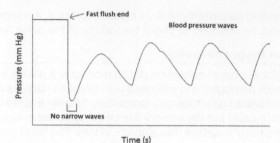

Fig. 1. An overdamped arterial line waveform.

with inspiration and expiration. This change in pressure will change the patients' pre-load, change the amount of blood in the pulmonary vasculature, and change the size of the ventricles in diastole, which in turn will change the patients' blood pressure slightly. This variability can be seen in the arterial line tracing (**Figs. 4** and **5**). The ability to see this in the tracing helps determine if someone may be fluid responsive. The more variability in patients' blood pressure during a respiratory cycle, the more the blood pressure should increase for a given fluid bolus. When there is no variability, patients will probably not be very fluid responsive.[11]

One of the newer benefits of arterial lines is the ability to infer the cardiac index with a device called the FloTrac (Edwards Lifesciences Corp, Irvine, CA, USA). The FloTrac sensor is attached to the arterial line and connected to its corresponding monitor. It takes 2000 blood pressure measurements every 20 seconds. This information, along with patient demographic information, is used to calculate the stroke volume index and cardiac index. This device correlates well with pulmonary artery (PA) catheter measurements for stroke volume index and cardiac index when patients have normal hemodynamics. Unfortunately, this correlation degrades as patients' hemodynamics become more abnormal.[12]

Complications from arterial lines tend to be low. There is always a possibility of infection similar to any invasive vascular line. The risk of infection is one infection for every 1000 line days, which breaks down to about 1% of lines developing an infection.[13] The more common complication is arterial insufficiency, which can occur in 25% of radial artery catheters. Arterial insufficiency is a complete spectrum from emboli to partial or complete arterial occlusion. The bleeding risk from an arterial line site is approximately 3%.[14]

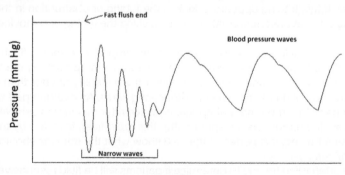

Fig. 2. An underdamped arterial line waveform.

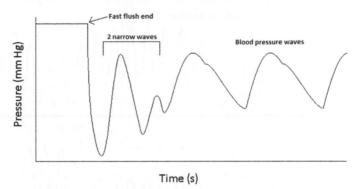

Fig. 3. An appropriately damped arterial line waveform.

Central Venous Pressure

Central venous lines have a long history of use in the ICU. They are used for good intravenous access, total parenteral nutrition, and central venous pressure (CVP) monitoring. CVP measurement is used to help determine patients' fluid status. In a person with normal hemodynamics, a higher CVP indicates a higher preload and, therefore, a higher intravascular volume, with the contrary also being true. Low CVPs usually indicate that someone is volume depleted and their blood pressure will increase with fluid boluses. Placing a central venous line and monitoring CVP is the easiest method to obtain a snapshot of patients' volume status. Current surviving sepsis guidelines recommend getting the CVP of patients with sepsis between 8 and 12 mm Hg[15] by fluid resuscitation. However, CVP monitoring is not always as reliable as we wish it to be.[16] Many comorbidities make CVP monitoring unreliable. Many disease processes elevate CVP, yet patients may still need volume expansion. These disease processes include pulmonary embolism, pulmonary hypertension, right heart failure, and right heart valve disease. Ascites and abdominal hypertension are 2 other conditions that can falsely elevate CVP measurements. Most problems with CVP interpretation occur when the CVP is elevated and when the CVP is low, and it almost always means that patients' are volume depleted and more fluid is needed. Another way to interpret CVP values is to remember that the trend over time is the most valuable aspect of CVP monitoring.[17]

If the CVP changes during the respiratory cycle or with a fluid challenges it usually indicates that patients are intravascularly depleted. Intrapleural pressures should be equal to atmospheric pressure at end expiration whether patients are on positive pressure ventilation or breathing room air. This observation suggests that the CVP should

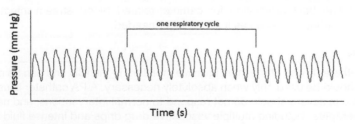

Fig. 4. Stroke volume variability.

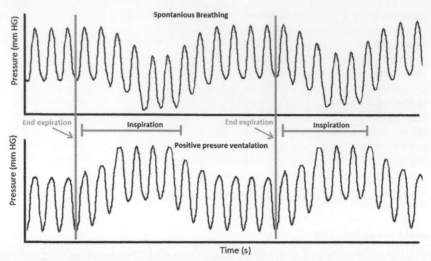

Fig. 5. Respiratory variation in CVP in patients with spontaneous breathing and on positive pressure ventilation.

be measured at end expiration. In a spontaneously breathing patient CVP is higher at end expiration where in a ventilated patient CVP is lowest at end expiration (see **Fig. 5**).

As with any invasive device, there are complications associated with the central line used to measure CVP. Complications are commonly divided into those occurring during placement and those secondary to the catheter being maintained. Pneumothorax or arterial injuries are the 2 most common types of complications when placing a central line. The risk of any complication on insertion is between 6% and 12%.[18] The most common complication is arterial puncture, which can be reduced for jugular insertion with ultrasound.[19,20] Pneumothorax is more common with subclavian access and is reported to occur 1% to 3% of the time. Femoral central line placement is not recommended for CVP monitoring and has the highest complication rate of any access site.[21,22] A chest radiograph is needed after placement to make sure the central line is at the superior vena cava–right atria junction before accurate measurements can be made.

Maintaining the catheter is also associated with complications. Ventricular perforation is an uncommon complication associated with a catheter that is placed too deep so that the tip resides at the atrial ventricular junction or actually into the ventricle. Arm movement can make this catheter move and puncture the ventricle. The major complication during catheter maintenance is blood stream infection. The risk of a blood stream infection from a central line in the jugular or subclavian position is 2 per 1000 patient-days. This risk goes up with increasing length of time the catheter is in place.[23,24] The best prevention for catheter-related blood stream infection is to remove the catheter as soon as it is no longer needed.

PA Catheter

The PA catheter is one of the most invasive monitors in the ICU and can be difficult to place. It should be used only when absolutely necessary. A PA catheter is used when patients are in severe shock; do not respond to normal interventions; and need more intense therapies, including multiple vasoactive drug drips and intense fluid management. With the introducer catheter ideally placed in the right jugular vein or left subclavian vein, the catheter is floated through the right side of the heart and placed into the PA and then wedged into a terminal branch of the PA.

Placing the PA catheter is a bedside procedure that requires an understanding of the pressure waveforms as the catheter is passed from the superior vena cava to the pulmonary artery (**Figs. 6–9**). The catheter is floated with the aid of a balloon at its tip, which allows the catheter to be guided by the blood flow and helps avoid irritating the heart as the catheter is passed through the right ventricle into the PA. The waveforms are followed, and advancement is stopped when the wedge pressure is visualized. The balloon is deflated and the pressure tracing should revert to the PA pressure waveform. If the wedge pressure persists, the catheter should be withdrawn slightly and the balloon inflated again to achieve a wedge pressure. Deflating the balloon should give the PA pressures at this time.

When properly placed and verified by chest radiograph, the PA catheter will give you a massive amount of information about patients' CV function. The main parameter is the cardiac output. The cardiac output is determined by a thermodilution technique and is normalized to patients' body surface area giving the cardiac index. Most manipulations we use are used to optimize the cardiac output or index. Our goal with fluids and vasoactive drugs is to improve cardiac output, which should improve tissue perfusion and organ function.

Other parameters obtained via the PA catheter include the CVP, the PA pressures, and the wedge pressure. The catheter can also be used to obtain a mixed venous gas, or some PA catheters can actually measure mixed venous oxygen saturation (SvO_2) continuously. Other calculated parameters include stroke volume and systemic vascular resistance. The wedge pressure is used to assess left atrial filling pressure and, by inference, the left-sided filling volume. This relationship is usually correlated, and low values indicate the need for fluid administration. High values commonly indicate cardiac dysfunction, which suggests that the treatment should be aimed at improving myocardial function and not administering more fluid. Mixed venous oxygen content is used with peripheral arterial oxygen content to determine how much oxygen the body is consuming. Stroke volume, which is calculated, is used by some to determine how efficient each beat of the heart is. Systemic vascular resistance is calculated by using Ohm's law ([mean arterial pressure – central venous pressure]/cardiac output). It can be used to communicate how well a vasoactive drug is working.

Because the catheter tip of the PA catheter sits in the PA, it is an ideal instrument to obtain SvO_2 readings. This reading can either be done by taking a blood sample from the tip or by using a PA catheter that is equipped to directly measure the oxygen saturation at the tip fiber optically. An SvO_2 reading is very useful in determining how well

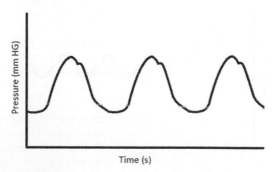

Time (s)

Fig. 6. CVP pressure waveform.

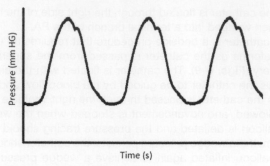

Fig. 7. Right ventricular pressure waveform.

the body tissues are receiving and using oxygen. The normal SvO_2 is between 65% and 75%.[25,26] A decrease in this number usually means that not enough oxygen is being delivered to tissue or more oxygen than normal is being taken out of the blood.

The extraction ratio is a relatively quick calculation that helps determine if patients are getting and using an adequate amount of oxygen. The extraction ratio is calculated using the SvO_2 and the arterial oxygen saturation. The following set of equations show how the extraction ratio equation is derived.

The oxygen delivery equation is as follows:

$$(DO_2)\ (mL/min) = (CO) \times \text{blood oxygen content}$$

$$DO_2 = CO \times \left(13.4 \times Hgb \times \frac{S_aO_2}{100} + 0.031 \times P_aO_2 \right)$$

where CO is cardiac output, DO_2 is oxygen delivery, Hgb is the patients' hemoglobin, S_aO_2 is arterial oxygen saturation in percent, and 13.4 and 0.031 are conversion factors for oxygen carried by hemoglobin and plasma A normal cardiac output is 5 L/min, hemoglobin is 15, arterial oxygen saturation is 97%, and P_aO_2 is 100. This calculation gives a normal oxygen delivery of 1000 mL/min. The body only uses or consumes about 250 mL/min.

The oxygen consumption equation is as follows:

$$VO_2 = CO \times (C_aO_2 - C_vO_2)$$

where CO is cardiac output, C_aO_2 is arterial oxygen content, C_vO_2 is mixed venous oxygen content, and VO_2 is oxygen consumption

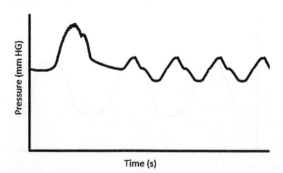

Fig. 8. Wedged pressure waveform.

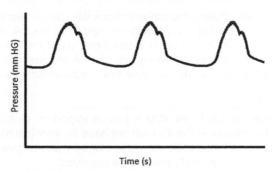

Fig. 9. Pulmonary artery pressure waveform.

$$VO_2 = CO \times (13.4 \times Hgb \times S_aO_2 - 13.4 \times Hgb \times S_vO_2)$$

where CO is cardiac output, Hgb is the patients' hemoglobin, S_aO_2 is arterial oxygen saturation in percent, S_vO_2 is mixed venous oxygen saturation, and VO_2 is oxygen consumption

or

$$VO_2 = CO \times 13.4 \times Hgb \times (S_aO_2 - S_vO_2)$$

where CO is cardiac output, Hgb is the patients' hemoglobin, S_aO_2, is arterial oxygen saturation in percent, S_vO_2 is mixed venous oxygen saturation, and VO_2 is oxygen consumption

The S_vO_2 is normally about 75%.

By combining oxygen delivery and consumption, an oxygen extraction ratio can be calculated. The equation is as follows:

$$OER = VO_2/DO_2$$

where DO_2 is oxygen delivery, OER is oxygen extraction ratio, and VO_2 is oxygen consumption

Plugging in the aforementioned equations for oxygen consumption and oxygen delivery are canceling terms, the following simplified equation based solely on mixed venous saturation and arterial oxygen saturation is reached:

$$OER = (S_aO_2 - S_vO_2)/S_aO_2$$

where OER is oxygen extraction ratio, S_aO_2, is arterial oxygen saturation in percent, and S_vO_2 is mixed venous oxygen saturation

An extraction ratio of 25% to 30% is normal. Anything less may indicate a need for intervention. Treatment is either to increase delivery by increasing cardiac output, increasing oxygen in blood, or increasing hemoglobin or to decrease consumption by decreasing the work of breathing, sedation, decreasing heart rate, eliminating fever, or even paralyzing patients.

The PA catheter is a very useful tool in the treatment of critically ill patients if used properly and on carefully selected patients. It carries the same general complications that a central venous line has, including mechanical complications during placement and catheter-related blood stream infection during maintenance. It has other complications because it passes through the heart. It causes multiple types of arrhythmias as a result of irritating the conducting system of the heart. The most alarming is asystole, which happens if patients already have baseline left heart block and the PA catheter causes right heart block. Pulling the catheter back will usually resolve this situation. Another potentially devastating complication is rupture of the PA This complication happens if the catheter tip is too far in a distal branch of the PA and the balloon ruptures the small vessel it is in. A free rupture of a PA requires quick attention from a surgeon adept in thoracic surgery because this is a potentially fatal problem.

Pulmonary Monitors

Monitoring respiratory status in the ICU is just as important as monitoring the CV system. Most of the patients in the ICU will not have an endotracheal tube in place, at least at some point. In these patients, pulse oximetry and respiratory rate are the only continuous monitors that really need to be observed.

Transthoracic impedance measuring is the technique that is used most commonly to continuously measure respiratory rate in ICU patients. This measuring is done with the telemetry leads. A small current is passed from one of the left-sided leads to one of the right-sided leads and the voltage is measured. This voltage will change with each breath as a result of the change in electrical resistance of the chest with each breath. The resulting rate of voltage cycles then corresponds to the patients' respiratory rate.

Capnography

The ventilator has many monitors to help care for intubated patients. Continuous capnography measures the amount of carbon dioxide that is exhaled with each breath. It is displayed as a waveform and looks like a square wave (**Fig. 10**). The plateau of the wave measures the amount of carbon dioxide made, and the shape of the wave corresponds more to the flow of air through the lungs. The more the wave looks like a square, the less restrictive the airway; the more the wave looks like a shark fin, the more obstructed the airway is, as in asthma[27] (**Fig. 11**). Changes in the amount of exhaled carbon dioxide can be one of the first signs of a change in physiologic status in critically ill patients. A decrease in exhaled carbon dioxide could indicate decreased production or increased minute ventilation. An increase in the difference between the expired carbon dioxide and the partial pressure of carbon dioxide measured in an arterial blood gas indicates an increase in dead space ventilation (**Figs. 10–12**).[28] Continuous capnography is not commonly used in ventilated patients but is used to confirm the placement of an endotracheal tube using a simple carbon dioxide monitor attached to the endotracheal tube after intubation.

GASTRIC TONOMETRY

Gastric tonometry is used to measure the mucosal carbon dioxide levels of the mucosa in the stomach. As blood flow to the stomach decreases, the carbon dioxide

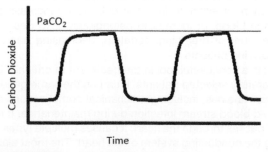

Fig. 10. Normal capnography.

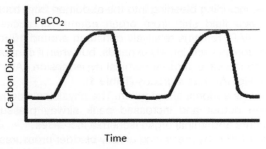

Fig. 11. Restrictive capnography (shark-fin wave).

levels of the tissues will increase. The theory is that by measuring this increase in carbon dioxide and reacting to its change, interventions can be done to improve the patient outcome.

The probe of the device is similar to a nasogastric tube and it is inserted in the same way. It measures mucosal carbon dioxide by allowing it to diffuse through a semipermeable membrane into a balloon that is on the distal part of the nasogastric tube. The machine then continuously measures the partial pressure of carbon dioxide in the balloon. If the partial pressure of carbon dioxide has increased by more than 8 mm Hg compared with an arterial blood gas, there is some form of mucosal ischemia.[29]

There are only a small number of studies that investigate this device. Of these studies, there are a few that are observational and show that patients who have a worse outcome do have an increase in gastric carbon dioxide concentrations.[30,31] There are few randomized trials using gastric tonometry. One trial showed that if gastric carbon dioxide was normal on admission to the ICU, patients that had care with gastric tonometry had better outcomes than those without. However, the same study showed no difference in the groups if gastric carbon dioxide was high on admission to the ICU.[32] No other randomized trials showed any difference, but there are trends toward gastric tonometry being another helpful tool in your ICU monitoring arsenal especially in extremely sick patients.[33–35]

ABDOMINAL COMPARTMENT PRESSURE MONITORING

Abdominal compartment hypertension and subsequent compartment syndrome are ominous entities and are a result of a few pathologic processes. While the intra-abdominal contents remain consistent, the volume of fluid in the abdomen can increase. An increase in fluid within the abdominal compartment occurs secondarily

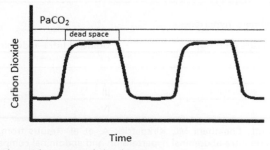

Fig. 12. Capnography with increased dead space.

to several situations, including bleeding into the abdomen from trauma or a ruptured aneurysm, third space fluid shift from organ edema, or ascites. Normal intra-abdominal pressure (IAP) remains relatively constant, around 10 mm Hg.[36] As fluid accumulates, the abdominal wall initially expands, but when it cannot stretch anymore the pressure starts to increase. Intra-abdominal hypertension (IAH) is defined as IAP greater than 12 mm Hg. IAH has 4 grades (**Table 1**).

The first sign of IAH is abdominal distention. The physiologic consequences of IAH are decreased urine output and increased peak airway pressures in ventilated patients. As IAH occurs abdominal organ ischemia increases.

The way to monitor IAP is by measuring urinary bladder pressures via a Foley catheter. The IAP is measured directly through the Foley catheter. The catheter is attached to a standard pressure transducer; 50 mL of saline are injected through the catheter into the bladder, and then the catheter is clamped so that the transducer will measure the pressure in the bladder. This procedure is done every hour for patients whose pressure is greater than 15 mm Hg. Medical management is recommended until IAP reaches 25 mm Hg. It is currently recommended that once the IAP is greater than 25 mm Hg, the abdomen needs decompression.[37]

Intracranial Pressure Monitoring

Cerebral blood flow depends on both blood pressure and intracranial pressure (ICP). For blood to circulate through the brain the pressure in the skull has to be less than mean arterial pressure. Cerebral perfusion pressure (CPP) is calculated as mean arterial pressure minus ICP. If ICP increases to approximate mean arterial pressure, blood will not flow into the brain and brain death will begin. There are many conditions that will cause an increase in ICP. Traumatic brain injury is the most common reason in the surgical ICU, but other causes include hydrocephalus, meningitis, brain tumor, stroke, or reperfusion of the brain after anoxia. If an increase in ICP is suspected by disease process, physiologic signs, or imaging and patients have altered mental status, an ICP monitor might be warranted.[38,39] These monitors are placed at the bedside by drilling a hole through the skull. A bolt is placed snugly through the hole and a transducer is then placed through the bolt into the subdural space to directly transduce ICP.

ICP in supine patients should be less than 20 mm Hg. Once ICP pressures start to exceed 20 mm Hg, complication rates start to increase. Maintaining a lower ICP is more important in patients with unilateral mass effect from tumors or trauma because these patients are more likely to herniate their brain compared with those patients with global brain edema. CPP is what is really important, so as ICP increases one can attempt to increase mean arterial pressure to maintain CPP.[38]

An external ventricular drain is a type ICP monitor where a catheter is placed through the previously mentioned bolt into one of the lateral ventricles of the brain.

Table 1	
Grades of intra-abdominal hypertension	
Intra-abdominal Pressure (mm Hg)	**Grade of Intra-abdominal Hypertension**
12–15	I
16–20	II
21–25	III
>25	IV

Data from Malbrain ML, Cheatham ML, Kirkpatrick A, et al. Results from the international conference of experts on intra-abdominal hypertension and abdominal compartment syndrome. I. Definitions. Intensive Care Med 2006;32(11):1722–32.

In this position, it can measure ICP but can also be used to drain cerebral spinal fluid (CSF). By draining CSF, one can directly reduce ICP.[40] This reduction can be of great importance, especially if that ventricle cannot drain naturally as a result of blood or some other obstruction.

TRANSCRANIAL DOPPLER ULTRASONOGRAPHY

Transcranial Doppler monitoring is a noninvasive monitoring technique used to measure the velocity of blood flow through the major blood vessels off of the circle of Willis. The transducer is placed on the side of the head and can determine the velocity, direction, and the depth of the artery that it is transducing. It is mainly used to monitor vasospasm, stenosis flow, flow in a subarachnoid hemorrhage, or to determine flow in possible brain death.[41] A major drawback to transcranial Doppler monitoring is the requirement of a skilled technician to perform the examination and a skilled person to interpret the results.

The transducer uses a 2 MHz wave. This frequency is relatively low for ultrasound, but this is required to penetrate the bone and have a signal that can be received from 3 major arteries in the brain. The normal velocities from the middle cerebral artery, anterior cerebral artery, and posterior cerebral artery are 62, 51, and 44 cm/s, respectively.[42] Once the velocities start to increase more than 120 cm/s, mild vasospasm is considered, and severe vasospasm is considered after 200 cm/s.[43,44] However, these velocities are arbitrary, and clinical assessment is key to determining if the results indicate ischemia. Some investigators advocate using flow acceleration and the pulsatility index as more accurate measurements.[45]

Transcranial Doppler examination can also be used to confirm brain death.[46] The caveat is that a prior transcranial Doppler study is required because 8% of patients do not have an acoustic window where flow can be obtained.[47]

Jugular Venous Bulb Oximetry

Jugular venous bulb oximetry is a technique to measure the mixed venous oxygen content in the blood leaving the brain. It is used to help determine if there is enough oxygen being delivered to the brain or if too much oxygen is being used. A catheter is placed in the jugular vein and directed cephalad to the jugular venous bulb. The catheter should be placed on the side with the dominant venous drainage. This side is usually the right side and can be determined if an intracranial bolt is present by occluding each side with manual pressure. The jugular occlusion should increase the ICP, and the side with the greatest pressure increase is the dominant side.[48] Mixed venous blood gases can be acquired via the catheter, or continuous jugular bulb venous oximetry can be used.[49] Common practice is to treat a mixed venous jugular saturation of less than 50% either by decreasing oxygen demand or by increasing oxygen delivery to the brain.[49]

Continuous Transesophageal Echocardiography

Transesophageal echocardiography is a very useful tool to determine the functionality of the heart. It is commonly used in the operating room during cardiac surgery.[50,51] It can be used to determine the cardiac parameters and fluid status of patients in the ICU, similar to the information obtained from a PA catheter; however, this was historically seen as a single-point-in-time invasive test.[52] Continuous transesophageal echocardiography has recently become available. The disposable probe is small and is placed in the esophagus and will continuously monitor cardiac function for up to 72 hours, at which time the probe is removed. This new technology may or may not change how we monitor patients in the ICU, but it does illustrate that there are many different ways to monitor patients in the ICU and there are probably many more to come.

REFERENCES

1. Tarditi DJ, Hollenberg SM. Cardiac arrhythmias in the intensive care unit. Semin Respir Crit Care Med 2006;27(3):221–9.
2. Polanczyk CA, Goldman L, Marcantonio ER, et al. Supraventricular arrhythmia in patients having noncardiac surgery: clinical correlates and effect on length of stay. Ann Intern Med 1998;129(4):279–85.
3. Walder LA, Spodick DH. Global T wave inversion. J Am Coll Cardiol 1991;17(7): 1479–85.
4. Walder LA, Spodick DH. Global T wave inversion: long-term follow-up. J Am Coll Cardiol 1993;21(7):1652–6.
5. Severinghaus JW, Honda Y. History of blood gas analysis. VII. Pulse oximetry. J Clin Monit 1987;3(2):135–8.
6. Benoit H, Costes F, Feasson L, et al. Accuracy of pulse oximetry during intense exercise under severe hypoxic conditions. Eur J Appl Physiol Occup Physiol 1997;76(3):260–3.
7. Santora RJ, Moore FA. Monitoring trauma and intensive care unit resuscitation with tissue hemoglobin oxygen saturation. Crit Care 2009;13(Suppl 5):S10.
8. Baetz MD, Pylypchuk G, Baetz M. A complication of ambulatory blood pressure monitoring. Ann Intern Med 1994;121(6):468–9.
9. Alford JW, Palumbo MA, Barnum MJ. Compartment syndrome of the arm: a complication of noninvasive blood pressure monitoring during thrombolytic therapy for myocardial infarction. J Clin Monit Comput 2002;17(3–4):163–6.
10. Low LL, Harrington GR, Stoltzfus DP. The effect of arterial lines on blood-drawing practices and costs in intensive care units. Chest 1995;108(1):216–9.
11. Marx G, Cope T, McCrossan L, et al. Assessing fluid responsiveness by stroke volume variation in mechanically ventilated patients with severe sepsis. Eur J Anaesthesiol 2004;21(02):132–8.
12. Monnet X, Anguel N, Jozwiak M, et al. Third-generation FloTrac/Vigileo does not reliably track changes in cardiac output induced by norepinephrine in critically ill patients. Br J Anaesth 2012;108(4):615–22.
13. Lucet JC, Bouadma L, Zahar JR, et al. Infectious risk associated with arterial catheters compared with central venous catheters. Crit Care Med 2010;38(4): 1030–5.
14. Stafford R. Placement of arterial line. Operat Tech Gen Surg 2003;5(3):7.
15. Dellinger RP, Levy MM, Carlet JM, et al. Surviving sepsis campaign: international guidelines for management of severe sepsis and septic shock: 2008. Crit Care Med 2008;36(1):296–327.
16. Marik PE. Techniques for assessment of intravascular volume in critically ill patients. J Intensive Care Med 2009;24(5):329–37.
17. Izakovic M. Central venous pressure–evaluation, interpretation, monitoring, clinical implications. Bratisl Lek Listy 2008;109(4):185–7.
18. McGee DC, Gould MK. Preventing complications of central venous catheterization. N Engl J Med 2003;348(12):1123–33.
19. Randolph AG, Cook DJ, Gonzales CA, et al. Ultrasound guidance for placement of central venous catheters: a meta-analysis of the literature. Crit Care Med 1996; 24(12):2053–8.

20. Hind D, Calvert N, McWilliams R, et al. Ultrasonic locating devices for central venous cannulation: meta-analysis. BMJ 2003;327(7411):361.
21. Litmanovitch M, Hon H, Luyt DK, et al. Comparison of central venous pressure measurements in the intrathoracic and the intra-abdominal vena cava in critically ill children. Anaesthesia 1995;50(5):407–10.
22. Joynt GM, Gomersall CD, Buckley TA, et al. Comparison of intrathoracic and intra-abdominal measurements of central venous pressure. Lancet 1996;347(9009): 1155–7.
23. McLaws ML, Berry G. Nonuniform risk of bloodstream infection with increasing central venous catheter-days. Infect Control Hosp Epidemiol 2005;26(8): 715–9.
24. Maki DG, Kluger DM, Crnich CJ. The risk of bloodstream infection in adults with different intravascular devices: a systematic review of 200 published prospective studies. Mayo Clin Proc 2006;81(9):1159–71.
25. Kandel G, Aberman A. Mixed venous oxygen saturation. Its role in the assessment of the critically ill patient. Arch Intern Med 1983;143(7):1400–2.
26. Nelson LD. Continuous venous oximetry in surgical patients. Ann Surg 1986; 203(3):329–33.
27. You B, Peslin R, Duvivier C, et al. Expiratory capnography in asthma: evaluation of various shape indices. Eur Respir J 1994;7(2):318–23.
28. Ahrens T, Sona C. Capnography application in acute and critical care. AACN Clin Issues 2003;14(2):123–32.
29. Bennett-Guerrero E. Gastric tonometry. In: Reich DL, editor. Monitoring in anesthesia and perioperative care. Cambridge (United Kingdom): Cambridge University Press; 2011. p. 95–7.
30. Riddington DW, Venkatesh B, Boivin CM, et al. Intestinal permeability, gastric intramucosal pH, and systemic endotoxemia in patients undergoing cardiopulmonary bypass. JAMA 1996;275(13):1007–12.
31. Kavarana MN, Frumento RJ, Hirsch AL, et al. Gastric hypercarbia and adverse outcome after cardiac surgery. Intensive Care Med 2003;29(5):742–8.
32. Gutierrez G, Palizas F, Doglio G, et al. Gastric intramucosal pH as a therapeutic index of tissue oxygenation in critically ill patients. Lancet 1992;339(8787): 195–9.
33. Ivatury RR, Simon RJ, Islam S, et al. A prospective randomized study of end points of resuscitation after major trauma: global oxygen transport indices versus organ-specific gastric mucosal pH. J Am Coll Surg 1996;183(2):145–54.
34. Heard SO. Gastric tonometry: the hemodynamic monitor of choice (Pro). Chest 2003;123(Suppl 5):469S–74S.
35. Hamilton MA, Mythen MG. Gastric tonometry: where do we stand? Curr Opin Crit Care 2001;7(2):122–7.
36. Sanchez NC, Tenofsky PL, Dort JM, et al. What is normal intra-abdominal pressure? Am Surg 2001;67(3):243–8.
37. Malbrain ML, Cheatham ML, Kirkpatrick A, et al. Results from the international conference of experts on intra-abdominal hypertension and abdominal compartment syndrome. I. Definitions. Intensive Care Med 2006;32(11):1722–32.
38. Stefini R, Rasulo FA. Intracranial pressure monitoring. Eur J Anaesthesiol Suppl 2008;42:192–5.
39. March K. Intracranial pressure monitoring: why monitor? AACN Clin Issues 2005; 16(4):456–75.
40. Roitberg BZ, Khan N, Alp MS, et al. Bedside external ventricular drain placement for the treatment of acute hydrocephalus. Br J Neurosurg 2001;15(4):324–7.

41. White H, Venkatesh B. Applications of transcranial Doppler in the ICU: a review. Intensive Care Med 2006;32(7):981–94.

42. Aaslid R, Markwalder TM, Nornes H. Noninvasive transcranial Doppler ultrasound recording of flow velocity in basal cerebral arteries. J Neurosurg 1982;57(6):769–74.

43. Aaslid R, Huber P, Nornes H. A transcranial Doppler method in the evaluation of cerebrovascular spasm. Neuroradiology 1986;28(1):11–6.

44. Aaslid R, Huber P, Nornes H. Evaluation of cerebrovascular spasm with transcranial Doppler ultrasound. J Neurosurg 1984;60(1):37–41.

45. Tsivgoulis G, Alexandrov A, Sloan M. Advances in transcranial Doppler ultrasonography. Curr Neurol Neurosci Rep 2009;9(1):46–54.

46. Feri M, Ralli L, Felici M, et al. Transcranial Doppler and brain death diagnosis. Crit Care Med 1994;22(7):1120–6.

47. Maeda H, Matsumoto M, Handa N, et al. Reactivity of cerebral blood flow to carbon dioxide in various types of ischemic cerebrovascular disease: evaluation by the transcranial Doppler method. Stroke 1993;24(5):670–5.

48. Robertson CS, Narayan RK, Gokaslan ZL, et al. Cerebral arteriovenous oxygen difference as an estimate of cerebral blood flow in comatose patients. J Neurosurg 1989;70(2):222–30.

49. Schell RM, Cole DJ. Cerebral monitoring: jugular venous oximetry. Anesth Analg 2000;90(3):559–66.

50. Shanewise JS, Cheung AT, Aronson S, et al. ASE/SCA guidelines for performing a comprehensive intraoperative multiplane transesophageal echocardiography examination: recommendations of the American Society of Echocardiography Council for Intraoperative Echocardiography and the Society of Cardiovascular Anesthesiologists Task Force for Certification in Perioperative Transesophageal Echocardiography. Anesth Analg 1999;89(4):870–84.

51. Mishra M, Chauhan R, Sharma KK, et al. Real-time intraoperative transesophageal echocardiography-how useful? Experience of 5,016 cases. J Cardiothorac Vasc Anesth 1998;12(6):625–32.

52. Tousignant CP, Walsh F, Mazer CD. The use of transesophageal echocardiography for preload assessment in critically ill patients. Anesth Analg 2000;90(2):351–5.

Hypovolemic Shock Resuscitation

Leslie Kobayashi, MD, Todd W. Costantini, MD,
Raul Coimbra, MD, PhD*

KEYWORDS

- Hemorrhagic shock • Septic shock • Massive transfusion • Blood loss • Crystalloid

KEY POINTS

- Hypovolemic shock is defined as inadequate tissue perfusion caused by decreased intravascular circulating volume.
- Early transfusion with a 1:1:1 ratio of fresh frozen plasma to platelets to packed red blood cells has been associated with improved outcomes in patients requiring massive transfusion.
- Monitoring coagulation function with thromboelastography or rotational thromboelastometry may be superior to conventional coagulation assays in patients with hypovolemic shock.

DEFINITION OF SHOCK

Shock is the inability of the body to maintain adequate end-organ perfusion. Hypovolemic shock caused by blood loss is frequently encountered after severe injury.[1] Hemorrhagic shock should be assumed to be the cause of hypotension in all trauma patients until proven otherwise. Shock is a strong predictor of mortality, and is a major risk factor for the development of complications, particularly multiple organ dysfunction. Hence, it is important to rapidly identify patients in shock so that appropriate resuscitation can begin as soon as possible. Indicators of shock include elevated heart rate, low blood pressure, narrowed pulse pressure, decreased capillary refill, cool clammy extremities, pale skin, increased skin turgor, low urine output, dry mucus membranes, and alterations in mental status. In certain patients, clinicians must keep in mind that significant blood loss can occur with little effect on vital signs. In particular, pediatric patients have excellent cardiovascular reserve, preventing a drop in blood pressure even in the presence of large volume blood loss. Conversely, elderly patients are often unable to mount a tachycardic response to hemorrhage, or may be on medications that blunt or prohibit normal response to blood loss. Elderly patients often also

The authors have nothing to disclose.
Division of Trauma, Surgical Critical Care, and Burns, Department of Surgery, University of California San Diego School of Medicine, 200 West Arbor Drive ##8896, San Diego, CA 92103, USA
* Corresponding author.
E-mail address: rcoimbra@ucsd.edu

have chronic underlying hypertension, and apparently normal blood pressure may, for them, be relative hypotension.

CLASSIFICATION OF HEMORRHAGIC SHOCK

Hemorrhagic shock is classified according to severity from class I to IV shock (**Table 1**). Class I shock is minor blood loss, often resulting in no significant derangement of vital signs or findings on clinical examination. Severity increases with increasing volumes of blood loss, with class IV shock caused by loss of more than 40% of circulating blood volume and resulting in hypotension, tachycardia, and severe multisystem organ derangements.

MASSIVE BLOOD LOSS AND MASSIVE TRANSFUSION

In addition to the traditional classifications of shock, a subset of patients with extensive injuries causing rapid hemorrhage develop massive blood loss (MBL) (**Box 1**). These patients often require alterations in goals of care from definitive management to damage control, and may require different resuscitation strategies and monitoring. Patients with MBL often require massive transfusion in response to their hemorrhage. Massive transfusion (MT) is typically defined as 10 or more units of packed red blood cells (PRBCs) in a 24-hour period.[2–7] At this level of transfusion, hemodilution of fibrinogen, platelets, and clotting factors can occur as whole blood continues to be lost, and is replaced with only crystalloid or PRBCs. These patients are at high risk for developing acidosis and hypothermia from blood loss, injury burden, and associated need for multicavitary surgery. This acidosis and hypothermia can further exacerbate coagulopathy, resulting in the "bloody vicious triad."[8]

Of all trauma admissions, 8% to 11% of patients will require a blood transfusion during their hospital stay.[5] Only approximately 3% of trauma patients will have blood loss requiring MT, although this percentage may increase to 8% to 15% among busy urban trauma centers and among military casualties.[9–13] As many as 24% of patients presenting in shock will require MT, and those with MT account for up to 60% to 70% of all PRBCs used.[14,15] Mortality increases in a linear fashion with PRBC transfusions and can be as high as 60% to 100% (**Table 2**).[3,9,13–19]

CLASSICAL RESUSCITATION OF SHOCK STATES

The most important step in resuscitation of hemorrhagic shock is identification and rapid control of the source of bleeding, which can be accomplished with direct pressure, application of a tourniquet, suture ligation, or surgery. Although maneuvers to

Table 1
Classes of hemorrhagic shock

	Class I	Class II	Class III	Class IV
Blood loss (mL)	≤750	750–1500	1500–2000	≥2000
Blood loss (% blood volume)	≤15%	15%–30%	30%–40%	≥40%
Pulse rate (BPM)	<100	>100	>120	>140
Blood pressure	Normal	Normal	↓	↓
Pulse pressure	Normal or ↑	↓	↓	↓
Capillary refill	Normal	Delayed	Delayed	Delayed

Abbreviation: BPM, beats per minute.

Box 1
Definitions of massive blood loss
Loss of entire blood volume within 24 hours
Loss of 50% of blood volume within 3 hours
Ongoing blood loss of 150 mL/min
Ongoing blood loss of 1.5 mL/kg/min
Rapid blood loss leading to circulatory failure
Data from Fraga GP, Bansal V, Coimbra R. Transfusion of blood products in trauma: an update. J Emerg Med 2010;39(2):253–60.

control bleeding are ongoing, attempts should be made to ensure adequate intravenous access, which can be accomplished by placing 2 large-bore peripheral intravenous lines, or an intraosseous or central line.

Once access is secured, resuscitation should begin with immediate infusion of warmed fluids to restore circulating blood volume replacing losses from hemorrhage. Classical resuscitation strategies for hemorrhagic shock, taught by Advanced Trauma Life Support (ATLS), suggest bolus infusion of 2 L of warmed crystalloid if hypotension is present, followed by replacement of ongoing fluid or blood losses with isotonic fluids in a 3:1 ratio to accommodate losses into the interstitial space.[1,20]

Choice of fluid for resuscitation is an area of ongoing research. Resuscitation fluids should be considered medications, and as with any medication, may be associated with deleterious side effects, including exacerbation of cellular injury, immunosuppression, and inflammation.[20–22] Resuscitation fluids may result in significant acid base and electrolyte derangements. The ideal resuscitation fluid should be cheap, safe, easy to store, and portable; increase oxygen carrying capacity; have beneficial immuno-inflammatory properties; and be able to rapidly and effectively increase intravascular volume.

Crystalloids

Normal saline and lactated Ringer solution are the most commonly used resuscitation fluids in hypovolemic and hemorrhagic shock. Although lactated Ringer solution may theoretically be preferable because of its ability to buffer metabolic acidosis and prevent hyperchloremic acidosis associated with normal saline infusions, this

Table 2			
Stepwise increase in mortality with transfusion			
	Mortality		
PRBCs (Units)	Como et al,[15] 2004	Huber-Wagner et al,[17] 2007	Inaba et al,[142] 2008 *Uncross-Matched
1–10	22%	14.8%	<7 = 30% >7 = 54%
11–20	30%	35.1%	<15 = 78% ≥15 = 95%
21–40	50%	20–29 = 53.7% ≥30 = 60.4%	
>40	59%		

* This study includes patients given uncross-matched blood.

beneficial effect is seen only with massive infusions. Studies comparing normal saline and lactated Ringer solution in minimal and moderate hemorrhage show equivalent outcomes.[1,23,24] Because of its composition, a theoretical risk of hyperkalemia is associated with the use of lactated Ringer solution, which may be exacerbated in patients with acute kidney injury or chronic renal insufficiency. Additionally, the D isomer of lactate may have adverse inflammatory and immunomodulatory properties.[1,23]

Colloids

Colloids are theoretically retained in the intravascular space to a greater extent than crystalloids, which may have several benefits during resuscitation. First, intravascular volume can be expanded more rapidly. Second, a smaller total volume of fluid may be used to achieve adequate perfusion. Third, because there is potentially less third-spacing, the risk of complications such as bowel edema, abdominal compartment syndrome (ACS), and acute respiratory distress syndrome (ARDS) may be decreased. However, numerous studies examining the use of colloids in resuscitation of the critically ill and injured have failed to demonstrate a statistically significant benefit. A Cochrane review in 2002 comparing albumin with crystalloid resuscitation among a mixed intensive care unit (ICU) population found that the relative risk (RR) of death was higher with albumin than the comparison group (RR, 1.52; CI, 1.17–1.99), with a 5% absolute increase in the overall risk of death (14% compared with 9%).[25]

The Saline versus Albumin Fluid Evaluation (SAFE) Study, the largest randomized controlled trial to date, compared 3497 patients who received 4% albumin with 3500 patients receiving normal saline and found no significant difference in mortality, days on the ventilator, need for renal replacement therapy, or hospital length of stay.[26] Subsequent meta-analyses that included the SAFE Study have confirmed overall equivalence in outcomes when comparing albumin with crystalloid for hypovolemic critically ill patients.[27,28] Given the relative expense and lack of beneficial effects, albumin as a primary resuscitation fluid cannot be recommended. One should also keep in mind that some patients may be harmed by albumin resuscitation. A subgroup analysis of patients with traumatic brain injury (TBI) in the SAFE Study found that albumin resulted in significantly higher mortality in these patients (RR, 1.63; CI, 1.17–2.26; $P = .003$). This risk was even more pronounced among patients with severe TBI (RR, 1.88; CI, 1.31–2.7; $P<.001$).[29] Increased mortality associated with albumin resuscitation has also been noted in trauma and burn patients.[26,28,29]

In addition to albumin, multiple trials of synthetic colloids have also been conducted, including a variety of hydroxyethyl starch formulations. Synthetic colloids are appealing as a resuscitation fluid because they can be manufactured cheaply, avoid risks of blood borne pathogens, and theoretically increase circulating blood volume to a greater extent than crystalloids. However, significant evidence shows that their use may be associated with coagulopathy and an increased risk of acute kidney injury. Animal studies demonstrate significantly increased bleeding and clinical coagulopathy with hydroxyethyl starch compared with albumin and blood products. Even more concerning is that the coagulopathy in these animals manifested as increased bleeding and hemorrhagic death but was not associated with derangements in traditional laboratory measures of clotting, such as prothrombin time (PT) and activated partial thromboplastin time (aPTT).[30–32] Meta-analysis of both in vitro and in vivo studies involving several hydroxyethyl starch formulations confirmed these results, finding significant hypocoagulatory effects of hydroxyethyl starch as measured by thromboelastography (TEG) or rotation thromboelastometry (ROTEM).[33] Multiple meta-analyses have confirmed the association between acute kidney injury and hydroxyethyl starch administration with odds ratios for acute kidney injury ranging from 1.5–1.92.[34,35]

This association seems particularly strong when hydroxyethyl starch is used in resuscitating patients with sepsis and septic shock.[34]

Among humans, a meta-analysis of hydroxyethyl starch compared with other resuscitation fluids found no significant difference in mortality with the use of hydroxyethyl starch, but found insufficient data to determine overall affect of hydroxyethyl starch on coagulopathy and acute kidney injury.[36] A randomized controlled trial of severely injured trauma patients comparing hydroxyethyl starch and normal saline found that patients given hydroxyethyl starch required significantly more blood transfusions; however, they were also more severely injured. No difference in mortality was found between the groups.[37] A retrospective review of 2225 trauma patients found that those who received hydroxyethyl starch were more likely to develop acute kidney injury (RR, 1.73; CI, 1.3–2.28). Hydroxyethyl starch was also associated with increased risk of mortality (RR, 1.84; CI, 1.48–2.29) and was an independent predictor for death.[38]

HYPERTONIC SALINE

Hypertonic saline has anti-inflammatory and laudable immunomodulatory effects in animal models of hemorrhagic shock. These animal models demonstrate decreased lung and intestinal injury after hypertonic saline resuscitation.[21,22,39] Similar anti-inflammatory effects are also seen in small human trials.[39] In trauma patients, hypertonic saline has the additional benefit of acting as an osmotic agent to decrease cerebral edema in patients with TBI.[40,41] Because hypertonic solutions are retained more in the intravascular space, they have the potential to decrease risks of ACS and ARDS. Unfortunately, human clinical trials to date have not consistently found a benefit to hypertonic saline over isotonic fluids in the prehospital or acute resuscitation phase after traumatic injury.[42–45] Although an analysis of blunt trauma patients receiving hypertonic saline in conjunction with MT showed an improvement in ARDS-free survival (HR, 2.18; CI, 1.09–4.36),[42] a larger follow-up multicenter randomized controlled trial in trauma patients with hypovolemic shock found no survival or morbidity benefit compared with normal saline.[43] Subgroup analysis also revealed significantly increased mortality among the subset of patients who did not require a blood transfusion in the first 24 hours.[43] Additional studies of trauma patients with TBI also failed to demonstrate any improvement in mortality or neurologic outcomes.[46,47]

Blood Products

ATLS suggests transfusion of PRBCs only if patients fail to respond to crystalloid bolus.[48] Use of blood components, such as fresh frozen plasma (FFP), platelets, and fibrinogen, were not classically part of the initial trauma resuscitation. These components were typically only given if laboratory evidence of deficiencies were noted during ongoing resuscitation. Classical triggers of component therapy include FFP transfusion for PT and aPTT greater than 1.5 to 1.8 times normal; platelet transfusion for platelets less than 50×10^9/L; and cryoprecipitate transfusion if fibrinogen less than 0.8 g/L.

DAMAGE CONTROL RESUSCITATION
Problems with Classical Resuscitation

Classical resuscitation strategies present several problems in patients with hemorrhagic shock after trauma. First, immediate fluid resuscitation to normal goal blood pressures may increase the blood flow to injuries and perfusion pressures, increasing the risk of "popping the clot," causing recurrent bleeding, or increasing ongoing blood loss.[49] Additionally, the large volumes of fluid given in aggressive resuscitation strategies may result in significant third-spacing, causing complications such as bowel edema and anastomotic leaks, ACS, and ARDS.[50,51] Classical resuscitation strategies also presume that coagulopathy is a late complication after trauma. However, several studies have challenged this paradigm and demonstrated that coagulopathy is present in up to 24% to 74% of patients on admission.[4,5,52–57] Far from treating or preventing this complication, traditional resuscitation strategies may exacerbate bleeding through inducing a dilutional coagulopathy and exacerbating hypothermia. Several studies show a stepwise increase in coagulopathy associated with the volume of crystalloid administered.[6,54] Good evidence also suggests that resuscitation of MBL with PRBCs alone results in significant derangements of coagulation and thrombocytopenia as PRBC replacement approaches 12 units, or one circulating blood volume.[58,59] Even in the absence of documented coagulopathy, patients with MBL or requiring MT have poor outcomes in response to classic resuscitation strategies, with mortality ranging from 36% to 62%; this increases to 46% to 77% when coagulopathy is present.[7,53,60–62] Because of the potential for exacerbation of coagulopathy, increased bleeding, and potential complications associated with classical resuscitation, newer "damage control resuscitation strategies" are proposed. Damage control resuscitation (DCR), similar to damage control laparotomy, applies to patients with overwhelming injury burden and MBL. The tenets of DCR include selective use of permissive hypotension, early aggressive use of blood transfusions in a 1:1:1 ratio of PRBCs to FFP to platelets, and selective use of hemostatic adjuncts. The goals of DCR are to minimize bleeding, increase end organ perfusion, prevent coagulopathy, and minimize risks of multisystem organ dysfunction.

Permissive Hypotension

Permissive hypotension strategies withhold or minimize fluids as long as cerebral perfusion is evident and systolic blood pressures remain above a threshold value of 70 to 80 mm Hg. This low-volume strategy should be maintained until bleeding is controlled. Proponents of permissive hypotension suggest that administration of crystalloid may aggravate the inflammatory response, increase blood loss before definitive hemostasis, and increase transfusion requirements, which could further exacerbate early inflammation and late immunosuppression. Studies have examined the safety of permissive hypotension or restrictive resuscitation strategies in the prehospital, emergency department, and intraoperative phases of care. The landmark study by Bickell and colleagues[63] compared victims of penetrating torso trauma randomized to traditional fluid resuscitation or delayed resuscitation in the field and emergency department. The delayed group received no more than 100 mL of fluid before arrival in the operating room. Patients in the delayed group demonstrated a significant survival benefit (70% vs 62%), fewer complications, and a shorter hospital length of stay when compared with the traditional resuscitation group. Another prehospital study of patients with traumatic amputation found that restrictive prehospital fluid resuscitation strategies resulted in improved survival.[64] A study by Morrison and colleagues[65] compared low (50) versus traditional (65) mean arterial pressure goals to guide intraoperative resuscitation. The lower mean arterial pressure group experienced significantly less blood loss, had fewer transfusions, and had less crystalloid administered compared with the traditional group. The lower group had significantly improved early survival (98% vs 83%) and maintained a trend toward improved mortality at 30 days. As with the study by Bickell and colleagues,[63] the beneficial effects were most significant for victims of penetrating trauma. Unfortunately, few other studies have been able to replicate these positive effects, and active debate continues regarding the benefits of permissive hypotension. Its application, if used, should be limited to penetrating torso trauma victims.

Blood products

Evidence supporting early aggressive use of blood products for resuscitation came from work performed by the military. Austere combat settings limited access to large volumes of crystalloid and separated blood components; however, "walking blood banks" and fresh whole blood (FWB) were available. Studies of these patients revealed improved survival when FWB rather than PRBCs or traditional component therapy was used for resuscitation, and FWB was found to be associated with minimal infectious risk in these military populations.[18,66,67] Unlike the military, the civilian trauma patient is unlikely to have access to a reliable, homogenous, and immediately available "walking blood bank," and therefore, studies have focused on the effect of increasing the FFP-to-PRBC and platelets-to-PRBC ratios in an effort to mimic the composition of FWB for resuscitation of patients with MT. Two studies from the military revealed decreased mortality in a stepwise fashion with increasing plasma-to-PRBC ratios, with optimal results approaching a ratio of 1:1.[68–70] Civilian literature has also reflected improved mortality, with FFP-to-PRBC ratios approaching 1:1 (**Table 3**).[4,62,71–77] Unfortunately, most of these studies have been retrospective in nature and handicapped by the potential for survivor bias. A group in Germany has tried to compensate for this bias by performing a time-dependent covariate analysis among blunt trauma patients requiring MT, and found that even after correcting for survivor bias, an FFP-to-PRBC ratio of 1:1.5 or greater was associated with improved survival.[78] Studies of platelets-to-PRBC ratios have shown similar improvements in mortality, with higher ratios among patients undergoing MT (**Table 4**).[71,77,79–82] Lastly, studies of fibrinogen replacement have also supported both protocolized and TEG/ROTEM-guided supplementation of fibrinogen in the resuscitation of patients undergoing MT.[80,81,83–85] In contrast to FFP and platelets, which are available as single and pooled donor units only, fibrinogen can be supplemented using cryoprecipitate for transfusion or through administration of a concentrate derived from human plasma. Each vial contains between 900 and 1300 mg of lyophilized fibrinogen, which is reconstituted in as little as 50 mL of saline. Overall, a benefit does appear to be demonstrated from higher FFP-to-PRBC, platelets-to-PRBC, and fibrinogen-to-PRBC ratios during acute resuscitation of the MBL/MT patient. Although the ideal ratio

Table 3 FFP-to-PRBC ratio and outcomes		
Study	**FFP-to-PRBC Ratio**	**Outcome**
Military		
Borgman et al,[70] 2007	1:1.4	Improved mortality
Van et al,[69] 2010	<1:4	Improved mortality, no change MSOF
Civilian		
Sperry et al,[73] 2008	≥1:1.5	Improved mortality, increased ARDS
Kashuk et al,[72] 2008	1:2–1:3	Improved mortality
Holcomb et al,[71] 2008	≥1:2	Improved mortality
Gunter et al,[77] 2008	≥2:3	Improved mortality
Teixeira et al,[74] 2009	>1:3	Improved mortality
Snyder et al,[76] 2009	>1:2	Improved mortality
Duchesne et al,[4] 2009	1:1 vs 1:4	Improved mortality
Lustenberger et al,[78] 2011	≥1:1.5	Improved mortality

Abbreviations: ARDS, acute respiratory distress syndrome; MSOF, multisystem organ failure.

Table 4 Platelets-to-PRBC ratio and outcomes		
Study	Platelets-to-PRBC	Outcome
Military		
Perkins et al,[80] 2009	≥1:8	Improved mortality
Civilian		
Gunter et al,[77] 2008	≥1:5	Improved mortality
Holcomb et al,[71] 2008	≥1:2	Improved mortality
Zink et al,[82] 2009	≥1:4	Improved mortality
Inaba et al,[79] 2010	≥1:6	Improved mortality
Shaz et al,[81] 2010	≥1:2	Improved mortality

of each component is still unknown, 2 prospective trials are currently enrolling patients in an attempt to further delineate the ideal ratio of blood components for resuscitation and to answer definitively the question of survivor bias.[86,87]

Hemostatic adjuncts

In addition to a balanced transfusion strategy, several pharmacologic agents can be used as adjuncts to treat coagulopathy, including tranexamic acid, recombinant human factor VIIa, and prothrombin complex, which contains factors II, VII, IX, X, C, and S. Some evidence shows that use of these agents may decrease mortality, transfusion requirements, and rates of transfusion-related organ failure among certain trauma patients.

Factor VIIa

Initially developed for treatment of hemophilia, activated factor VIIa has been used to treat several trauma scenarios, including trauma-induced coagulopathy and reversal of anticoagulation in patients with brain injury. A randomized controlled trial of recombinant factor VIIa showed a decrease in PRBC transfusions and the percentage of patients requiring MT after blunt trauma.[88] A follow-up study from the same group confirmed the benefit of decreased transfusion requirements, and demonstrated lower rates of multisystem organ failure and ARDS associated with factor VIIa.[89] Although neither study found any increase in complications associated with factor VIIa, both studies were unable to confirm a mortality benefit. A study by Morse and colleagues[90] examining the protocolized use of factor VIIa as an adjunct in MT confirmed that it resulted in significantly decreased transfusion requirements, and also found a benefit in early mortality in the subset of patients receiving 30 units or greater of PRBCs (24-hour mortality, 26% vs 64%). Unfortunately, this benefit did not persist at 30 days. Subsequent studies, including a large multinational randomized controlled trial (CONTROL trial) also failed to confirm any significant mortality benefit in a variety of patient groups.[90–93] Additionally, concerns have been raised regarding increased thromboembolic complications, particularly those affecting the arterial circulation, associated with the use of factor VIIa.[92,94,95] Although factor VIIa is likely safe among patients with MBL, it is unlikely to be beneficial and therefore its use in DCR cannot be recommended.

Prothrombin complex

Prothrombin complex comes in a variety of formulations, all of which contain some combination of vitamin K–dependent coagulation factors. Three-factor prothrombin complex formulations contain factor II, IX, and X. Four-factor prothrombin complex formulations contain factor II, VII, IX, and X. Both 3- and 4-factor formulations also contain variable amounts of protein C and S. Several studies have compared PCC with FFP and vitamin K for reversal of pharmacologic coagulopathy after injury or in anticipation of emergent surgery or invasive procedures. These studies uniformly found that prothrombin complex was faster and more efficacious than FFP and vitamin K at correcting international normalized ratio (INR) without any significant increase in complications.[96–100] Normalization of laboratory values of coagulation was achieved in as quickly as 30 minutes after administration of prothrombin complex, although in some instances reversal was not as durable as that achieved with vitamin K.[98,100] Recent studies examining prothrombin complex in trauma patients revealed trends toward improved mortality, decreased transfusion requirements, fewer complications, and shorter lengths of stay. In particular, the risk of multiorgan failure and need for mechanical ventilation were diminished with the use of prothrombin complex.[84,85,101–103] Concern exists over the potential for prothrombin complex to increase the risks of thromboembolic complications similar to factor VIIa. A recent meta-analysis of the studies of prothrombin complex to date found a rate of thromboembolic events of 1.4%.[104] However, no statistically significant increases in thrombotic events over controls have been noted in studies of trauma patients to date.[102,103,105]

Tranexamic acid

Tranexamic acid is a synthetic derivative of lysine. Tranexamic acid inhibits plasminogen activation and plasmin activity through bonding to the lysine binding site, blocking binding to fibrin. Unlike factor VIIa and prothrombin complex, its effects occur primarily through preventing fibrinolysis rather than promoting coagulation.[106] Two large prospective trials, one among civilian trauma patients and one among more severely injured military trauma victims, both found significant benefit from use of tranexamic acid. The CRASH-2 trial was a prospective randomized controlled trial of 20,211 trauma patients randomized to tranexamic acid infusion or placebo. Tranexamic acid was associated with an absolute decrease in all-cause mortality (14.5% vs 16%), with an RR of 0.91 (CI, 0.85–0.97; $P = .0035$). Mortality from bleeding was also decreased (4.9% vs 5.7%), with an RR of 0.85 (CI, 0.76–0.96; $P = .0077$). No statistically significant increases in either venous or arterial thromboembolic complications were noted. However, benefit was only found if tranexamic acid was given within 3 hours of injury; administration after 3 hours was associated with increased mortality.[107] The Military Application of Tranexamic Acid in Traumatic Emergency and Resuscitative Surgery (MATTERs) study examined a group of severely injured military trauma patients, of which 26% required MT. Tranexamic acid was administered within 1 hour of injury to 293 patients. Despite a higher injury severity, patients who received tranexamic acid had a significantly decreased unadjusted mortality (17.4% vs 23.9%). This benefit was even more pronounced among patients who received MT, with mortality decreased 13.7% (14.4% vs 28.1%). After multivariate logistic regression analysis, tranexamic acid was found to be an independent predictor of survival. Although an increase in venous thromboembolic complications was associated with tranexamic acid, it was not an independent predictor of thromboembolic complications in either the group as a whole or among patients who received MT.[108]

Massive transfusion protocols

Standardizing transfusion ratios with institutional massive transfusion protocols (MTP) has increased in popularity. The goal of an MTP is to standardize the replacement of platelets and clotting factors in an optimum ratio to PRBCs, and increase speed and efficiency of transfusion. An MTP may include protocolized use of hemostatic adjuncts, such as tranexamic acid, prothrombin complex, and factor VIIa.

Carefully selected triggers of MTPs are important for 2 key reasons. First, rapid identification of patients likely to require MT and early aggressive transfusion of blood, FFP, and platelets has been associated with improved mortality.[109–111] Second, aggressive resuscitation and administration of higher ratios of FFP and platelets, when given to patients who are not massively bleeding, causes an unnecessary expenditure of resources and may result in worse outcomes for patients.[112–115] Indications for MTP include transfusion and clinical triggers. Transfusion triggers generally range between 6 and 10 units of PRBCs as a threshold to initiate MTP. Transfusion triggers are easily defined and adhered to, but may lead to delays in administration of FFP/platelets, because significant blood loss must have occurred before protocol initiation. Clinical variables commonly associated with MT include multicavitary trauma, penetrating mechanism, systolic blood pressure less than 90 mm Hg, heart rate greater than 120, anemia (hemoglobin <10) or coagulopathy (INR >1.5) at admission, and free fluid on focused assessment with sonography for trauma (FAST).[9,13,116,117] Clinical triggers are likely to result in earlier initiation of MTPs but use of any single element may be inaccurate. Therefore, several scoring systems have been created using multiple elements, including the trauma-associated severe hemorrhage (TASH) score, the McLaughlin score, and the assessment of blood consumption (ABC) score.[13,14,117] The TASH and McLaughlin scores include laboratory data such as hematocrit, pH, and base deficit, whereas the ABC score uses only clinical data immediately available on admission, which may make it a more useful tool. The ABC score consists of 4 elements: penetrating mechanism, positive FAST, blood pressure less than 90 mm Hg, and heart rate 120 or greater (**Table 5**). A score of 2 or more predicts MT with a sensitivity of 75% to 90% and specificity of 67% to 88% in initial studies.[9,13] When compared with the more complex TASH and McLaughlin scores, the ABC score was as or more accurate in predicting which patients would require MT.[12,13]

Initiation of an MTP is meant to increase communication among the surgeon/anesthesia team, laboratory, and blood bank, and increase ease and efficiency in ordering blood products. A growing body of evidence supports the efficacy of MTPs in the civilian trauma population. First and foremost, MTPs seem to be effective in achieving their primary goal of high FFP- and platelets-to-PRBC ratios, and significantly decreased crystalloid infusion.[10,118–120] Use of MTPs seems to decrease overall blood product use.[11,121] This finding may be because of prevention or more rapid treatment of coagulopathy, resulting in decreased total blood losses. Several studies show that the initiation of an MTP significantly decreases the time from admission to first transfusion, and the turnaround time for subsequent transfusions.[118,122] Meeting these goals of DCR decreases mortality and the percentage of patients developing acoagulopathy.[11,111,118–121] Although randomized controlled trials are lacking, multivariate analysis identifies DCR and MTP initiation as independent predictors of survival.[11,111,120,121] Additionally, a study performed solely after initiation of an institutional MTP found that compliance with all measures of the protocol improved survival (86.7% vs 45%; P<.001), and multivariate analysis identified compliance with MTP as an independent predictor of survival.[121] Efficacy in achieving high FFP-to-PRBC ratios and high survival rates is found with the use of MTPs among military personnel.[123] Analysis of survivors of MTP shows that decrease in mortality does not come at the cost of increased morbidity. Use of MTPs seems to result in significantly lower rates of ACS; decreased need for open abdomens; decreased rates of sepsis, particularly pneumonia; decreased rates of multiorgan failure, particularly respiratory failure;

Table 5 MTP predictive models			
Scoring System	ABC	TASH[117]	McLaughlin[14]
Variables	ED SBP $\leq$90 mm Hg (1 pnt) ED HR $\geq$120 BPM (1 pnt) Penetrating trauma (1 pnt) +FAST (1 pnt)	SBP <100 mm Hg (4 pnts) SBP <120 mm Hg (1 pnt) HR >120 BPM (2 pnts) Hgb <7 (8 pnts) Hgb <9 (6 pnts) Hgb <10 (4 pnts) Hgb <11 (3 pnts) +ΓAST (3 pnts) Complex fracture AIS 3–4 (3 pnts) AIS 5 (6 pnts) BE <−10 (4 pnts) BE <−6 (3 pnts) BE <−2 (1 pnt) Gender (male = 1 pnt)	SBP <110 mm Hg HR >105 BPM pH <7.25 Hct <32%
Predictive value	Score 2 = 38% MTP Score 3 = 45% MTP Score 4 = 100% MTP	Score $\geq$16 = 50% MTP Score $\geq$27 = 100% MTP	Score 1 = 20% MTP Score 4 = 80% MTP
Comparative accuracy Nunez et al,[13] 2009 Krumrei et al,[12] 2012	AROC = 0.842 AROC = 0.86	AROC = 0.842 AROC = 0.51	AROC = 0.846 AROC = 0.56

Abbreviations: AIS, abbreviated injury score; AROC, area under the receiver operating characteristic; BE, base excess; BPM, beats per minute; ED, emergency department; Hct, hematocrit; Hgb, hemoglobin; HR, heart rate; pnt, point; SBP, systolic blood pressure.

and decreased hospital length of stay. Lastly, some evidence shows that MTPs may significantly decrease hospital costs.[122]

Role of Laboratory Guidance

Classical measures of coagulopathy, such as PT/INR and aPTT, which are warmed to standard body temperature (37°C) before analysis, may falsely normalize results and lead to underdiagnosis of coagulopathy. These tests do not address platelet dysfunction caused by medications, hypothermia, or fibrinolysis, further underestimating coagulopathy. In fact, several studies that reported clinically evident coagulopathy found that these traditional laboratory values correlate poorly with clinical evidence of medical bleeding in humans and animals.[19,124] Additionally PT, aPTT, and complete blood cell counts often require 30 minutes to more than an hour before results are available, potentially delaying treatment of trauma-related coagulopathy.[57,125] These limitations of traditional measures of coagulopathy have led to a resurgence in the use of alternative measures of clotting and clot strength, including TEG or ROTEM. TEG and ROTEM work similarly and measure the viscoelastic properties of a patient's blood sample. TEG/ROTEM have the benefit of rapidly providing detailed information on clot formation and strength, and are run at patient temperatures, potentially improving accuracy in diagnosing coagulopathy. In the resuscitation of trauma patients in severe hemorrhagic shock, TEG/ROTEM can have 2 potential applications: results drawn at admission can be used to predict and trigger MTPs, and serial results can be used to direct ongoing blood component therapy. Persuasive evidence currently shows that TEG/ROTEM are beneficial in both roles. Several studies have proven TEG/ROTEM to be good predictors of the need for transfusion and MT, and of mortality.[10,56,125-128] Additionally, several of these studies compared TEG/ROTEM results with standard laboratory findings (PT/INR and aPTT) and found them to have a higher sensitivity for detecting coagulopathy on admission and an improved accuracy in predicting transfusion, MT, and mortality.[10,56,125,128]

TEG/ROTEM results are available to the clinician running the resuscitation significantly quicker than traditional laboratory measures of coagulopathy, with initial results available within 5 minutes.[10,125] When used in ongoing resuscitation or as part of an MTP, TEG/ROTEM was associated with shorter time to first transfusion, higher FFP-to-PRBC ratios, and increased platelet transfusion.[52,129] Effect of TEG/ROTEM use on mortality is unclear, but some evidence suggests a survival benefit. In a study of trauma patients, ROTEM-guided resuscitation resulted in mortality significantly less than that predicted by the trauma score–injury severity score, or TRISS (24.4% vs 33.7%; $P = .032$). This survival benefit was even more dramatic after excluding patients with isolated TBI (14% vs 27.8%; $P = .0018$).[84] Another study of patients requiring MT treated before and after initiation of MTP with TEG found that MTP with TEG guidance was associated with a significant improvement in 30-day (20.4% vs 31.5%; $P = .0002$) and 90-day mortality (22.4% vs 34.6%; $P<.0001$).[129]

Efficacy

Damage control resuscitation, including permissive hypotension, early use of blood products, more aggressive coagulation factor replacement, and MTPs, seems to have had a beneficial effect on outcomes. A study reviewing patients with MBL who were resuscitated with classical techniques within the period of 1970 to 1990 showed that they experienced very poor outcomes, with mortality ranging from 61% to 90%.[7,19,60,61,130] These findings improved somewhat in later studies conducted from 1990 to the 2000s, but survival was still poor, ranging from 45% to 87%.[3,4,111,118,119,130] In contrast, current mortality rates after initiation of DCR and MTPs range from 8% to 34%.[3,4,54,55,111,118,123]

VASOACTIVE AGENTS

Because of the morbidity associated with excessive fluid administration and the paucity of evidence supporting permissive hypotension outside of penetrating trauma, many investigators have begun examining the role of early vasopressor use in patients with hypovolemic shock. Early use of vasopressors, particularly before definitive hemostasis, has the theoretical benefit of allowing the surgeon to maintain an acceptable mean arterial pressure while avoiding the need for large volume fluid administration. Several animal models show that endogenous vasopressin is required to maintain blood pressure in response to hemorrhage, and exogenous vasopressin can act as an effective vasopressor, reversing advanced hemorrhagic shock more effectively than other agents or fluid administration.[131-134] Vasopressin use resulted in significantly decreased blood loss and improved survival in several of these studies.[131,134] Data suggest a deficit of endogenous vasopressin after hemorrhagic shock in association with TBI.[135,136] Human data supporting the use of vasopressin in the acute resuscitation period are lacking. A single prospective randomized controlled trial of patients who experienced hypotensive trauma randomized to standard fluid resuscitation or resuscitation with bolus then infusion of vasopressin after trauma found a nonsignificant improvement in mortality (13% vs 25%; $P = .19$). This study also found that the vasopressin group received significantly less fluid in the first 5 days; however, this did not translate into any benefit in terms of 30-day mortality, morbidity, or organ dysfunction.[137] Another small study of patients experiencing blunt traumatic arrest found that the addition of vasopressin and hydroxyethyl starch to standard cardiopulmonary resuscitation resulted in increased return of spontaneous circulation and 24-hour survival.[138] However, 3 large retrospective studies of severely injured and hypotensive trauma patients found the administration of vasopressin was associated with significantly increased risk of death regardless of volume status.[139–141] Evidence is currently insufficient to recommend the use of vasopressin or other vasoactive agents as a substitute for aggressive fluid resuscitation in the acute period after trauma.

SUMMARY

Patients with MBL resulting in hemorrhagic shock requiring an MT account for a small percentage of total trauma admissions. However, they account for a significant percentage of potentially preventable deaths. DCR techniques, including selective use of permissive hypotension, avoidance of overly aggressive crystalloid resuscitation, and early aggressive transfusion strategies with higher FFP-to-platelets-to-PRBC ratios have improved mortality over previous decades. MTPs are useful institutional tools for improving communication between the blood bank and the clinician. MTPs improve availability of blood products, decrease times to transfusion, likely improve mortality, and may decrease cost. Tranexamic acid and prothrombin complex may be beneficial adjuncts to resuscitation of patients in hemorrhagic shock. Viscoelastic testing using TEG/ROTEM is useful in predicting and triggering MTPs and in guiding ongoing resuscitation.

REFERENCES

1. Moore FA, McKinley BA, Moore EE, et al. Inflammation and the Host Response to Injury, a large-scale collaborative project: patient-oriented research core–standard operating procedures for clinical care. III. Guidelines for shock resuscitation. J Trauma 2006;61(1):82–9.
2. Malone DL, Hess JR, Fingerhut A. Massive transfusion practices around the globe and a suggestion for a common massive transfusion protocol. J Trauma 2006;60(Suppl 6):S91–6.
3. Duchesne JC, Hunt JP, Wahl G, et al. Review of current blood transfusions strategies in a mature level I trauma center: were we wrong for the last 60 years? J Trauma 2008;65(2):272–6 [discussion: 276–8].
4. Duchesne JC, Islam TM, Stuke L, et al. Hemostatic resuscitation during surgery improves survival in patients with traumatic-induced coagulopathy. J Trauma 2009;67(1):33–7 [discussion: 37–9].
5. Fraga GP, Bansal V, Coimbra R. Transfusion of blood products in trauma: an update. J Emerg Med 2010;39(2):253–60.
6. Hewson JR, Neame PB, Kumar N, et al. Coagulopathy related to dilution and hypotension during massive transfusion. Crit Care Med 1985;13(5):387–91.
7. Harvey MP, Greenfield TP, Sugrue ME, et al. Massive blood transfusion in a tertiary referral hospital. Clinical outcomes and haemostatic complications. Med J Aust 1995;163(7):356–9.
8. Cosgriff N, Moore EE, Sauaia A, et al. Predicting life-threatening coagulopathy in the massively transfused trauma patient: hypothermia and acidoses revisited. J Trauma 1997;42(5):857–61 [discussion: 861–2].

9. Cotton BA, Dossett LA, Haut ER, et al. Multicenter validation of a simplified score to predict massive transfusion in trauma. J Trauma 2010;69(Suppl 1):S33–9.

10. Cotton BA, Faz G, Hatch QM, et al. Rapid thrombelastography delivers real-time results that predict transfusion within 1 hour of admission. J Trauma 2011;71(2): 407–14 [discussion: 414–7].

11. Cotton BA, Reddy N, Hatch QM, et al. Damage control resuscitation is associated with a reduction in resuscitation volumes and improvement in survival in 390 damage control laparotomy patients. Ann Surg 2011;254(4):598–605.

12. Krumrei NJ, Park MS, Cotton BA, et al. Comparison of massive blood transfusion predictive models in the rural setting. J Trauma Acute Care Surg 2012;72(1): 211–5.

13. Nunez TC, Voskresensky IV, Dossett LA, et al. Early prediction of massive transfusion in trauma: simple as ABC (assessment of blood consumption)? J Trauma 2009;66(2):346–52.

14. McLaughlin DF, Niles SE, Salinas J, et al. A predictive model for massive transfusion in combat casualty patients. J Trauma 2008;64(Suppl 2):S57–63 [discussion: S63].

15. Como JJ, Dutton RP, Scalea TM, et al. Blood transfusion rates in the care of acute trauma. Transfusion 2004;44(6):809–13.

16. Brakenridge SC, Phelan HA, Henley SS, et al. Early blood product and crystalloid volume resuscitation: risk association with multiple organ dysfunction after severe blunt traumatic injury. J Trauma 2011;71(2):299–305.

17. Huber-Wagner S, Qvick M, Mussack T, et al. Massive blood transfusion and outcome in 1062 polytrauma patients: a prospective study based on the Trauma Registry of the German Trauma Society. Vox Sang 2007;92(1):69–78.

18. Spinella PC. Warm fresh whole blood transfusion for severe hemorrhage: U.S. military and potential civilian applications. Crit Care Med 2008;36(Suppl 7): S340–5.

19. Wilson RF, Dulchavsky SA, Soullier G, et al. Problems with 20 or more blood transfusions in 24 hours. Am Surg 1987;53(7):410–7.

20. Cervera AL, Moss G. Dilutional re-expansion with crystalloid after massive hemorrhage: saline versus balanced electrolyte solution for maintenance of normal blood volume and arterial pH. J Trauma 1975;15(6):498–503.

21. Coimbra R, Hoyt DB, Junger WG, et al. Hypertonic saline resuscitation decreases susceptibility to sepsis after hemorrhagic shock. J Trauma 1997; 42(4):602–6 [discussion: 606–7].

22. Angle N, Hoyt DB, Coimbra R, et al. Hypertonic saline resuscitation diminishes lung injury by suppressing neutrophil activation after hemorrhagic shock. Shock 1998;9(3):164–70.

23. Schreiber MA. The use of normal saline for resuscitation in trauma. J Trauma 2011;70(Suppl 5):S13–4.

24. Healey MA, Davis RE, Liu FC, et al. Lactated ringer's is superior to normal saline in a model of massive hemorrhage and resuscitation. J Trauma 1998;45(5): 894–9.

25. Alderson P, Bunn F, Lefebvre C, et al. Human albumin solution for resuscitation and volume expansion in critically ill patients. Cochrane Database Syst Rev 2002;(1):CD001208.

26. Finfer S, Bellomo R, Boyce N, et al. A comparison of albumin and saline for fluid resuscitation in the intensive care unit. N Engl J Med 2004;350(22):2247–56.

27. Liberati A, Moja L, Moschetti I, et al. Human albumin solution for resuscitation and volume expansion in critically ill patients. Intern Emerg Med 2006;1(3):243–5.

28. Roberts I, Blackhall K, Alderson P, et al. Human albumin solution for resuscitation and volume expansion in critically ill patients. Cochrane Database Syst Rev 2011;(11):CD001208.

29. SAFE Study Investigators, Australian and New Zealand Intensive Care Society Clinical Trials Group, Australian Red Cross Blood Service, et al. Saline or albumin for fluid resuscitation in patients with traumatic brain injury. N Engl J Med 2007;357(9):874–84.

30. Cabrales P, Tsai AG, Intaglietta M. Resuscitation from hemorrhagic shock with hydroxyethyl starch and coagulation changes. Shock 2007;28(4):461–7.

31. Kheirabadi BS, Crissey JM, Deguzman R, et al. Effects of synthetic versus natural colloid resuscitation on inducing dilutional coagulopathy and increasing hemorrhage in rabbits. J Trauma 2008;64(5):1218–28 [discussion: 1228–9].

32. Sondeen JL, Prince MD, Kheirabadi BS, et al. Initial resuscitation with plasma and other blood components reduced bleeding compared to hetastarch in anesthetized swine with uncontrolled splenic hemorrhage. Transfusion 2011; 51(4):779–92.

33. Hartog CS, Reuter D, Loesche W, et al. Influence of hydroxyethyl starch (HES) 130/0.4 on hemostasis as measured by viscoelastic device analysis: a systematic review. Intensive Care Med 2011;37(11):1725–37.

34. Dart AB, Mutter TC, Ruth CA, et al. Hydroxyethyl starch (HES) versus other fluid therapies: effects on kidney function. Cochrane Database Syst Rev 2010;(1):CD007594.

35. Wiedermann CJ, Dunzendorfer S, Gaioni LU, et al. Hyperoncotic colloids and acute kidney injury: a meta-analysis of randomized trials. Crit Care 2010; 14(5):R191.

36. Gattas DJ, Dan A, Myburgh J, et al. Fluid resuscitation with 6% hydroxyethyl starch (130/0.4) in acutely ill patients: an updated systematic review and meta-analysis. Anesth Analg 2012;114(1):159–69.

37. James MF, Michell WL, Joubert IA, et al. Resuscitation with hydroxyethyl starch improves renal function and lactate clearance in penetrating trauma in a randomized controlled study: the FIRST trial (Fluids in Resuscitation of Severe Trauma). Br J Anaesth 2011;107(5):693–702.

38. Lissauer ME, Chi A, Kramer ME, et al. Association of 6% hetastarch resuscitation with adverse outcomes in critically ill trauma patients. Am J Surg 2011; 202(1):53–8.

39. Rizoli SB, Rhind SG, Shek PN, et al. The immunomodulatory effects of hypertonic saline resuscitation in patients sustaining traumatic hemorrhagic shock: a randomized, controlled, double-blinded trial. Ann Surg 2006;243(1):47–57.

40. Vassar MJ, Fischer RP, O'Brien PE, et al. A multicenter trial for resuscitation of injured patients with 7.5% sodium chloride. The effect of added dextran 70. The Multicenter Group for the Study of Hypertonic Saline in Trauma Patients. Arch Surg 1993;128(9):1003–11 [discussion: 1011–3].

41. DuBose JJ, Kobayashi L, Lozornio A, et al. Clinical experience using 5% hypertonic saline as a safe alternative fluid for use in trauma. J Trauma 2010;68(5): 1172–7.

42. Bulger EM, Jurkovich GJ, Nathens AB, et al. Hypertonic resuscitation of hypovolemic shock after blunt trauma: a randomized controlled trial. Arch Surg 2008;143(2):139–48 [discussion: 149].

43. Bulger EM, May S, Kerby JD, et al. Out-of-hospital hypertonic resuscitation after traumatic hypovolemic shock: a randomized, placebo controlled trial. Ann Surg 2011;253(3):431–41.

44. Mattox KL, Maningas PA, Moore EE, et al. Prehospital hypertonic saline/dextran infusion for post-traumatic hypotension. The U.S.A. Multicenter Trial. Ann Surg 1991;213(5):482–91.

45. Younes RN, Aun F, Accioly CQ, et al. Hypertonic solutions in the treatment of hypovolemic shock: a prospective, randomized study in patients admitted to the emergency room. Surgery 1992;111(4):380–5.

46. Bulger EM, May S, Brasel KJ, et al. Out-of-hospital hypertonic resuscitation following severe traumatic brain injury: a randomized controlled trial. JAMA 2010;304(13):1455–64.

47. Cooper DJ, Myles PS, McDermott FT, et al. Prehospital hypertonic saline resuscitation of patients with hypotension and severe traumatic brain injury: a randomized controlled trial. JAMA 2004;291(11):1350–7.

48. American College of Surgeons Committee on Trauma. Advanced trauma life support for doctors: student course manual. 8th edition. Chicago: American College of Surgeons; 2008.

49. McSwain N Jr, Barbeau J. Potential use of prothrombin complex concentrate in trauma resuscitation. J Trauma 2011;70(Suppl 5):S53–6.

50. Schnuriger B, Inaba K, Wu T, et al. Crystalloids after primary colon resection and anastomosis at initial trauma laparotomy: excessive volumes are associated with anastomotic leakage. J Trauma 2011;70(3):603–10.

51. Cotton BA, Guy JS, Morris JA Jr, et al. The cellular, metabolic, and systemic consequences of aggressive fluid resuscitation strategies. Shock 2006;26(2):115–21.

52. Dirks J, Jorgensen H, Jensen CH, et al. Blood product ratio in acute traumatic coagulopathy–effect on mortality in a Scandinavian level 1 trauma centre. Scand J Trauma Resusc Emerg Med 2010;18:65.

53. Brohi K, Singh J, Heron M, et al. Acute traumatic coagulopathy. J Trauma 2003;54(6):1127–30.

54. Maegele M, Lefering R, Yucel N, et al. Early coagulopathy in multiple injury: an analysis from the German Trauma Registry on 8724 patients. Injury 2007;38(3):298–304.

55. Niles SE, McLaughlin DF, Perkins JG, et al. Increased mortality associated with the early coagulopathy of trauma in combat casualties. J Trauma 2008;64(6):1459–63 [discussion: 1463–5].

56. Plotkin AJ, Wade CE, Jenkins DH, et al. A reduction in clot formation rate and strength assessed by thrombelastography is indicative of transfusion requirements in patients with penetrating injuries. J Trauma 2008;64(Suppl 2):S64–8.

57. Rugeri L, Levrat A, David JS, et al. Diagnosis of early coagulation abnormalities in trauma patients by rotation thrombelastography. J Thromb Haemost 2007;5(2):289–95.

58. Leslie SD, Toy PT. Laboratory hemostatic abnormalities in massively transfused patients given red blood cells and crystalloid. Am J Clin Pathol 1991;96(6):770–3.

59. Murray DJ, Olson J, Strauss R, et al. Coagulation changes during packed red cell replacement of major blood loss. Anesthesiology 1988;69(6):839–45.

60. Phillips TF, Soulier G, Wilson RF. Outcome of massive transfusion exceeding two blood volumes in trauma and emergency surgery. J Trauma 1987;27(8):903–10.

61. Kivioja A, Myllynen P, Rokkanen P. Survival after massive transfusions exceeding four blood volumes in patients with blunt injuries. Am Surg 1991;57(6):398–401.

62. Brown LM, Aro SO, Cohen MJ, et al. A high fresh frozen plasma: packed red blood cell transfusion ratio decreases mortality in all massively transfused

trauma patients regardless of admission international normalized ratio. J Trauma 2011;71(2 Suppl 3):S358–63.

63. Bickell WH, Wall MJ Jr, Pepe PE, et al. Immediate versus delayed fluid resuscitation for hypotensive patients with penetrating torso injuries. N Engl J Med 1994;331(17):1105–9.

64. Owens TM, Watson WC, Prough DS, et al. Limiting initial resuscitation of uncontrolled hemorrhage reduces internal bleeding and subsequent volume requirements. J Trauma 1995;39(2):200–7 [discussion: 208–9].

65. Morrison CA, Carrick MM, Norman MA, et al. Hypotensive resuscitation strategy reduces transfusion requirements and severe postoperative coagulopathy in trauma patients with hemorrhagic shock: preliminary results of a randomized controlled trial. J Trauma 2011;70(3):652–63.

66. Spinella PC, Perkins JG, Grathwohl KW, et al. Warm fresh whole blood is independently associated with improved survival for patients with combat-related traumatic injuries. J Trauma 2009;66(Suppl 4):S69–76.

67. Spinella PC, Perkins JG, Grathwohl KW, et al. Risks associated with fresh whole blood and red blood cell transfusions in a combat support hospital. Crit Care Med 2007;35(11):2576–81.

68. Spinella PC, Perkins JG, Grathwohl KW, et al. Effect of plasma and red blood cell transfusions on survival in patients with combat related traumatic injuries. J Trauma 2008;64(Suppl 2):S69–77 [discussion: S77–8].

69. Van PY, Sambasivan CN, Wade CE, et al. High transfusion ratios are not associated with increased complication rates in patients with severe extremity injuries. J Trauma 2010;69(Suppl 1):S64–8.

70. Borgman MA, Spinella PC, Perkins JG, et al. The ratio of blood products transfused affects mortality in patients receiving massive transfusions at a combat support hospital. J Trauma 2007;63(4):805–13.

71. Holcomb JB, Wade CE, Michalek JE, et al. Increased plasma and platelet to red blood cell ratios improves outcome in 466 massively transfused civilian trauma patients. Ann Surg 2008;248(3):447–58.

72. Kashuk JL, Moore EE, Johnson JL, et al. Postinjury life threatening coagulopathy: is 1:1 fresh frozen plasma:packed red blood cells the answer? J Trauma 2008;65:261–70.

73. Sperry JL, Ochoa JB, Gunn SR, et al. An FFP: PRBC transfusion ratio >/=1:1.5 is associated with a lower risk of mortality after massive transfusion. J Trauma 2008;65(5):986–93.

74. Teixeira PG, Inaba K, Shulman I, et al. Impact of plasma transfusion in massively transfused trauma patients. J Trauma 2009;66(3):693–7.

75. Wafaisade A, Maegele M, Lefering R, et al. High plasma to red blood cell ratios are associated with lower mortality rates in patients receiving multiple transfusion (4</=red blood cell units<10) during acute trauma resuscitation. J Trauma 2011;70(1):81–8 [discussion: 88–9].

76. Snyder CW, Weinberg JA, McGwin G Jr, et al. The relationship of blood product ratio to mortality: survival benefit or survival bias? J Trauma 2009;66(2):358–62 [discussion: 362–4].

77. Gunter OL Jr, Au BK, Isbell JM, et al. Optimizing outcomes in damage control resuscitation: identifying blood product ratios associated with improved survival. J Trauma 2008;65(3):527–34.

78. Lustenberger T, Frischknecht A, Bruesch M, et al. Blood component ratios in massively transfused, blunt trauma patients–a time-dependent covariate analysis. J Trauma 2011;71(5):1144–50 [discussion: 1150–1].

79. Inaba K, Lustenberger T, Rhee P, et al. The impact of platelet transfusion in massively transfused trauma patients. J Am Coll Surg 2010;211(5):573–9.
80. Perkins JG, Cap AP, Spinella PC, et al. An evaluation of the impact of apheresis platelets used in the setting of massively transfused trauma patients. J Trauma 2009;66(Suppl 4):S77–84 [discussion: S84–5].
81. Shaz BH, Dente CJ, Nicholas J, et al. Increased number of coagulation products in relationship to red blood cell products transfused improves mortality in trauma patients. Transfusion 2010;50(2):493–500.
82. Zink KA, Sambasivan CN, Holcomb JB, et al. A high ratio of plasma and platelets to packed red blood cells in the first 6 hours of massive transfusion improves outcomes in a large multicenter study. Am J Surg 2009;197(5): 565–70 [discussion: 570].
83. Stinger HK, Spinella PC, Perkins JG, et al. The ratio of fibrinogen to red cells transfused affects survival in casualties receiving massive transfusions at an army combat support hospital. J Trauma 2008;64(Suppl 2):S79–85 [discussion: S85].
84. Schochl H, Nienaber U, Hofer G, et al. Goal-directed coagulation management of major trauma patients using thromboelastometry (ROTEM)-guided adminis-tration of fibrinogen concentrate and prothrombin complex concentrate. Crit Care 2010;14(2):R55.
85. Schochl H, Nienaber U, Maegele M, et al. Transfusion in trauma: thromboelastometry-guided coagulation factor concentrate-based therapy versus standard fresh frozen plasma-based therapy. Crit Care 2011;15(2):R83.
86. Nascimento B, Rizoli S, Rubenfeld G, et al. Design and preliminary results of a pilot randomized controlled trial on a 1:1:1 transfusion strategy: the trauma formula-driven versus laboratory-guided study. J Trauma 2011;71(5 Suppl 1): S418–26.
87. Rahbar MH, Fox EE, Del Junco DJ, et al. Coordination and management of multicenter clinical studies in trauma: experience from the PRospective Obser-vational Multicenter Major Trauma Transfusion (PROMMTT) Study. Resuscitation 2012;83(4):459–64.
88. Boffard KD, Riou B, Warren B, et al. Recombinant factor VIIa as adjunctive therapy for bleeding control in severely injured trauma patients: two parallel randomized, placebo-controlled, double-blind clinical trials. J Trauma 2005; 59(1):8–15 [discussion: 15–8].
89. Rizoli SB, Boffard KD, Riou B, et al. Recombinant activated factor VII as an adjunctive therapy for bleeding control in severe trauma patients with coagulop-athy: subgroup analysis from two randomized trials. Crit Care 2006;10(6):R178.
90. Morse BC, Dente CJ, Hodgman EI, et al. The effects of protocolized use of recombinant factor VIIa within a massive transfusion protocol in a civilian level I trauma center. Am Surg 2011;77(8):1043–9.
91. Hauser CJ, Boffard K, Dutton R, et al. Results of the CONTROL trial: efficacy and safety of recombinant activated Factor VII in the management of refractory trau-matic hemorrhage. J Trauma 2010;69(3):489–500.
92. Hsia CC, Chin-Yee IH, McAlister VC. Use of recombinant activated factor VII in patients without hemophilia: a meta-analysis of randomized control trials. Ann Surg 2008;248(1):61–8.
93. Woodruff SI, Dougherty AL, Dye JL, et al. Use of recombinant factor VIIA for control of combat-related haemorrhage. Emerg Med J 2010;27(2):121–4.
94. Thomas GO, Dutton RP, Hemlock B, et al. Thromboembolic complications asso-ciated with factor VIIa administration. J Trauma 2007;62(3):564–9.

95. Levi M, Levy JH, Andersen HF, et al. Safety of recombinant activated factor VII in randomized clinical trials. N Engl J Med 2010;363(19):1791–800.
96. Boulis NM, Bobek MP, Schmaier A, et al. Use of factor IX complex in warfarin-related intracranial hemorrhage. Neurosurgery 1999;45(5):1113–8 [discussion: 1118–9].
97. Cartmill M, Dolan G, Byrne JL, et al. Prothrombin complex concentrate for oral anticoagulant reversal in neurosurgical emergencies. Br J Neurosurg 2000; 14(5):458–61.
98. Pabinger I, Brenner B, Kalina U, et al. Prothrombin complex concentrate (Beriplex P/N) for emergency anticoagulation reversal: a prospective multinational clinical trial. J Thromb Haemost 2008;6(4):622–31.
99. Schick KS, Fertmann JM, Jauch KW, et al. Prothrombin complex concentrate in surgical patients: retrospective evaluation of vitamin K antagonist reversal and treatment of severe bleeding. Crit Care 2009;13(6):R191.
100. Yasaka M, Sakata T, Minematsu K, et al. Correction of INR by prothrombin complex concentrate and vitamin K in patients with warfarin related hemorrhagic complication. Thromb Res 2002;108(1):25–30.
101. Schochl H, Cotton B, Inaba K, et al. FIBTEM provides early prediction of massive transfusion in trauma. Crit Care 2011;15(6):R265.
102. Nienaber U, Innerhofer P, Westermann I, et al. The impact of fresh frozen plasma vs coagulation factor concentrates on morbidity and mortality in trauma-associated haemorrhage and massive transfusion. Injury 2011;42(7):697–701.
103. Chapman SA, Irwin ED, Beal AL, et al. Prothrombin complex concentrate versus standard therapies for INR reversal in trauma patients receiving warfarin. Ann Pharmacother 2011;45(7–8):869–75.
104. Dentali F, Marchesi C, Pierfranceschi MG, et al. Safety of prothrombin complex concentrates for rapid anticoagulation reversal of vitamin K antagonists. A meta-analysis. Thromb Haemost 2011;106(3):429–38.
105. Bruce D, Nokes TJ. Prothrombin complex concentrate (Beriplex P/N) in severe bleeding: experience in a large tertiary hospital. Crit Care 2008;12(4):R105.
106. Cap AP, Baer DG, Orman JA, et al. Tranexamic acid for trauma patients: a critical review of the literature. J Trauma 2011;71(Suppl 1):S9–14.
107. CRASH-2 trial collaborators, Shakur H, Roberts I, Bautista R, et al. Effects of tranexamic acid on death, vascular occlusive events, and blood transfusion in trauma patients with significant haemorrhage (CRASH-2): a randomised, placebo-controlled trial. Lancet 2010;376(9734):23–32.
108. Morrison JJ, Dubose JJ, Rasmussen TE, et al. Military application of tranexamic acid in trauma emergency resuscitation (MATTERs) study. Arch Surg 2012; 147(2):113–9.
109. Moore FA, Nelson T, McKinley BA, et al. Is there a role for aggressive use of fresh frozen plasma in massive transfusion of civilian trauma patients? Am J Surg 2008;196(6):948–58 [discussion: 958–60].
110. Gonzalez EA, Moore FA, Holcomb JB, et al. Fresh frozen plasma should be given earlier to patients requiring massive transfusion. J Trauma 2007;62(1): 112–9.
111. Cotton BA, Au BK, Nunez TC, et al. Predefined massive transfusion protocols are associated with a reduction in organ failure and postinjury complications. J Trauma 2009;66(1):41–8 [discussion: 48–9].
112. Inaba K, Branco BC, Rhee P, et al. Impact of plasma transfusion in trauma patients who do not require massive transfusion. J Am Coll Surg 2010;210(6): 957–65.

113. Mitra B, Cameron PA, Gruen RL. Aggressive fresh frozen plasma (FFP) with massive blood transfusion in the absence of acute traumatic coagulopathy. Injury 2012;43(1):33–7.
114. Sambasivan CN, Kunio NR, Nair PV, et al. High ratios of plasma and platelets to packed red blood cells do not affect mortality in nonmassively transfused patients. J Trauma 2011;71(2 Suppl 3):S329–36.
115. Watson GA, Sperry JL, Rosengart MR, et al. Fresh frozen plasma is independently associated with a higher risk of multiple organ failure and acute respiratory distress syndrome. J Trauma 2009;67(2):221–7 [discussion: 228–30].
116. Schreiber MA, Perkins J, Kiraly L, et al. Early predictors of massive transfusion in combat casualties. J Am Coll Surg 2007;205(4):541–5.
117. Yucel N, Lefering R, Maegele M, et al. Trauma Associated Severe Hemorrhage (TASH)-Score: probability of mass transfusion as surrogate for life threatening hemorrhage after multiple trauma. J Trauma 2006;60(6):1228–36 [discussion: 1236–7].
118. Riskin DJ, Tsai TC, Riskin L, et al. Massive transfusion protocols: the role of aggressive resuscitation versus product ratio in mortality reduction. J Am Coll Surg 2009;209(2):198–205.
119. Dente CJ, Shaz BH, Nicholas JM, et al. Improvements in early mortality and coagulopathy are sustained better in patients with blunt trauma after institution of a massive transfusion protocol in a civilian level I trauma center. J Trauma 2009;66(6):1616–24.
120. Duchesne JC, Barbeau JM, Islam TM, et al. Damage control resuscitation: from emergency department to the operating room. Am Surg 2011;77(2):201–6.
121. Cotton BA, Dossett LA, Au BK, et al. Room for (performance) improvement: provider-related factors associated with poor outcomes in massive transfusion. J Trauma 2009;67(5):1004–12.
122. O'Keeffe T, Refaai M, Tchorz K, et al. A massive transfusion protocol to decrease blood component use and costs. Arch Surg 2008;143(7):686–90 [discussion: 690–1].
123. Allcock EC, Woolley T, Doughty H, et al. The clinical outcome of UK military personnel who received a massive transfusion in Afghanistan during 2009. J R Army Med Corps 2011;157(4):365–9.
124. Martini WZ, Cortez DS, Dubick MA, et al. Thrombelastography is better than PT, aPTT, and activated clotting time in detecting clinically relevant clotting abnormalities after hypothermia, hemorrhagic shock and resuscitation in pigs. J Trauma 2008;65(3):535–43.
125. Davenport R, Manson J, De'Ath H, et al. Functional definition and characterization of acute traumatic coagulopathy. Crit Care Med 2011;39(12): 2652–8.
126. Leemann H, Lustenberger T, Talving P, et al. The role of rotation thromboelastometry in early prediction of massive transfusion. J Trauma 2010;69(6): 1403–8 [discussion: 1408–9].
127. Nystrup KB, Windelov NA, Thomsen AB, et al. Reduced clot strength upon admission, evaluated by thrombelastography (TEG), in trauma patients is independently associated with increased 30-day mortality. Scand J Trauma Resusc Emerg Med 2011;19:52.
128. Tauber H, Innerhofer P, Breitkopf R, et al. Prevalence and impact of abnormal ROTEM(R) assays in severe blunt trauma: results of the 'Diagnosis and Treatment of Trauma-Induced Coagulopathy (DIA-TRE-TIC) study'. Br J Anaesth 2011;107(3):378–87.

129. Johansson PI, Stensballe J. Effect of Haemostatic Control Resuscitation on mortality in massively bleeding patients: a before and after study. Vox Sang 2009;96(2):111–8.
130. Cinat ME, Wallace WC, Nastanski F, et al. Improved survival following massive transfusion in patients who have undergone trauma. Arch Surg 1999;134(9): 964–8 [discussion: 968–70].
131. Stadlbauer KH, Wagner-Berger HG, Raedler C, et al. Vasopressin, but not fluid resuscitation, enhances survival in a liver trauma model with uncontrolled and otherwise lethal hemorrhagic shock in pigs. Anesthesiology 2003;98(3): 699–704.
132. Schwartz J, Reid IA. Effect of vasopressin blockade on blood pressure regulation during hemorrhage in conscious dogs. Endocrinology 1981;109(5): 1778–80.
133. Errington ML, Rocha e Silva M Jr. The secretion and clearance of vasopressin during the development of irreversible haemorrhagic shock. J Physiol 1971; 217(Suppl):43P–5P.
134. Voelckel WG, Raedler C, Wenzel V, et al. Arginine vasopressin, but not epinephrine, improves survival in uncontrolled hemorrhagic shock after liver trauma in pigs. Crit Care Med 2003;31(4):1160–5.
135. Behan LA, Phillips J, Thompson CJ, et al. Neuroendocrine disorders after traumatic brain injury. J Neurol Neurosurg Psychiatry 2008;79(7):753–9.
136. Morales D, Madigan J, Cullinane S, et al. Reversal by vasopressin of intractable hypotension in the late phase of hemorrhagic shock. Circulation 1999;100(3): 226–9.
137. Cohn SM, McCarthy J, Stewart RM, et al. Impact of low-dose vasopressin on trauma outcome: prospective randomized study. World J Surg 2011;35(2): 430–9.
138. Grmec S, Strnad M, Cander D, et al. A treatment protocol including vasopressin and hydroxyethyl starch solution is associated with increased rate of return of spontaneous circulation in blunt trauma patients with pulseless electrical activity. Int J Emerg Med 2008;1(4):311–6.
139. Collier B, Dossett L, Mann M, et al. Vasopressin use is associated with death in acute trauma patients with shock. J Crit Care 2010;25(1):173.e9–173.e14.
140. Plurad DS, Talving P, Lam L, et al. Early vasopressor use in critical injury is associated with mortality independent from volume status. J Trauma 2011;71(3): 565–70 [discussion: 570–2].
141. Sperry JL, Minei JP, Frankel HL, et al. Early use of vasopressors after injury: caution before constriction. J Trauma 2008;64(1):9–14.
142. Inaba K, Teixeira PG, Shulman I, et al. The impact of uncross-matched blood transfusion on the need for massive transfusion and mortality: analysis of 5,166 uncross-matched units. J Trauma 2008;65(6):1222–6.

Epidemiology of Sepsis in Surgical Patients

Laura J. Moore, MD[a],*, Frederick A. Moore, MD[b]

KEYWORDS

• Sepsis • Surgical critical care • Evidence-based care • Patient outcomes

KEY POINTS

• Surgical patients account for nearly one-third of sepsis cases in the United States.
• Sepsis remains the leading cause of death in noncardiac intensive care units.
• Early identification of patients and timely implementation of evidence-based therapies continue to represent significant clinical challenges for care providers.
• The implementation of a sepsis screening program in conjunction with protocol for the delivery of evidence-based care and rapid source control can improve patient outcomes.

INTRODUCTION

Despite advances in surgical critical care, sepsis among surgical patients continues to be a common and serious problem. As the population ages, the incidence of sepsis in the United States continues to rise. It is estimated that in the United States, there are greater than 1.1 million cases of sepsis per year[1] at an annual cost of $24.3 billion.[2] Sepsis remains the leading cause of death in noncardiac ICUs.[2] In spite of extensive research, sepsis-related mortality remains prohibitively high (>40%).[1–4]

Among surgical patients, sepsis is a leading cause of morbidity and mortality. Surgical patients account for nearly one-third of sepsis cases in the United States.[5] A recent analysis of the American College of Surgeons National Surgical Quality Improvement Project Database determined that sepsis and septic shock are 10 times more common than perioperative myocardial infarction and pulmonary embolism.[4] In addition, the mortality rate for septic shock in the perioperative period exceeds that of both myocardial infarction and pulmonary embolism.[4] These findings underscore the importance of studying sepsis specifically in general surgery patients.

Risk factors for both the development of sepsis and death from sepsis included age older than 60 years, the need for emergency surgery, and the presence of comorbid

[a] Department of Surgery, The University of Texas Health Science Center, 6431 Fannin Street, MSB 4292, Houston, TX 77030, USA; [b] Department of Surgery, The University of Florida, 1600 South West Archer Road, Gainesville, FL 32608, USA
* Corresponding author.
E-mail address: laura.j.moore@uth.tmc.edu

Surg Clin N Am 92 (2012) 1425–1443
http://dx.doi.org/10.1016/j.suc.2012.08.009
0039-6109/12/$ – see front matter © 2012 Published by Elsevier Inc.

surgical.theclinics.com

conditions.[6] Intraabdominal infection is the most common source of sepsis among surgical patients, accounting for approximately two-thirds of all cases.[3] Among intra-abdominal causes of sepsis, colon perforation is the predominant source of intraabdominal sepsis.[7] When septic shock follows sepsis, there is a 39% mortality rate among emergent surgical patients and a 30% mortality rate among elective surgical patients.

DEFINITION OF SURGICAL SEPSIS

A clear and accurate definition of surgical sepsis is critical for clinicians and researchers. Standard definitions allow us to identify patients, lead to a better understanding of the disease process, and facilitate clinical research. Roger Bone first defined the sepsis syndrome in the literature in 1989.[8] This was followed by the American College of Chest Physicians and the Society of Critical Care Medicines (ACCP/SCCM) Consensus Conference in 1991 that defined the systemic inflammatory response syndrome (SIRS) and multiple organ dysfunction syndrome (MODS).[9] A second consensus conference was convened in 2001 to revise the original definitions. The updated consensus conference definitions expanded the list of signs and symptoms of sepsis.[10] Although the 2001 definitions are widely accepted, they do not specifically define surgical sepsis. The consensus conference definitions remain nonspecific and allow variability, especially in defining organ dysfunction.

In an attempt to better define the categories of sepsis, severe sepsis, and septic shock the authors have modified the ACCP/SCCM Consensus Conference definitions. The modified definition of surgical sepsis is SIRS plus an infection requiring surgical intervention for source control or SIRS plus an infection within 14 days of a major surgical procedure.[3] A major surgical procedure is defined as any procedure requiring general anesthesia for more than 1 hour. Severe sepsis is defined as SIRS plus infection plus acute organ dysfunction. The types of acute organ dysfunction are further defined. Neurologic is identified as a Glasgow Coma Scale (GCS) less than 13 on recognition of sepsis or deteriorating GCS to less than 13 during the first 24 hours. Pulmonary dysfunction includes a Pao_2 to fraction of inspired oxygen ratio less than 250 (<200 if lung is primary site of infection) and pulmonary capillary wedge pressure (PCWP), if available, not suggestive of fluid overload. Renal dysfunction is defined as one of the following criteria: (1) urine output less than 0.5 mL/kg for greater than or equal to 1 hour despite adequate volume resuscitation, (2) increase in serum creatinine greater than or equal to 0.5 mg/dL from baseline (measured within 24 hrs of starting sepsis resuscitation) despite adequate volume resuscitation, or (3) increase in serum creatinine greater than or equal to 0.5 mg/dL during first 24 hours of sepsis management despite adequate volume resuscitation. Adequate volume resuscitation is defined as a minimum intravenous (IV) fluid infusion of 20 mL/kg of ideal body weight or central venous pressure (CVP) greater than or equal to 8 mm Hg or PCWP greater than or equal to 12 mm Hg. Coagulation dysfunction is also described by any one of these criteria: international normalized ratio greater than 1.5, platelet count less than 80,000 or greater than or equal to 50%, or decreased platelets compared with 24 hours before instituting sepsis resuscitation or in the 24 hours after starting sepsis resuscitation in the absence of chronic liver disease. Hypoperfusion is defined by a lactate level greater than 4 mmol/L. Cardiac dysfunction is defined by the presence of an IV fluid challenge greater than or equal to 20 mL/kg of ideal body weight of isotonic crystalloid infusion, CVP greater than or equal to 8 mm Hg, or PCWP greater than or equal to 12 mm Hg and the requirement for vasopressors to increase mean arterial pressure (MAP) greater than or equal to 65 mm Hg. Septic shock is defined as SIRS plus infection plus acute cardiac dysfunction.

SEPSIS SCREENING

The early identification and management of sepsis remains a significant challenge to health care providers. Multiple organizations have focused their efforts on providing evidence-based guidelines (EBGs) in an attempt to decrease the morbidity and mortality associated with sepsis. Identifying patients in the early stages of sepsis is imperative if mortality rates are to be improved. If patients are allowed to progress from sepsis into septic shock, their mortality is prohibitively high (>40%) despite aggressive interventions. The interventions demonstrated to improve survival in patients with sepsis are time-sensitive. The use of early goal-directed therapy (EGDT) for patients with severe sepsis and septic shock improves survival rates.[11] Administration of empiric, broad-spectrum, antibiotic therapy is recommended within 1 hour of recognition of sepsis-induced hypotension.[12] Each hour of delay in the administration of antibiotic therapy is associated with an increased mortality rate.[13] However, early intervention requires early identification of sepsis. A recently published study by Kumar and colleagues[13] demonstrated a significant correlation between time to appropriate antibiotic administration and patient survival.

In spite of strong evidence that the early implementation of evidence-based, sepsis-specific therapies saves lives, the early identification of sepsis remains challenging. The signs and symptoms of sepsis are nonspecific, particularly in the early phases of sepsis. Because health care providers focus on multiple priorities and tasks, early signs of sepsis are often missed, resulting in delays for the time-sensitive interventions that improve patient outcomes. In the surgical patient, some of the early signs of sepsis are often attributed to other common problems seen in the postoperative period. For example, altered mental status is often attributed to the administration of narcotic pain medication or sundowning, particularly in the elderly patient. Oliguria is often attributed to underresuscitation. Although many nurses notify physicians of hyperthermia, hypothermia, which is also an early sign of sepsis, is often not reported. Likewise, acute hypoxia on the surgical wards spurs a workup for pulmonary embolism. However, it may also herald the onset of severe sepsis or septic shock. Identifying patients in these early stages of sepsis is imperative. Considering these factors, the benefit of routine, accurate screening of patients for sepsis quickly becomes apparent.

An audit of ward nurses demonstrated that fewer than 40% were able to recognize a patient with sepsis.[14] Physicians also struggle with the early identification and evidence-based management of sepsis. A recent survey of 917 physicians showed that only 27.3% of physicians were able to recognize sepsis.[15] Recognition of severe sepsis and septic shock was slightly improved, but still unsatisfactory, at 56.7% and 81%, respsectively.[15] The reasons listed for missing the diagnosis of sepsis included lack of monitoring, lack of a common definition for sepsis, and lack of knowledge. Of the 1058 physicians surveyed, only 140 (13.2%) were able to give the definition of sepsis from the ACCP/SCCM Consensus Conference statement. These results are confirmed in other studies reporting similar findings.[16,17]

Little attention has been dedicated to the topic of sepsis screening. The use of SIRS score to identify patients with sepsis has been largely abandoned because of lack of sensitivity and specificity.[18] The Early Warning Score and Modified Early Warning Score can predict illness severity and in-hospital mortality but are not helpful in the early recognition of sepsis.[19–21] Attempting to increase the early identification of sepsis, a sepsis screening tool was developed at the author's Surgical Intensive Care Unit (SICU).[22] The initial portion of this sepsis screening tool (**Fig. 1**) focuses on assessing SIRS severity and is completed by the bedside nurse. A score of greater

Sepsis Screening Score

Current Heart Rate: _____

Temperature Minimum (prior 24hours): _____

Temperature Maximum (prior 24hours): _____

Current Respiratory Rate: _____

WBC (most recent): _____

	0	1	2	3	4
Heart Rate	70-109		55-69 110-139	40-54 140-179	≤ 39 ≤ 180
Temp (°C)	36 – 38.4	34-35.9 38.5-38.9	32 – 33.9	30 – 31.9 39 – 40.9	≤ 29.9 ≥ 41
Temp (°F)	96.8 – 101.1	93.1-96.7 101.2-102.0	89.6-93.0	86 – 89.5 102.1 – 105.6	≤ 85.9 ≥ 105.7
Respiratory Rate	12-24	10-11 25-34	6-9	35-49	≤5 ≥50
Latest WBC Count	3-14.9	15-19.9	1 – 2.9 20-39.9		< 1 ≥ 40
Acute change in mental status	No	Yes			
SIRS Score (total points)		*If the SIRS Score is ≥ 4 please notify the mid level provider or resident physician to complete the assessment for infection.*			

Fig. 1. Sepsis screening score.

than or equal to 4 is considered to be a positive score and prompts the nurse to call a clinician to evaluate the patient for a possible infection (**Fig. 2**). Initial experience with this mandatory sepsis screening tool in the SICU showed promising results. The screening tool yielded a sensitivity of 96.5%, a specificity of 96.7%, a positive predictive value of 80.2%, and a negative predictive value of 99.5%. In addition, sepsis-related mortality decreased from 35.1% to 23.3%. Subsequently, the institution has implemented and validated the sepsis screening tool on the inpatient surgical ward. The screening tool yielded a sensitivity of 99.9%, specificity of 91.3%, a positive predictive value of 16.3%, and a negative predictive value of 99.9%. The sepsis-related mortality in those patients who screened positive for sepsis was 6.3%. Subsequent implementation and validation of this sepsis screening tool among trauma patients yielded similar results with a sensitivity of 97.9%, specificity of 91.8%, positive predictive value of 51%, and negative predictive value of 99.8%. It is important to emphasize the extremely high negative predictive value (99.5%–99.9%) of this sepsis screening tool across a broad range of surgical patients. These results emphasize the importance of sepsis screening for the early identification of sepsis.

PRACTICAL CONSIDERATIONS FOR THE MANAGEMENT OF SURGICAL SEPSIS
Initial Assessment

A clinical suspicion of sepsis should prompt further evaluation of the patient. This initial evaluation should focus on determining the degree of physiologic derangement exhibited by the patient. It is especially important to assess for the presence and

Midlevel/Physician Sepsis Screening
Assessment for Source of Infection

1. Vascular access?

					Yes	No	Suspicion of:
type	dialysis	triple / quad	PICC	port	tunneled	other (IV, art)	line infection?
date placed							
site							Yes No
local finding							
blood culture finding							

2. Clinical pulmonary infection score (CPIS)

Variable		points	score		pneumonia?
temperature (°C)	time (hhmm)				
36.5 – 38.4		0	Intubated /		Yes No
38.5 – 38.9		1	mech vent		
> 39.0 or < 36.0		2	support?		
blood leukocyte count (# per mm³) time (hhmm)					
4,000 – 11,000		0	Yes No		
< 4,000 or > 11,000		1			
tracheal secretions time (hhmm)			date intubated:		
small		0			
moderate		1			
large		2			
purulent (add 1 point if purulent)		+1			
oxygenation (PaO₂/FiO₂) time (hhmm)					
≥ 240 or presence of ARDS		0			
< 240 and absence of ARDS		2			
chest radiograph time (hhmm)					
no infiltrate		0			
patchy or diffuse infiltrate		1			
localized infiltrate		2			

3. Abdomen

recent abdominal surgery?	Yes	No	abdominal
abdominal pain?	Yes	No	infection?
abdominal distention?	Yes	No	
purulent drainage from surgical drains?	Yes	No	Yes No
intolerance to enteral nutrition?	Yes	No	

4. Skin / soft tissue

erythema / drainage from other surgical site?	Yes	No	cellulitis / soft tissue infection?
site			
			Yes No

5. Urinary tract

urinary catheter?	Yes	No	UTI?
date placed			
latest urinalysis / urine culture results			Yes No

6. Other site

site	other infection?
	Yes No

Fig. 2. Sepsis screening tool: assessment for source of infection.

degree of tissue hypoperfusion. There are several clinical and laboratory variables that can be used to evaluate the state of tissue perfusion. The following indicate that the patient is experiencing tissue hypoperfusion: (1) urine output less than 0.5 mL/kg of ideal body weight, (2) MAP less than 65 mm Hg, (3) GCS less than 12, and (4) serum lactate greater than or equal to 4 mmol/L. Tissue hypoperfusion should prompt aggressive resuscitative measures focused on restoring tissue perfusion. Patients who do not have evidence of tissue hypoperfusion fall into the category of sepsis using current definitions. Patients who do have evidence of tissue hypoperfusion are categorized as having severe sepsis and/or septic shock.

Initial Resuscitation of Sepsis

The initial resuscitation phase begins immediately on recognition of sepsis. Initiation of resuscitation should not wait until the patient is transferred to a higher level of care.

The goals of the resuscitation include restoration of intravascular volume, diagnosis of the source of infection, initiation of broad spectrum antimicrobial therapy, and source control. Many institutions have developed sepsis order sets that specifically address each of these issues. The use of standardized protocols for the initial management of sepsis improves patient outcomes in multiple settings.[7,23–27]

The major tenets of initial resuscitation can be initiated in any area of the hospital and should not be delayed pending transfer to the ICU. Establishing IV access is a critical first step because this allows for the administration of resuscitative IV fluid and antimicrobials. For those patients without evidence of tissue hypoperfusion, a large-bore peripheral IV should be sufficient. If peripheral IV access is not attainable, a large-bore central venous line should be inserted in a timely fashion to facilitate fluid resuscitation.

Fluid resuscitation should be guided with the following goals in mind: (1) CVP, if available, 8 to 12 mm Hg in nonintubated patients and a target CVP 12 to 15 mm Hg in mechanically ventilated patients,[28] (2) MAP greater than or equal to 65 mm Hg,[29] (3) urine output greater than or equal to 0.5 mL/kg/h, and (4) central venous oxygen saturation (ScvO$_2$) greater than or equal to 70% or mixed venous oxygen saturation (SvO2), if available, greater than or equal to 65%.[11] These endpoints of resuscitation should be achieved within 6 hours of the recognition of sepsis. In addition, a baseline serum lactate is sent on the identification of sepsis. A repeat serum lactate level is sent 4 hours later to monitor the progress of the initial resuscitation.

The initial resuscitation fluid of choice remains extremely controversial. There are no prospective, randomized, controlled trials evaluating crystalloid versus colloid resuscitation in surgical patients with sepsis. If colloids are given, the initial fluid bolus should be 300 to 500 mL of colloid over 30 minutes. If crystalloids are given, the initial fluid challenge should be 1000 cc of crystalloid over 30 minutes. The patient's response to fluid bolus will dictate the need for additional resuscitation. The Saline versus Albumin Fluid Evaluation (SAFE) study randomized nearly 7000 critically ill patients requiring fluid resuscitation to receive albumin or normal saline and no difference in mortality was identified. Interestingly, a subgroup analysis of the 1218 patients with severe sepsis documented that albumin was associated with a trend toward reduced mortality (relative risk of death 0.87; 95% CI 0.74–1.02).[30] Currently, two randomized trials are ongoing to investigate this finding. They are, in Italy, the Volume Replacement with Albumin in Severe Sepsis (ALBIOS) trial [31] and, in France, the Early Albumin Resuscitation during Septic Shock trial.[32]

Initial Resuscitation of Severe Sepsis and Septic Shock

For patients presenting with severe sepsis and septic shock, the timely correction of tissue hypoperfusion is critical. The concept of EGDT in severe sepsis and septic shock was initially developed and validated in the emergency department (ED) setting in a single-center trial.[11] The ED is frequently the point of entry for many septic patients into the hospital. Unfortunately, many of these patients may wait for prolonged periods of time in the ED. The end result is often a delay in the implementation of early sepsis resuscitation.

The implementation of EGDT improves survival in patients presenting with severe sepsis and septic shock.[11,26,33,34] The basic principles of EGDT are to recognize tissue hypoperfusion and initiate therapies to reverse global tissue hypoxia by optimizing oxygen delivery. Tissue perfusion can be monitored by measuring SvO$_2$, ScvO$_2$, or peripheral muscle hemoglobin oxygen saturation (StO$_2$). A SvO2 of less than or equal to 65%, a ScvO2 of less than or equal to 70%, or a StO2 of less than or equal to 75% are considered indicators of tissue hypoperfusion. Once tissue hypoperfusion is identified, specific therapies are instituted to reverse tissue hypoxia by restoring adequate perfusion. The factors affecting oxygen delivery are cardiac output, hemoglobin, and percent arterial hemoglobin oxygen saturation (SaO_2). EGDT attempts to restore tissue perfusion by addressing these variables. The evidence-based Sepsis Resuscitation Bundle (SRB) was established with a goal to accomplish all indicated tasks, 100% of the time, within 6 hours of the diagnosis of sepsis The elements of the 6 hour SRB include measurement of serum lactate, obtaining blood cultures before the initiation of antibiotics, administration of broad-spectrum antibiotics within 1 hour of sepsis recognition, and fluid resuscitation for the treatment of hypotension.

To restore intravascular volume and enhance cardiac output, an initial crystalloid fluid bolus of 20 mL/kg of ideal body weight is recommended. This fluid bolus can be administered initially through existing peripheral IVs; however, placement of a central venous line for monitoring of CVP Is recommended. An arterial line should be placed in patients with unresponsive hypotension. The use of noninvasive blood pressure monitoring for patients in septic shock often produces inaccurate measurements and should be avoided for titration of vasoactive medications. A Foley catheter is inserted to allow for close monitoring of urine output. Bladder pressures should be monitored in patients requiring aggressive volume loading to recognize abdominal compartment syndrome (ACS). The goals of resuscitation remain the same as those listed above. In the event that a ScvO2 of greater than or equal to 70% or SvO2 greater than or equal to 65% cannot be achieved with restoration of intravascular volume and MAP of 65 to 90 mm Hg, red blood cells should be transfused to achieve of hematocrit of greater than or equal to 30%.

Multiple international randomized controlled trials of early goal-directed therapy for patients with severe sepsis are underway to validate the findings of the single-center Rivers trial. These include ProCESS (Protocolized Care for Early Septic Shock), ARISE (Australian Resuscitation in Sepsis Evaluation), and ProMISe (Protocolized Management in Sepsis). The ProCESS trial will randomize 1950 subjects who present to the ED in septic shock to three arms: (1) the EGDT Rivers protocol described above, (2) a less complicated, less invasive protocol using esophageal Doppler monitor and no blood transfusion, and (3) usual care.[35] The ARISE trial will randomize 1600 subjects to EGDT versus standard care and assess 90-day mortality in subjects presenting to the ED with severe sepsis.[36] The ProMISe trial will randomize 1260 subjects to EGDT versus standard care and assess 90-day mortality in subjects presenting to the ED with septic shock.[37] Furthermore, an individual, subject data meta-analysis will be performed across the three trials.

Having achieved the goal CVP, the goal MAP, and the goal hematocrit, if there is still evidence of tissue hypoperfusion, inotropic agents should be administered to improve cardiac output. In patients presenting with septic shock, the initial fluid bolus may not restore their MAP to greater than or equal to 65 mm Hg. A repeat fluid bolus of 20 mL/kg of ideal body weight can be given to correct hypovolemia. However, transient vasopressors therapy may need to be initiated, even if volume resuscitation is still ongoing.

Vasopressor therapy

Septic shock is primarily a vasodilatory shock, associated with a high cardiac output and a low systemic vascular resistance. Therefore, initial vasopressors therapy should be targeted at restoring vascular tone. Both norepinephrine and dopamine are acceptable first-line agents for treatment of septic shock, and should be administered through a central venous catheter. Norepinephrine is primarily an α-receptor agonist that promotes widespread vasoconstriction and has little effect on heart rate or stroke volume. Dopamine has dose-dependent effects on α-, β-, and dopaminergic receptors. The initial increase in blood pressure seen with dopamine is related to increasing cardiac output. At higher doses (>7.5 μg/kg/min), dopamine does activate α-receptors with resultant vasoconstriction.

In patients with septic shock that is refractory to first-line vasopressors, the addition of vasopressin may be beneficial. Vasopressin is a stress hormone that has vasoactive effects. The use of vasopressin is supported by suggestive data indicating that in states of septic shock there is a relative deficiency of vasopressin.[38] The administration of vasopressin in this patient population improves responsiveness to catecholamines and potentially reduces the amount of catecholamine needed to maintain blood pressure.[39]

The Vasopressin and Septic Shock Trial (VASST) randomized 779 subjects in septic shock requiring norepinephrine (5 μg/min) for at least 6 hours and at least one organ system dysfunction present for less than 24 hours to vasopressin (0.01–0.03 U/min) versus higher dose norepinephrine (5–15 μg/min).[40] No difference in 28-day or 90-day mortality was identified. In the prospectively defined stratum of less severe septic shock, the mortality rate was lower in the vasopressin group than in the norepinephrine group at 28 days (26.5% vs 35.7%, $P = .05$) which persisted to 90-day mortality (35.8% vs 46.1%, $P = .04$). A post hoc analysis of the VASST study identified that the combination of low-dose vasopressin and corticosteroids was associated with decreased mortality and organ dysfunction compared with norepinephrine and corticosteroids.[41] Based on the results of studies to date, clinicians should consider the addition of low-dose continuous infusion vasopressin (up to 0.03 U/min) in individual septic shock patients who, despite adequate resuscitation, are still requiring high doses of vasopressors. It is the author's current practice to initiate a vasopressin drip at a rate of 0.04 U/min in patients requiring norepinephrine infusion at greater than or equal to 15 μg/min. The dose of vasopressin should not exceed 0.04 U/min because of the possibility of decreased cardiac output and myocardial ischemia at higher doses.[42]

Although most patients with sepsis initially present with increased cardiac output, a subset of patients will develop myocardial depression from sepsis. The exact mechanism for this reversible myocardial dysfunction is still under investigation. B-type natriuretic peptide (BNP) is secreted in response to stretching of myocardium and is used clinically to assess volume overload and predict death in acute congestive heart failure. BNP is elevated in early septic shock and elevations are associated with increased death. BNP increases with initial sepsis severity and is associated with early left ventricular dysfunction that, in itself, is associated with later death.[43] Monitoring BNP in early sepsis to identify occult left ventricular dysfunction may prompt earlier use of inotropes, which are not commonly used in early sepsis resuscitation.

For patients with suspected or known cardiac dysfunction, the addition of inotropic therapy is recommended. Dobutamine is the first-line agent for treatment of cardiac dysfunction in patients with sepsis. The management of patients with a cardiac component to their shock state presents a unique challenge to the clinician because they require the titration of vasopressors and inotropic agents. In this subset of patients, the use of a pulmonary artery catheter can be extremely useful. This allows for the specific titration of vasopressors based on systemic vascular resistance and inotropic agents based on cardiac output. There is no evidence to support increasing cardiac index to supranormal levels.

Steroids in Septic Shock

The use of steroids for the management of septic shock has been debated for several decades. In recent years, the concept of relative adrenal insufficiency in septic shock has received renewed interest. Despite several large clinical trials addressing the issue of steroid use in patients with septic shock, the topic remains controversial. The ongoing debate is primarily on the definition of relative adrenal insufficiency in critically ill patients and the gold standard for diagnosing adrenal insufficiency in this population.

Previously, it was common practice to perform a low-dose ACTH (cosyntropin) stimulation test on all patients with septic shock as a means to identify those patients with relative adrenal insufficiency. To perform the cosyntropin stimulation test, a baseline serum cortisol is drawn which represents time zero (T_0). The patient is then given 250 µg of IV cosyntropin. Subsequent serum cortisol levels are measured at 30 (T_{30}) and 60 (T_{60}) minutes after the cosyntropin. If the delta cortisol is less than or equal to 9 µg/dL then the patient is considered to have relative adrenal insufficiency and steroids are initiated. Based on the current evidence to date, it is now recognized that the ACTH stimulation test is not recommended to be used in this fashion among septic patients. Several factors interfere with the ACTH stimulation test, and current diagnostic tests are not accurate. Etomidate, which is commonly used for intubation causes a temporary suppression of the hypothalamic-pituitary-adrenal axis, resulting in transient adrenal insufficiency. In addition, patients that have received steroids at any time during the previous 6 months should not undergo testing of their adrenal function. Instead, these patients should be empirically initiated on steroid therapy. The current edition (2008) of the Surviving Sepsis Campaign Guidelines recommends that IV hydrocortisone should be considered for adult septic shock when hypotension responds poorly to adequate fluid resuscitation and vasopressors. The literature indicates that low-dose corticosteroids decrease the time to cessation of vasopressors,[44] increase the systemic vascular resistance and MAP,[45] and decrease the risk of death.[46] The dose of hydrocortisone should be less than or equal to 300 mg/d. The author currently gives hydrocortisone 50 mg IV every 6 hours. The duration of steroid administration also remains controversial. The current recommendation is that steroids be discontinued once vasopressors are no longer required.

Identifying the Source of Infection

Identifying the source of infection is essential to sepsis management. Whenever possible, cultures should be obtained before initiation of empiric antimicrobial therapy. Current recommendations include obtaining a minimum of two blood cultures, including one blood culture from each vascular access device and one blood culture from a peripheral puncture. Additional cultures from other sites (eg, respiratory, urinary tract) and radiographic imaging are dictated by clinical suspicion. In the surgical population this may include obtaining cultures from surgical drains and performing pertinent imaging to identify an undrained abscess. Despite the importance of source identification, difficulty in the collection of cultures should not generate a significant delay in the administration of antimicrobial therapy.

To improve the chances of detecting bacteremia it is crucial to obtain the appropriate volume of blood for the culture medium. Several studies demonstrate that the volume of blood cultured is the single-most important factor in the detection of bacteremia.[47–49] The recommend volume of blood per culture tube is greater than or equal to 10 mL. Obtaining blood cultures from all vascular access devices along with simultaneous collection of blood cultures from a peripheral site is beneficial in diagnosing catheter-related infections. The concept of differential time to positivity is well described.[50,51] Differential time to positivity is defined as the difference in time necessary for blood cultures drawn simultaneously from a peripheral site and a central venous catheter to become positive. The differential time to positivity is considered to be positive if the blood culture that is drawn through the vascular access device becomes positive at least 120 minutes before the peripheral culture. If a patient has an indwelling vascular access device and the cultures drawn from that device become positive at least 120 minutes before the peripheral cultures become positive, it is recommended that the device be removed because it is likely infected.[50]

Initiation of Empiric Antimicrobial Therapy

Another key component of the initial resuscitation of the septic patient is the administration of IV antimicrobial therapy. Antimicrobials should be administered after appropriate cultures are collected but within 1 hour of sepsis recognition. Difficulty with specimen collection should not delay the initiation of antibiotic therapy. The time to antimicrobial administration is a critical factor in survival of patients presenting with sepsis. A recent study by Kumar and colleagues[13] found that each hour in delay of antimicrobials was associated with an average decrease in survival of 7.6%. Delayed administration of antifungal therapy in subjects with *Candida* bloodstream infections was an independent predictor of hospital mortality.[52] Maintaining a supply of commonly used antimicrobials in the ED and ICU can assist in the timely administration of these agents. The Surviving Sepsis guidelines recommend initiation of IV broad-spectrum antibiotics within the first hour of recognizing severe sepsis and septic shock.

The selection of antimicrobial therapy should take into account the patient's history of drug allergies, recent antimicrobial exposure, suspected source of infection, and hospital-specific antibiograms. Within the author's surgical ICU, the multidisciplinary sepsis team has developed antimicrobial regimens based on suspected source of infection and the current institution specific antibiogram (see **Table 1**). When choosing empiric antimicrobial therapy, a few general rules should be applied. Chiefly, the initial antimicrobial coverage should be broad enough to cover all potential pathogens. Evidence suggests that administering inadequate initial antimicrobial coverage is associated with increased morbidity and mortality.[53–56] Any antimicrobial that the patient has recently received should be avoided. Vigilant monitoring of culture data and de-escalation of the antimicrobial regimen based on culture results and sensitivities will reduce the risk of superinfection and the emergence of resistant organisms.

Obtaining Source Control

The final component of the resuscitation bundle is identification and source control of the infection. This can be as simple as removing an infected vascular access device. However, in the author's experience, in surgical patients the abdomen is the site of infection in greater than or equal to 50% of cases. These patients often require diagnostic imaging to identify the source and an operative procedure to attain source control. This includes, but is not limited to, emergent debridement of necrotic tissues, abscess drainage, removal of infected vascular access devices, and exploratory laparotomy. In the setting of septic shock, these procedures, although necessary, can present a unique challenge to the surgical team.

The concept of damage control laparotomy (DCL) was first recognized for the care of critically injured trauma patients.[57–59] Damage control is defined as rapid, initial control of hemorrhage and contamination followed by intraperitoneal packing, as needed, and temporary abdominal closure. This concept was used on patients presenting with severe physiologic derangements such as coagulopathy, acidosis, and hypothermia. Instead of persisting for hours performing the definitive operation, these patients have their critical surgical issues addressed in an abbreviated manner so they may be taken to the ICU for continued resuscitation. Once the physiologic derangements are corrected, the patient is taken back to the operating room for a definitive surgical procedure. The decision to use DCL should not be viewed as a bailout. Instead, it is a deliberate decision to truncate the surgical procedure to complete resuscitation and restore organ function to as normal as possible. The decision to perform DCL is often made before arriving in the operating room and is based on the severity of the patient's physiologic derangements at the time of presentation.

The concept of DCL has evolved to include critically ill patients with surgical sepsis. Like the trauma patient with the lethal triad of acidosis, hypothermia, and coagulopathy, many patients with septic shock present in a similar fashion. For those patients presenting with septic shock and an identified source of infection requiring surgical intervention, the use of DCL can be life saving. As patients progress from sepsis with SIRS through severe sepsis with organ dysfunction into septic shock, the abdominal infection often turns into an abdominal catastrophe. The surgeon needs to recognize that these patients are in the persistent septic shock cycle (see **Fig. 3**). This is characterized by excessive proinflammation, which causes vasodilation, hypotension, and myocardial depression. This, combined with endothelial activation and diffused intravascular coagulopathy, causes ongoing endothelial leak, cellular shock, and microvascular thrombosis. The clinical manifestation is septic shock with progressive multiple organ failure. The crucial question for the managing surgeon is timing of the operative intervention for source control to break this persistent cycle. These patients are hemodynamically unstable and are clearly not optimal candidates for operative interventions. The traditional approach is to take the patient to the operating room and perform a definitive operation (see **Fig. 4**). However, this often results in a patient who is underresuscitated, hypoperfused, and in septic shock being treated for prolonged periods in the operating room with vasopressors being used to maintain blood pressure. The end result is early deaths from fulminant multiple organ failure or acute kidney injury. However, with the recent EBGs recommending source control within 6 hours, a paradigm shift was proposed (see **Fig. 4**).

The first priority is to initiate resuscitation. The patient needs to undergo preoperative optimization, during which time the airway is secured, central venous and arterial lines are placed, volume resuscitation and broad-spectrum antimicrobial agents are administered, and, if needed, vasopressors are titrated to the appropriate endpoints. Within 6 hours, the patient is taken to the operating room for emergent laparotomy and potential damage control procedures. The surgeon needs to assess the degree of physiologic derangement early in the operation and, if severe physiologic derangements exist, the operative interventions need to be abbreviated. The primary aim is to control the source of infection. Ostomies are not formed. Bowel resections remove necrotic or perforated bowel, but the bowel is left in discontinuity. Abdominal closure is with a temporary abdominal closure device and the patient is returned to the ICU for physiologic optimization. This includes optimizing volume resuscitation and mechanical ventilation, correction of coagulopathy and hypothermia, and monitoring for ACS. Over the next 24 to 48 hours, abnormal physiology is corrected so that the patient can safely return to the operating room for a definitive operation and abdominal closure.

One of the problems with this damage control strategy is that the midline abdominal fascia cannot be closed at the second operation because of bowel distention and edema. These patients require multiple additional laparotomies for definitive abdominal wall closure. The midline fascia is progressively closed with the use of a vacuum-assisted closure (VAC) device. For this technique to work it is important that the bowel not become adherent to peritoneum of the anterior abdominal wall or to the lateral paracolic gutters because, otherwise, the abdomen becomes "frozen" and the fascia cannot be brought to midline. The VAC device actively removes fluid and decreases

Table 1
Antibiotic agent selection for empiric treatment based on suspected site of infection

	Antibiotic Drug	Regimen
—	If vancomycin allergy (not intolerance), then use linezolid	600 mg IV q 12 h
Indication	1. Preferred therapy 2. Severe β-lactam allergy	—
Pneumonia	—	—
Community-acquired pneumonia (CAP)	1. Ceftriaxone + levofloxacin	1 g IV q 24 h ª750 mg IV q 24 h
	2. Aztreonam + levofloxacin	ª2 gm IV q 8 h ª750 mg IV q 24 h
Aspiration (not chemical pneumonitis)	Piperacillin or tazobactam	ª4.5 g IV q 6 h
Ventilator-associated pneumonia (VAP)	—	—
Early (<5 d)	1. Cefepime	ª2 g IV q 12 h
—	2. Ciprofloxacin	ª400 mg IV q 12 h
Late (≥5 d) Pseudomonas risk: previous hospital or broad-spectrum antibiotic exposure + pseudomonas culture	1. Cefepime + vancomycin + tobramycin	ª2 g IV q 8 h ª15 mg/kg IV q 12 h ª,b7 mg/kg IV
	2. Ciprofloxacin + vancomycin + tobramycin	ª400 mg IV q 8 h ª15 mg/kg IV q 12 h ª,b7 mg/kg IV
Catheter-related	—	—
Urinary catheter; UTI	1. Cefepime 2. Ciprofloxacin	ª1 gm IV q 12 h ª400 mg IV q 12 h
IV, Art cath; bloodstream	Vancomycin	ª1 gm IV q 12 h
Candidemia high-risk (TPN, steroid Tx, diabetes, hepatic failure)	Fluconazole	ª800 mg IV q 24 h
Wound/Soft tissue	—	—
Necrotizing fasciitis	1. Piperacillin or tazobactam + vancomycin + clindamycin 2. Ciprofloxacin + vancomycin + clindamycin	ª4.5 g IV q 6 h ª15 mg/kg IV q 12 h 900 mg IV q 8 h ª400 mg IV q 8 h ª15 mg/kg IV q 12 h 900 mg IV q 8 h
Surgical site	1. Ertapenem + vancomycin	ª1 gm IV q 24 h ª15 mg/kg IV q 12 h
	2. Ciprofloxacin + vancomycin	ª400 mg IV q 12 h ª15 mg/kg IV q 12 h
Intra-abdominal	—	—
Pseudomonas low-risk	1. Ertapenem + vancomycin	ª1 gm IV q 24 h ª15 mg/kg IV q 12 h
	2. Ciprofloxacin + metronidazole + vancomycin	ª400 mg IV q 8 h 500 mg IV q 8 h ª15 mg/kg IV q 12 h

(continued on next page)

Table 1 (continued)		
	Antibiotic Drug	**Regimen**
—	**If vancomycin allergy (not intolerance), then use linezolid**	**600 mg IV q 12 h**
Pseudomonas high-risk Previous hospitalization or broad-spectrum antibiotic exposure; + pseudomonas culture	1. Imipenem or cilastatin + vancomycin 2. Ciprofloxacin + metronidazole + vancomycin	[a]500 mg IV q 6 h [a]15 mg/kg IV q 12 h [a]400 mg IV q 8 h 500 mg IV q 8 h [a]15 mg/kg IV q 12 h
Candidiasis high risk (TPN, steroid Tx, diabetes, hepatic failure, upper GI perf + H2 blocker, age ≥75, prolonged antibiotic, long-term care)	Consider fluconazole	[a]800 mg IV q 24 h

Abbreviations: Art cath, arterial catheter; Dysfxn, dysfunction; GI perf, gastrointestinal perforation; H2, histamine type 2; TPN, total parenteral nutrition; Tx, therapy; UTI, urinary tract infection.
[a] Monitor; adjust if renal dysfunction.
[b] Kinetic monitoring.

edema, provides medial tension, which helps to minimize fascial retraction and loss of domain, and protects the abdominal contents by providing separation between abdominal wall and viscera, with no fascial damage because it does not require fascial suture placement. Traditionally, abdominal wall defects in these frozen abdomens were closed by mobilizing skin or subcutaneous tissue flaps to cover the defect (ie, accepting a large hernia defect and need for delayed reconstruction) or by bridging the defect with mesh with later split thickness skin grafting once granulation tissue has developed. This is associated with a 20% gastrointestinal fistula rate, which is an extremely morbid complication. Additionally, many of these patients required delayed complex abdominal wall reconstructions. Recently, there has been significant enthusiasm for acute reconstruction with biologic mesh. Unfortunately, long-term follow-up studies show that many of these patients still require delayed hernia repairs of large defects.[60] In the author's published experience of treating the open abdomen with the VAC device, primary fascia closure was achieved in 87% of cases at a mean 7 days with a 2% fistula rate and no intraabdominal abcesses.[61,62] These results are nearly identical to the results reported by Miller and colleagues[63] from Wake Forest University.

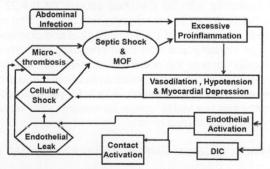

Fig. 3. The persistent septic shock cycle. DIC, diffused intravascular coagulopathy; MOF, multiple organ failure.

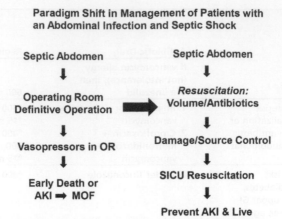

Paradigm Shift in Management of Patients with an Abdominal Infection and Septic Shock

Fig. 4. Paradigm shift for management of the septic abdomen. AKI, acute kidney injury; MOF, multiple organ failure.

More recently, Cothren and colleagues[64] have reported 100% primary fascial closure rate using a modified VAC device technique. The long-term outcomes are not known; however, in short-term follow-up (mean 180 days) ventral hernia was 2.3%. However, as is true with all emergency laparotomies, this rate will increase with time.

In addition to damage control scenarios, there are other reasons to leave the abdomen open and plan for a staged relaparotomy. Patients with ischemic bowel that have undergone a resection will be taken back the next day to assess viability of the remaining bowel before attempts at anastomosis or ostomy creation. The author has been successful in completing the small bowel to colon anastomosis at the second operation and, thus, these patients have avoided the need for a temporary ileostomy. For patients with necrotizing pancreatitis, the attempt is to avoid an operative intervention but, occasionally, it becomes necessary. Patients who have massive bowel distention that cannot be closed without causing significant intraabdominal hypertension will undergo temporary abdominal closure. Intraabdominal hypertension sets the stage of ACS, which occurs with subsequent ICU resuscitation.[65] Avoiding ACS significantly improves survival. Patients who develop ACS require a decompressive laparotomy. ACS is increasingly being recognized in nontrauma ICU patients, including those experiencing sepsis.[66–68]

The author's SICU has been using DCL for our patients with septic shock. Over 2 years, 22 patients underwent DCL for source control. Sources of intraabdominal infection were colon (11 patients), small bowel (4), stomach (2), and pancreas (1). Four patients had peritonitis with no identified source. Of the 22 patients, 6 died from multiple organ failure, for an actual mortality rate of 27%. The mean P-POSSUM (portsmouth predictor modification of the physiological and operative severity score for the enumeration of mortality and morbidity) predicted mortality was significantly higher at 69.4% ($P<.02$), as was the predicted mortality of 76% based on a mean APACHE (acute physiology and chronic health evaluation) II score of 31.8 ($P<.02$).[69] These data suggest that the implementation of DCL for patients with surgical sepsis is decreasing mortality and is a viable option for patients with septic shock and the need for immediate operative source control.

COMPUTERIZED CLINICAL DECISION SUPPORT TO HELP IMPLEMENT EBGS

In an attempt to improve sepsis-related outcomes, EBGs were developed for the management of sepsis.[12] When bedside clinicians are able to effectively implement these EBGs, patient outcomes improve significantly.[70–72] However, an alarmingly low percentage of patients with sepsis actually receive timely, evidence-based care.[71,72] The relationship between compliance with evidence-based guidelines for sepsis and mortality has been well established. A study by Gao and colleagues[70] demonstrated a twofold increase in hospital mortality in patients who did not receive the 6-hour sepsis bundle. In addition, noncompliance with the 24-hour sepsis bundle was associated with a 76% increase in risk for death. A recent multicenter, prospective study of over 15,000 subjects documented that only one-third of all subjects with sepsis receive appropriate evidence-based care.[72] This inability to consistently implement EBGs represents a significant gap between the best available evidence and the ability to effectively implement that knowledge at the patient's bedside. This gap can be bridged by leveraging technology in the form of computerized clinical decision support (CCDS) to aid bedside clinicians in consistently implementing EBGs at the bedside. Compliance with EBGs for the management of sepsis improves survival. However, achieving high levels of compliance remains extremely challenging. This is due to the complexity of the EBGs. The use of a CCDS program improves compliance with EBGs in multiple clinical settings, including the management of adult respiratory distress syndrome,[73] management of intracranial pressure,[74] and hemorrhagic shock resuscitation.[75] This investigative team has developed a CCDS program for the early identification of sepsis. The implementation of a CCDS program for the management of sepsis will dramatically improve compliance with the EBGs, thereby improving patient outcomes.

SUMMARY

Sepsis in the surgical patient continues to be a common and potentially lethal problem. Early identification of patients and timely implementation of evidence-based therapies continue to represent significant clinical challenges for care providers. The implementation of a sepsis screening program in conjunction with protocol for the delivery of evidence-based care and rapid source control can improve patient outcomes.

REFERENCES

1. Hall MJ, Williams SN, Defrances CJ, et al. Inpatient care for septicemia or sepsis: a challenge for patients and hospitals. NCHS Data Brief 2011;62:1–8.
2. Lagu T, Rothberg MB, Shieh MS, et al. Hospitalizations, costs, and outcomes of severe sepsis in the United States 2003 to 2007. Crit Care Med 2011. Available at: http://www.ncbi.nlm.nih.gov/pubmed/21963582. Accessed January 5, 2012.
3. Moore LJ, McKinley BA, Turner KL, et al. The epidemiology of sepsis in general surgery patients. J Trauma 2011;70(3):672–80.
4. Moore LJ, Moore FA, Todd SR, et al. Sepsis in general surgery: the 2005–2007 national surgical quality improvement program perspective. Arch Surg 2010; 145(7):695–700.
5. Angus DC, Linde-Zwirble WT, Lidicker J, et al. Epidemiology of severe sepsis in the United States: analysis of incidence, outcome, and associated costs of care. Crit Care Med 2001;29(7):1303–10.
6. Moore LJ, Moore FA, Jones SL, et al. Sepsis in general surgery: a deadly complication. Am J Surg 2009;198(6):868–74.
7. Moore LJ, Turner KL, Todd SR, et al. Computerized clinical decision support improves mortality in intra abdominal surgical sepsis. Am J Surg 2010;200(6): 839–43 [discussion: 843–4].

8. Balk RA, Bone RC. The septic syndrome. Definition and clinical implications. Crit Care Clin 1989;5(1):1–8.
9. Anon. American College of Chest Physicians/Society of Critical Care Medicine Consensus Conference: definitions for sepsis and organ failure and guidelines for the use of innovative therapies in sepsis. Crit Care Med 1992;20(6):864–74.
10. Levy MM, Fink MP, Marshall JC, et al. 2001 SCCM/ESICM/ACCP/ATS/SIS International Sepsis Definitions Conference. Intensive Care Med 2003;29(4):530–8.
11. Rivers E, Nguyen B, Havstad S, et al. Early goal-directed therapy in the treatment of severe sepsis and septic shock. N Engl J Med 2001;345(19):1368–77.
12. Dellinger RP, Levy MM, Carlet JM, et al. Surviving sepsis campaign: international guidelines for management of severe sepsis and septic shock: 2008. Crit Care Med 2008;36(1):296–327.
13. Kumar A, Roberts D, Wood KE, et al. Duration of hypotension before initiation of effective antimicrobial therapy is the critical determinant of survival in human septic shock. Crit Care Med 2006;34(6):1589–96.
14. Robson W, Beavis S, Spittle N. An audit of ward nurses' knowledge of sepsis. Nurs Crit Care 2007;12(2):86–92.
15. Assunção M, Akamine N, Cardoso GS, et al. Survey on physicians' knowledge of sepsis: do they recognize it promptly? J Crit Care 2010;25(4):545–52.
16. Fernandez R, Boque M, Rodriguez G. Sepsis: a study of physician's knowledge about the surviving sepsis campaign in Puerto Rico. Critical Care (London, England)2006;10:126.
17. Ziglam HM, Morales D, Webb K, et al. Knowledge about sepsis among training-grade doctors. J Antimicrob Chemother 2006;57(5):963–5.
18. Lai NA, Kruger P. The predictive ability of a weighted systemic inflammatory response syndrome score for microbiologically confirmed infection in hospitalised patients with suspected sepsis. Crit Care Resusc 2011;13(3):146–50.
19. Cei M, Bartolomei C, Mumoli N. In-hospital mortality and morbidity of elderly medical patients can be predicted at admission by the modified early warning score: a prospective study. Int J Clin Pract 2009;63(4):591–5.
20. Burch VC, Tarr G, Morroni C. Modified early warning score predicts the need for hospital admission and inhospital mortality. Emerg Med J 2008;25(10):674–8.
21. Gardner-Thorpe J, Love N, Wrightson J, et al. The value of Modified Early Warning Score (MEWS) in surgical in-patients: a prospective observational study. Ann R Coll Surg Engl 2006;88(6):571–5.
22. Moore LJ, Jones SL, Kreiner LA, et al. Validation of a screening tool for the early identification of sepsis. J Trauma 2009;66(6):1539–46 [discussion: 1546–7].
23. Sebat F, Johnson D, Musthafa AA, et al. A multidisciplinary community hospital program for early and rapid resuscitation of shock in nontrauma patients. Chest 2005;127(5):1729–43.
24. Shorr AF, Micek ST, Jackson WL, et al. Economic implications of an evidence-based sepsis protocol: can we improve outcomes and lower costs? Crit Care Med 2007;35(5):1257–62.
25. Nguyen HB, Corbett SW, Steele R, et al. Implementation of a bundle of quality indicators for the early management of severe sepsis and septic shock is associated with decreased mortality. Crit Care Med 2007;35(4):1105–12.
26. Shapiro NI, Howell MD, Talmor D, et al. Implementation and outcomes of the Multiple Urgent Sepsis Therapies (MUST) protocol. Crit Care Med 2006;34(4):1025–32.
27. Micek ST, Roubinian N, Heuring T, et al. Before-after study of a standardized hospital order set for the management of septic shock. Crit Care Med 2006; 34(11):2707–13.

28. Bendjelid K, Romand J-A. Fluid responsiveness in mechanically ventilated patients: a review of indices used in intensive care. Intensive Care Med 2003; 29(3):352–60.
29. Varpula M, Tallgren M, Saukkonen K, et al. Hemodynamic variables related to outcome in septic shock. Intensive Care Med 2005;31(8):1066–71.
30. Finfer S, Bellomo R, Boyce N, et al. A comparison of albumin and saline for fluid resuscitation in the intensive care unit. N Engl J Med 2004;350(22):2247–56.
31. Anon. Volume replacement with albumin in severe sepsis (ALBIOS). NCT00707122. Available at: http://www.clinicaltrials.gov/ct2/show/NCT00707122?term=albumin+sepsis&rank=1. Accessed February 3, 2012.
32. Anon. Early albumin resuscitation during septic shock. NCT00327704. Available at: http://www.clinicaltrials.gov/ct2/show/NCT00327704?term=albumin+sepsis&rank=10. Accessed February 3, 2012.
33. Kortgen A, Niederprüm P, Bauer M. Implementation of an evidence-based "standard operating procedure" and outcome in septic shock. Crit Care Med 2006; 34(4):943–9.
34. Trzeciak S, Dellinger RP, Abate NL, et al. Translating research to clinical practice: a 1-year experience with implementing early goal-directed therapy for septic shock in the emergency department. Chest 2006;129(2):225–32.
35. Anon. ProCESS. Available at: a. https://crisma.upmc.com/processtrial/index.asp; http://clinicaltrials.gov/ct2/show/NCT00510835. Accessed February 3, 2012.
36. Anon. ARISE Trial. Available at: http://www.anzicrc.monash.org/process.html; http://clinicaltrials.gov/ct2/show/NCT00975793. Accessed February 3, 2012.
37. Anon. ProMISe Trial. Available at: http://www.icnarc.org; https://www.icnarc.org/documents/ProMISe%20Information%20Sheet.pdf. Accessed February 3, 2012.
38. Landry DW, Levin HR, Gallant EM, et al. Vasopressin deficiency contributes to the vasodilation of septic shock. Circulation 1997;95(5):1122–5.
39. Russell JA. Vasopressin in vasodilatory and septic shock. Curr Opin Crit Care 2007;13(4):383–91.
40. Russell JA, Walley KR, Singer J, et al. Vasopressin versus norepinephrine infusion in patients with septic shock. N Engl J Med 2008;358(9):877–87.
41. Russell JA, Walley KR, Gordon AC, et al. Interaction of vasopressin infusion, corticosteroid treatment, and mortality of septic shock. Crit Care Med 2009;37(3):811–8.
42. Holmes CL, Walley KR, Chittock DR, et al. The effects of vasopressin on hemodynamics and renal function in severe septic shock: a case series. Intensive Care Med 2001;27(8):1416–21.
43. Turner K, Moore L, Todd S, et al. Identification of cardiac dysfunction in sepsis with B-Type natriuretic peptide. J Am Coll Surg 2011;213(1):139–46 [discussion: 146–7].
44. Oppert M, Schindler R, Husung C, et al. Low-dose hydrocortisone improves shock reversal and reduces cytokine levels in early hyperdynamic septic shock. Crit Care Med 2005;33(11):2457–64.
45. Keh D, Boehnke T, Weber-Cartens S, et al. Immunologic and hemodynamic effects of "low-dose" hydrocortisone in septic shock: a double-blind, randomized, placebo-controlled, crossover study. Am J Respir Crit Care Med 2003; 167(4):512–20.
46. Annane D, Sebille V, Charpentier C, et al. Effect of treatment with low doses of hydrocortisone and fludrocortisone on mortality in patients with septic shock. JAMA 2002;288(7):862–71.
47. Arpi M, Bentzon MW, Jensen J, et al. Importance of blood volume cultured in the detection of bacteremia. Eur J Clin Microbiol Infect Dis 1989;8(9):838–42.

48. Mermel LA, Maki DG. Detection of bacteremia in adults: consequences of culturing an inadequate volume of blood. Ann Intern Med 1993;119(4): 270–2.

49. Bouza E, Sousa D, Rodríguez-Créixems M, et al. Is the volume of blood cultured still a significant factor in the diagnosis of bloodstream infections? J Clin Microbiol 2007;45(9):2765–9.

50. Blot F, Schmidt E, Nitenberg G, et al. Earlier positivity of central-venous- versus peripheral-blood cultures is highly predictive of catheter-related sepsis. J Clin Microbiol 1998;36(1):105–9.

51. Blot F, Nitenberg G, Chachaty E, et al. Diagnosis of catheter-related bacteraemia: a prospective comparison of the time to positivity of hub-blood versus peripheral-blood cultures. Lancet 1999;354(9184):1071–7.

52. Morrell M, Fraser VJ, Kollef MH. Delaying the empiric treatment of candida blood-stream infection until positive blood culture results are obtained: a potential risk factor for hospital mortality. Antimicrob Agents Chemother 2005;49(9):3640–5.

53. Kreger BE, Craven DE, McCabe WR. Gram-negative bacteremia. IV. Re-evaluation of clinical features and treatment in 612 patients. Am J Med 1980;68(3):344–55.

54. Ibrahim EH, Sherman G, Ward S, et al. The influence of inadequate antimicrobial treatment of bloodstream infections on patient outcomes in the ICU setting. Chest 2000;118(1):146–55.

55. Leibovici L, Shraga I, Drucker M, et al. The benefit of appropriate empirical anti-biotic treatment in patients with bloodstream infection. J Intern Med 1998;244(5): 379–86.

56. Fitousis K, Moore LJ, Turner KL, et al. Evaluation of emperic antibiotic use in surgical sepsis. Am J Surg 2010;200(6):776–82 [discussion: 782].

57. Cué JI, Cryer HG, Miller FB, et al. Packing and planned reexploration for hepatic and retroperitoneal hemorrhage: critical refinements of a useful technique. J Trauma 1990;30(8):1007–11 [discussion: 1011–3].

58. Rotondo MF, Schwab CW, McGonigal MD, et al. "Damage control": an approach for improved survival in exsanguinating penetrating abdominal injury. J Trauma 1993;35(3):375–82 [discussion: 382–3].

59. Burch JM, Ortiz VB, Richardson RJ, et al. Abbreviated laparotomy and planned reoperation for critically injured patients. Ann Surg 1992;215(5): 476–83 [discussion: 483–4].

60. de Moya MA, Dunham M, Inaba K, et al. Long-term outcome of acellular dermal matrix when used for large traumatic open abdomen. J Trauma 2008;65(2): 349–53.

61. Garner GB, Ware DN, Cocanour CS, et al. Vacuum-assisted wound closure provides early fascial reapproximation in trauma patients with open abdomens. Am J Surg 2001;182(6):630–8.

62. Suliburk JW, Ware DN, Balogh Z, et al. Vacuum-assisted wound closure achieves early fascial closure of open abdomens after severe trauma. J Trauma 2003; 55(6):1155–60 [discussion: 1160–1].

63. Miller PR, Thompson JT, Faler BJ, et al. Late fascial closure in lieu of ventral hernia: the next step in open abdomen management. J Trauma 2002;53(5):843–9.

64. Cothren CC, Moore EE, Johnson JL, et al. One hundred percent fascial approx-imation with sequential abdominal closure of the open abdomen. Am J Surg 2006;192(2):238–42.

65. Balogh Z, McKinley BA, Cox CS Jr, et al. Abdominal compartment syndrome: the cause or effect of postinjury multiple organ failure. Shock 2003;20(6):483–92.

66. Cothren CC, Moore EE, Johnson JL, et al. Outcomes in surgical versus medical patients with the secondary abdominal compartment syndrome. Am J Surg 2007; 194(6):804–7 [discussion: 807–8].
67. McNelis J, Marini CP, Jurkiewicz A, et al. Predictive factors associated with the development of abdominal compartment syndrome in the surgical intensive care unit. Arch Surg 2002;137(2):133–6.
68. Malbrain ML, Chiumello D, Pelosi P, et al. Incidence and prognosis of intraabdominal hypertension in a mixed population of critically ill patients: a multiple-center epidemiological study. Crit Care Med 2005;33(2):315–22.
69. Turner KL, Moore LJ, Sucher JF, et al. Damage Control Laparotomy: beyond trauma. Poster session presented at the American Association for the Surgery of Trauma, 71st Annual Meeting. Pittsburg September 17–21, 2009.
70. Gao F, Melody T, Daniels DF, et al. The impact of compliance with 6-hour and 24-hour sepsis bundles on hospital mortality in patients with severe sepsis: a prospective observational study. Crit Care 2005;9(6):R764–70.
71. Levy MM, Dellinger RP, Townsend SR, et al. The surviving sepsis campaign: results of an international guideline-based performance improvement program targeting severe sepsis. Intensive Care Med 2010;36(2):222–31.
72. McKinley BA, Moore LJ, Sucher JF, et al. Computer protocol facilitates evidence-based care of sepsis in the surgical intensive care unit. J Trauma 2011;70(5): 1153–66 [discussion: 1166–7].
73. McKinley BA, Moore FA, Sailors RM, et al. Computerized decision support for mechanical ventilation of trauma induced ARDS: results of a randomized clinical trial. J Trauma 2001;50(3):415–24 [discussion: 425].
74. McKinley BA, Parmley CL, Tonneson AS. Standardized management of intracranial pressure: a preliminary clinical trial. J Trauma 1999;46(2):271–9.
75. Sucher JF, Moore FA, Sailors RM, et al. Performance of a computerized protocol for trauma shock resuscitation. World J Surg 2010;34(2):216–22.

The Value of Critical Care

Philip S. Barie, MD, MBA[a],*, Vanessa P. Ho, MD, MPH[b]

KEYWORDS

• Critical care • Cost-effectiveness • Cost analysis • Value definitions

KEY POINTS

• The rapid growth in health care expenditure has engendered careful scrutiny of the practice of medicine with regard not only to effectiveness but also to efficiency.
• Physicians must understand the effectiveness of their interventions and the cost at which this effectiveness is obtained.
• As physicians and policy-makers encounter cost-effectiveness analyses in the literature, they must evaluate such studies as they would any clinical study—with caution, skepticism, and attention to the methods used.
• There is a growing interest in the application of emerging methodology to quantify the value of health care interventions by applying the methods of economics.
• Specific critical care inventions have been demonstrated to be cost-effective.

NOTE TO THE READER

Your humble correspondents, in seeking editorial guidance as to the scope of this essay, were advised to interpret our charge as we see fit. Whereas your essayists generally feel no qualms regarding what to write, the term "value" has many meanings and connotations. At the risk of imposing our own "values" (biases) on the reader, it is hoped that the reader will find "value" from the reading of this contribution.

INTRODUCTION

"Value" has many connotations (**Box 1, Fig. 1**).[1] Applied to critical care, the meaning may be economic (is this a "reasonable" use of resources?), ethical (is this something that the patient wants?), or philosophic (the old cliché, "how do you put a value on a human life?"). The only aspect that can really be quantified is the former, and even then the numbers of studies are few that have brought analytical rigor to the question of the "value of critical care." With the predicates that lower mortality/better surgical outcomes and lower resource use are desirable, and that measuring and

[a] Department of Surgery and Public Health, Joan and Sanford I. Weill Medical College of Cornell University, 1300 York Avenue, New York, NY 10065, USA; [b] Department of Surgery, New Jersey Medical School, University of Medicine and Dentistry of New Jersey, 185 South orange Avenue, Newark, NJ 07103, USA
* Corresponding author. Department of Surgery, New York-Presbyterian Hospital, Weill Cornell Medical Center, 525 East 68 Street, P713A, New York, NY 10065.
E-mail address: pbarie@med.cornell.edu

Surg Clin N Am 92 (2012) 1445–1462
http://dx.doi.org/10.1016/j.suc.2012.09.001
0039-6109/12/$ – see front matter © 2012 Published by Elsevier Inc.
surgical.theclinics.com

Box 1
Dictionary definition of "value"

val·ue [val-yoo] noun, verb, val·ued, val·u·ing. Noun, verb.

c.1300, from Old French value "worth, value" (13c.), noun use of feminine past participle of *valoir* "be worth," from Latin valere "be strong, be well, be of value" (see valiant). The verb is recorded from late 15c.

noun

1. Relative worth, merit, or importance: the value of a college education; the value of a queen in chess.

2. Monetary or material worth, as in commerce or trade: This piece of land has greatly increased in value.

3. The worth of something in terms of the amount of other things for which it can be exchanged or in terms of some medium of exchange.

4. Equivalent worth or return in money, material, services, etc.: to give value for value received.

5. Estimated or assigned worth; valuation: a painting with a current value of $500,000.

6. Denomination, as of a monetary issue or a postage stamp.

7. (Mathematics). (A) Magnitude; quantity; number represented by a figure, symbol, or the like: the value of an angle; the value of x; the value of a sum. (B) A point in the range of a function; a point in the range corresponding to a given point in the domain of a function: The value of x^2 at 2 is 4.

8. Import or meaning; force; significance: the value of a word.

9. Liking or affection; favorable regard.

10. Values (Sociology). the ideals, customs, institutions, etc., of a society toward which the people of the group have an affective regard. These values may be positive, as cleanliness, freedom, or education, or negative, as cruelty, crime, or blasphemy.

11. (Ethics). any object or quality desirable as a means or as an end in itself.

12. (Fine Arts). (A) Degree of lightness or darkness in a color. (B) The relation of light and shade in a painting, drawing, or the like.

13. (Music). the relative length or duration of a tone signified by a note.

14. Values (Mining). the marketable portions of an ore body.

15. (Phonetics). (A) Quality. (B) The phonetic equivalent of a letter, as the sound of "a" in hat, sang, etc.

verb (used with object)

16. To calculate or reckon the monetary value of; give a specified material or financial value to; assess; appraise: to value their assets.

17. To consider with respect to worth, excellence, usefulness, or importance.

18. To regard or esteem highly: He values her friendship.

Adapted from Value. Dictionary.com. Dictionary.com unabridged. Random House, Inc. Available at: http://dictionary.reference.com/browse/value. Accessed June 03, 2012.

recording outcomes remains challenging,[2–7] especially for heterogeneous patient populations or when the interactions of multiple coexisting conditions may be confounding,[7] the primary focus of this review is on the cost-effectiveness of critical care.

Surgical mortality appears to be decreasing. Using the Nationwide Inpatient Sample, Semel and colleagues[8] compared deaths within 30 days of admission for patients

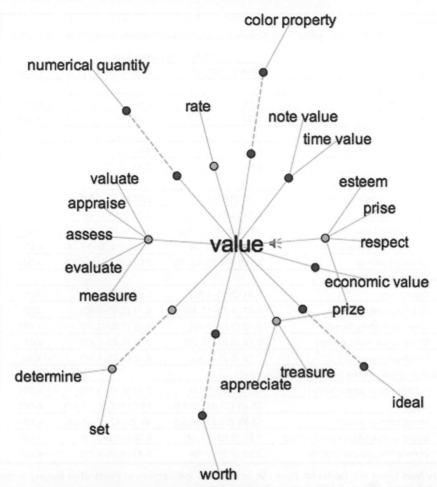

Fig. 1. Visual representation of the meaning of "value." (Image from the Visual Thesaurus, Copyright ©1998–2012 Thinkmap, Inc. All rights reserved.)

undergoing 2520 different surgical procedures in 1996 and 2006. The inpatient 30-day death rate was examined for all procedures, procedures with the most deaths, high-risk cardiovascular and cancer procedures, and patients who suffered a recorded complication. Logistic regression modeling was used to adjust 1996 mortality rates to the age and gender distributions for patients undergoing surgery in 2006. In 1996 there were 12,573,331 admissions with a surgical procedure (95% confidence interval [CI], 12,560,171–12,586,491) and 224,111 inpatient deaths within 30 days of admission (95% CI, 221,912–226,310). In 2006 there were 14,333,993 admissions with a surgical procedure (95% CI, 14,320,983–14,347,002) and 189,690 deaths (95% CI, 187,802–191,578). The inpatient 30-day mortality decreased from 1.78% in 1996 to 1.33% in 2006 ($P<.001$). Of the 21 procedures with the most deaths in 1996, 15 had significant decreases in adjusted mortality in 2006 (**Table 1**). Among these 15 procedures, 8 had significant decreases in operative volume. Comparing 1996 and 2006, the inpatient 30-day mortality rate for patients who suffered a complication decreased from 12.10% to 9.84% ($P<.001$). Although there are myriad factors that contribute to

Table 1
Surgical mortality, 2006 versus 1996. Selected outcomes of relevance to surgical critical care

Patient Group	30-Day Mortality Rate 1996% (95% CI)	2006% (95% CI)	P Value
Admission type			
Emergency	3.65	2.62	<.001
Urgent	1.83	1.48	<.001
Charlson Comorbidity Index			
3	4.73	3.27	<.001
≥4	6.94	4.84	<.001
High number of deaths			
Coronary artery bypass	2.80 (2.62–3.00)	1.67 (1.51–1.84)	<.001
Debridement wound/burn	4.04 (3.61–4.52)	2.23 (2.02–2.46)	<.001
Small bowel resection	10.38 (9.37–11.50)	6.83 (6.29–7.42)	<.001
Temporary tracheostomy	22.51 (20.92–24.21)	15.94 (14.80–17.14)	<.001
Ventriculostomy	38.09 (34.25–42.35)	29.21 (26.81–31.72)	<.001
High-risk operations			
Cystectomy	3.31 (2.50–4.39)	1.85 (1.38–2.47)	.045
Esophagectomy	9.07 (6.72–12.23)	4.77 (3.42–6.60)	.012
Lower extremity bypass	3.12 (2.84–3.42)	2.09 (1.82–2.33)	<.001
Mitral valve replacement	9.86 (8.62–11.29)	7.59 (6.83–8.42)	.001
Pancreatic resection	7.10 (5.21–9.68)	4.10 (3.37–4.97)	.016
Major complications (failure to rescue rate)			
Postoperative pneumonia	8.54 (7.93–9.19)	7.34 (6.93–7.77)	<.001
Sepsis	18.69 (17.81–19.61)	14.03 (13.40–14.68)	<.001
Shock/cardiac arrest	53.82 (51.72–56.02)	44.15 (42.07–46.26)	<.001
Upper gastrointestinal bleeding	9.96 (8.82–11.24)	6.86 (6.03–7.79)	<.001
Venous thromboembolism	8.69 (7.97–9.49)	5.43 (4.90–6.00)	<.001

Data from Semel ME, Lipsitz SR, Funk LM, et al. Rates and patterns of death after surgery in the United States, 1996 and 2006. Surgery 2012;151:171–82.

decreased surgical mortality, the decreases among elderly patients, after high-risk procedures, and after major complications suggest that the decreases in mortality are due in part to advances in surgical critical care. Note in particular the decreases in mortality from complications related to infection/sepsis (see **Table 1**).

Mortality in the intensive care unit (ICU) may also be decreasing. Although data from population-based samples are lacking, data are available from sequential reports from major centers,[9–14] and inferences can be drawn from results of clinical trials (eg, severe sepsis/septic shock).[15–19] Ironically, the decreased mortality from septic shock occasioned by the implementation of evidence-based best practices, perhaps unanticipated or of greater magnitude than believed possible, may be confounding ongoing clinical research in the field.[19,20]

METHODS FOR EVALUATING COST-EFFECTIVENESS
Quality of Life

Quality of life (QoL) is an amorphous concept that has usage across many disciplines, including health economics. It is a vague concept; it is multidimensional and theoretically incorporates all aspects of an individual's life. Research on valued states of existence has reported that health is the most valued state, and there is a rapidly expanding literature on health-related QoL (HRQoL). Patients' expectations of a morbidity-free life at older age have also increased, and have led to attempts to measure health expectancy. Moreover, purchasing debates in health care now focus on health care cost in relation to "health gain," or benefit from the treatments and interventions that are contracted for. The increasing emphasis on health care provision as a scarce resource has given impetus to this trend.

HRQoL, a subjective health status, is patient-based but focuses more on the impact of a perceived health state on the ability to live a fulfilling life. It is a double-sided concept, assessing positive as well as negative aspects of well-being and life by incorporating social, psychological, and physical health. It also includes some assessment of the patient's level of satisfaction with treatment, outcome, and health status, and with future prospects. It is distinct from QoL as a whole, which includes adequacy of housing, income, and perceptions of the immediate environment. It is also ultimately a dynamic (unstable?) concept, for as health status deteriorates, perspectives on life, roles, relationships, and experiences change.

Some investigators are skeptical about patient-based indicators, but others believe that it is important to include patient-based indicators in assessments of outcome because they do not necessarily correlate with objective measures of physical functioning. There is often poor agreement among physicians in relation to supposed objective clinical findings and variations in physicians' clinical judgments. Subjective indicators such as HRQoL are increasingly popular because of the recognition of the importance of patient satisfaction and how individuals feel, rather than what statistics imply they ought to feel. In this view, clinical indicators of outcome are no longer sufficient; assessment of QoL as a measure of outcome redirects clinicians from limiting the measurement of outcome to postintervention survival, complication rates, and various physical or biochemical indicators toward consideration of the impact of disease and therapy on the patient's emotional and physical functioning and lifestyle.

The measurement of health outcomes of clinical interventions has become a cornerstone of health services research, and is also linked to the assessment of the appropriateness of health care interventions. QoL assessment as a supplement to the documentation of symptom rates, toxicity, adverse effects, and survival patterns is given more urgency in the light of data that some surgery is inappropriate or ineffective. QoL assessment is also popular among pharmaceutical companies, with most reporting that they have used some type of QoL instrument in their clinical trials of drugs, but the US Food and Drug Administration (FDA) considers the state of the art of QoL measurement too immature to merit mandatory inclusion in clinical trials.

Cost-utility studies (see later discussion) need a common measurement of health outcome. With these cost-utility analyses, the cost of an intervention is related to the number of quality-adjusted life years (QALYs). A QALY is a year of full life quality; poor health may reduce the quality of a year (eg, from 1 to 0.5). In QALYs, improvements in the length and QoL are amalgamated into one single index. Each life-year is quality-adjusted with a utility value, where 1 = full health. The utility value aims to reflect the HRQoL. Thus, QALYs are not really measures of QoL per se, but rather are measures of units of benefit from a medical intervention, combining life expectancy with an index of, for example, disability and distress. That they are based on invalidated value judgments has led to criticism.

Values of QALYs can be derived by several different methods. The disadvantages of all these methods are their cost, the requirements for skilled interviewers, and complexity (leading to reliance on nonrandom or unrepresentative samples). One of the main debates surrounding the use of these techniques is who should provide the utility values: the general public, health care providers, or patients and their families? Bowling[21] provides a comprehensive discussion of QoL research, oriented toward the social sciences.

Defining "Value"

"Value" is a key parameter in determining whether the cost of something is "appropriate." Any level of spending may be acceptable, depending on the value provided by that expenditure. However, revelations about the prevalence of medical errors and their high cost,[22] as well as the challenges inherent in translating evidence into practice,[23] underscore that health care delivery can be excessive and wasteful. The practice of medicine is being scrutinized regarding the efficient allocation of resources, in the belief that optimal resource allocation may improve both clinical and economic outcomes.[24] Medical cost has been increasing for years at a rate exceeding the general rate of inflation, heightening the sense that translation of (often expensive) new diagnostics and therapeutics into practice must be done efficiently.

Conceptually, efficiency represents the attempt to obtain the most value and output for every dollar spent. Hence, there is a growing interest in the application of emerging methodology to quantify the value of health care interventions by applying the methods of economics.

Types of Cost

What is meant by "cost?" An important distinction exists between charges and costs. Charges reflect the desired reimbursement rates for a hospital or provider. Included in this value are the true expenditures for care and some measure of reasonable profit.[25] Charges are basically an accounting tool that may bear little relation to expected reimbursement from third-party payors (or cost, for that matter), except that they are set higher invariably to maximize reimbursement. Because of the variable nature of charges, cost is the preferred numerator for cost-effectiveness analyses (CEAs, see later discussion), as they are meant to represent actual resource consumption.

Costs can be derived from charges on the basis of the published hospital-specific cost:charge ratios from The Centers for Medicare and Medicaid Services (CMS). Costs may be direct, indirect, or intangible; or either fixed or variable. Direct costs are those of labor and goods used in the delivery of the intervention. Indirect costs, on the other hand, are those attributable to lost productivity resulting from illness (from the patient perspective), or those that are amortized (from the institutional perspective, eg, depreciation, debt service). Intangible costs incorporate the pain and suffering resulting from the disease or intervention. Fixed costs are those that remain the same regardless of the amount of production output. In a hospital setting, these include costs associated with running the physical plant and equipment, or the minimum level of staffing and inventory to remain open and functional for patient care. Variable costs are those that change in the short term with the changes in production output, such as costs of having to increase the number of nursing staff because of a temporary surge in ICU volume. There is controversy regarding whether CEA should address fixed, variable, or total (the sum of fixed and variable) cost. Although most studies analyze total cost, variable costs are influenced by externalities.[26] Fixed costs cannot be reduced short of closing the facility; they accrue no matter what transpires. However, fixed costs are also subject to external influences, albeit to a lesser degree and over longer periods of time.

Analyzing fixed versus variable costs can result in vastly different estimates of the cost of an illness. For example, Dasta and colleagues[27] estimated the total cost for a patient with respiratory failure on the first day of ICU care in the United States to be $8000, diminishing for subsequent days to $3600 to $3900 (2002 US dollars). By contrast, Kahn and colleagues[26] calculated the direct variable costs of the last ICU day in a cohort of similar patients who survived beyond ICU day 3 to be $400, with the first day on the ward costing only $280. By this reckoning, a hypothetical intervention that reduces the ICU length of stay (LOS) by 1 day saves the hospital only $120, which lacks face validity unless, for example, transfer out of the ICU is delayed by a lack of floor beds.

Types of Cost Analysis

There are 5 major types of cost analysis: (1) cost minimization; (2) cost-benefit; (3) cost-consequence; (4) cost-effectiveness; and (5) cost-utility; the last 2 being encountered most frequently in the medical literature. Cost minimization compares the infrequent situations in which 2 interventions produce identical effects. Cost-benefit analysis examines both cost and benefit in terms of monetary units, whereas cost-consequence analysis evaluates costs and consequences separately, allowing users to choose the costs and the consequences relevant to a specific circumstance.

In medicine generally, most economic research takes the form of either CEAs or cost-utility analyses. CEA examines the ratio of the cost of a particular intervention to a chosen unit of effectiveness. The need for a CEA or cost-utility analyses (these terms are sometimes used interchangeably) usually arises when the value proposition of a new intervention is unclear. (A value proposition is a business or marketing statement that summarizes why a consumer should buy a product or use a service. This statement should convince a potential consumer that one particular product or service will add more value or solve a problem better than other similar products. In practical terms, companies use the value proposition to target customers who will benefit most from using the company's products, and this helps maintain an economic "moat" [ie, imperviousness to competition]).

When a new therapy (A) is both less expensive and more effective than its comparator (B), it is said to "dominate" the comparator; in such a case (albeit rare in medicine) the decision to adopt therapy A is clear. Conversely, A is dominated by B if A is less effective and more costly than B. Ambiguity arises when either A is more effective and more costly than B or A is less effective and less costly than B. It is important to understand that being cost-effective does not necessarily mean cost-saving. Some effective therapies are expensive. Under these circumstances, it is important to articulate the resource expenditure per unit of effectiveness by a formal means for balancing the trade-offs between the 2 interventions, yielding a rational decision that maximizes outcome. Consensus-based recommendations for the conduct of CEAs have been published.[28]

Perspective

"Perspective" is the point of view taken when conducting a CEA. Perspective is crucial because it determines which costs and outcomes are likely to matter more than others. For example, in an ICU study, the cost of averting one case of ventilator-associated pneumonia (VAP) is borne almost completely by the hospital, and this is therefore an outcome that is important from the hospital's perspective. However, the development of VAP may affect morbidity but not necessarily the direct cost that the patient must pay. Other perspectives may represent those of payors, pharmacies, the ICU (as a cost center), or society as a whole. The costs and benefits of an intervention may not be borne equally; therefore, if the assessment is not made from a sufficiently broad perspective, the assessment of an intervention may be skewed and lead to potential bias. Moreover, cost shifting may be attractive to those whose costs would be diminished, but not to those who would bear the additional cost. This dilemma led to the principle in CEA that one should adopt whenever possible a societal perspective from which all costs may be incorporated, regardless of who bears the burden.

When considering CEAs, it can be ascertained quickly whether the investigators have used a societal perspective. In general, such articles describe results in terms of a reference case (baseline scenario) that is being explored, which serves as the frame of reference for other comparisons. The reference case incorporates QALYs in the denominator of the cost-effectiveness ratio. By definition, this represents the societal perspective, and is therefore most important for public health and overall resource allocation. The calculation of the reference case requires a long-term evaluation of both cost (lifetime health care cost) and effectiveness outcomes. Because some interventions may restore a person to perfect health, whereas others (while extending life) leave the person debilitated, not only are expected years of survival included in the denominator but also the quality of those years of life. The usual denominator in cost-utility studies is the QALY, and cost/QALY serves as the reference case. In addition, reference cases are useful because they provide a baseline scenario against which to compare alternative resource allocation decisions; it is valid to compare the costs per QALY in reference cases across unrelated conditions and interventions. In general, a cost/QALY of less than $100,000 is considered the threshold for determining that a therapy is cost-effective (the lower, the better).

Modeling

Whereas data regarding long-term outcomes for chronic conditions may be available for researchers to apply in CEA, those for acute and short-lived episodes may not exist, such as those that arise in the ICU. To circumvent this challenge, investigators may adopt the technique of decision modeling, in which assumptions about long-term outcomes, based on previous work in published populations, are entered into a mathematical formula to generate the outcome estimates of interest. This method is a preferred approach to building a reference case, as practical considerations, such as the urgency of the need for cost-effectiveness information and the enormous resources required, preclude real-time collection of actual long-term outcomes.

Incremental Cost-Effectiveness Ratio

Comparative effectiveness research (CER) represents a useful application of CEAs and cost-utility analyses. The purpose of CER is to compare explicitly the effectiveness of 2 interventions used for the same condition. The single value representing comparative cost-effectiveness is the incremental cost-effectiveness ratio (ICER). For example, Shorr and colleagues[29] examined the cost-effectiveness of linezolid as compared with vancomycin for the treatment of methicillin-resistant *Staphylococcus aureus* VAP. The ICER was calculated as the ratio of the differences in costs to the differences in effectiveness measures of the compared therapies. By definition, the lower the ICER, the better the cost-effectiveness profile. In the base-case analyses, the estimates were approximately $67,000, $22,000, and $30,000 for incremental costs per survivor, per life-year saved, and per QALY, respectively.[29]

Sensitivity Analysis

Because model inputs are based on assumptions, they invariably include some degree of uncertainty. Sensitivity analyses are designed to estimate how this uncertainty in the assumptions may affect the precision of the outcome estimates.[28] These sensitivity analyses usually include univariate (one input is varied at a time), 2-way (2 inputs with the strongest effect on the outcome variability are varied simultaneously), and multivariable analyses (all inputs are varied at the same time across their plausible ranges). The extent of uncertainty used in sensitivity analyses is most appropriate if derived from actual clinical data, and should represent the 95% CIs around various point estimates. In the literature the reader may encounter Markov analysis or Monte Carlo simulation, with which the reader should be familiar; these are described briefly in **Box 2**.

A CEA that does not report a sensitivity analysis should be viewed with skepticism. For example, a recent cost-effectiveness simulation of a silver-coated endotracheal tube as a preventive measure for VAP found the tube to be cost-saving in the base case.[30] Univariate analyses indicated that VAP costs and the risk reduction resulting from use of the novel endotracheal tube accounted for most of the model uncertainty. A 2-way sensitivity analysis revealed outcome estimates ranging from savings of $34,000 to an expenditure of $205 to prevent one case of VAP.[30]

Another useful type of sensitivity analysis is a worst-case scenario analysis, wherein all inputs are biased against one of the comparators (usually the novel intervention). In a study of the cost-effectiveness of micafungin as compared with fluconazole for empiric treatment of candidemia in the ICU, the calculated base-case cost/QALY was $35,000 (well below the traditional non–cost-effective threshold of >$100,000 per QALY). In the worst-case scenario, the cost-utility ratio gave a cost of $72,000 to save one additional QALY.[31] A threshold analysis suggested that when the prevalence of azole resistance reached 1.5%, micafungin was no longer cost-effective relative to fluconazole.[31]

Box 2
Descriptions of Markov analysis and Monte Carlo simulation

Definition of Markov Analysis

A method used to forecast the value of a variable whose future value is independent of its past history. The technique is named after Russian mathematician Andrei Andreyevich Markov, who pioneered the study of stochastic processes, which are processes that involve the operation of chance. The Markov Analysis introduces a method for forecasting random variables. Markov analysis has several applications in the business world. Two common applications are in estimating the proportion of a company's accounts receivable that will become bad debts, and forecasting future brand loyalty of current customers.

Read more:

http://www.investopedia.com/terms/m/markov-analysis.asp#ixzz1wjU5xcYi

http://en.wikipedia.org/wiki/Markov_chain

Definition of Monte Carlo Simulation

A problem-solving technique used to approximate the probability of certain outcomes by running multiple trial runs, called simulations, using random variables.

Monte Carlo simulation is named after the city in Monaco, where the primary attractions are casinos. Gambling games, such as roulette, dice, and slot machines, exhibit random behavior.

Read more:

http://www.investopedia.com/terms/m/montecarlosimulation.asp#ixzz1wjZ7w0sV

http://en.wikipedia.org/wiki/Monte_carlo_simulation

Inflation Adjustments and Discounting

Adjustment of costs for inflation, and to discount both future costs and effectiveness estimates, can be used as markers of study quality.[28] Inflation adjustment is necessary for several reasons. Medical cost inflation increases rapidly, therefore cost needs to be adjusted to the current time; a dollar spent today presumably has more value than a dollar spent in the future. Inflation adjustment to the same year confers uniformity and the ability to compare "apples with apples." Any analysis that quantifies future cost (eg, lifetime health care cost) and outcomes (eg, QALYs) needs adjustment for inflation in both the numerator and the denominator of any CER. The recommended annual base discount rate (the general inflation rate in the United States) is 3%, whereas medical cost inflation increases by at least twice that rate.

IS ICU CARE COST-EFFECTIVE?

Several rigorous examples do demonstrate that critical care is cost-effective. Among 937 critically ill patients treated in the critical care setting at a major European university teaching hospital, the influence was examined of using different HRQoL instruments on the calculation of the number of QALYs gained and the cost per QALY.[32] Two HRQoL tools were used at 6 and 12 months after the start of treatment, and QALYs were calculated using 4 different sets of assumptions (**Box 3**). Each of the 8 conditions (2 × 4 factorial) generated unique information regarding QALYs gained and cost/QALY, with the former ranging from 49 to 150 QALYs gained, and cost/QALY ranging from €38,405 to €118,668. Thus, critical care was considered to be cost-effective in 7 of the 8 scenarios.[32]

Box 3
Effect of health-related quality of life assessment and QoL calculation using several methodologies and assumptions

Assumption 1

Without treatment, patients would die (HRQoL = 0, QALYs gained = 0).

After treatment, HRQoL is increased to the 6-month time point, then changes linearly with QALY thereafter. Thus, for those who die before the first follow-up, the QALY gain is zero. The maximum number of QALYs to be gained is 1.

Assumption 2

Without treatment, patients would die (HRQoL = 0, QALYs gained = 0). After treatment, HRQoL increases linearly with QALY thereafter. The maximum number of QALYs to be gained is 0.75.

Assumption 3

Without treatment, patients would stay at their same baseline HRQoL for the entire follow-up period. Nontreated patients are not assumed to die. With treatment, the HRQoL changes immediately to the level measured at 6 months, after which it increases linearly to the 12-month follow-up period. The maximum number of QALYs gained depends on the baseline HRQoL score.

Assumption 4

The assumptions are those set forth in Assumption 3, except that with treatment the change in HRQoL increases linearly from baseline through all follow-up periods. The maximum number of QALYs gained depends on the baseline HRQoL score.

Data from Vainiola T, Roine RP, Pettila V, et al. Effect of health-related quality-of-life instrument and quality-adjusted life-year calculation method on the number of life years gained in the critical care setting. Value Health 2011;14:1130–4.

Edbrooke and colleagues[33] studied 7659 patients (11 hospitals, 7 European countries) referred to the ICU who were stratified by whether or not they were accepted for ICU admission. Stratified by age, Karnofsky score (one of the earliest of the QoL assessment tools, developed in 1948; it is limited by its exclusive emphasis on physical functioning), reason for admission, and severity of illness. The two groups were compared in terms of cost and mortality using multilevel regression. Admission to the ICU reduced the risk of mortality overall (relative risk [RR] 0.70, 95% CI 0.52–0.94), and was related inversely to the predicted risk of death (for 40% predicted mortality, RR 0.55, 95% CI 0.37–0.83). Cost per life-year (CPLY) was $7065 overall, and $4088 for 40% risk of death. Results were robust when subjected to sensitivity analysis. Thus not only did ICU care reduce mortality, but CPLY decreased with increasing severity of illness, underscoring the cost-effectiveness of critical care.

QoL and lifetime cost-utility for critically ill patients with acute respiratory failure were assessed in a nationwide prospective study of 958 consecutive patients treated with mechanical ventilation in 25 Finnish ICUs.[34] One-year mortality was 35% (95% CI 32%–36%). Of the 619 survivors, 288 completed a QoL questionnaire. For the survivors, QoL at 1 year was lower than that reported by an age-matched and gender-matched general population. Among the 288 survivors, the mean predicted lifetime QALYs were 15.4 and 11.3 after adjustment for the missing data (reflecting all 958 patients). The mean estimated cost was €20,739 per hospital survivor, and the mean predicted lifetime cost-utility for all patients was €1391/QALY. Among age subgroups (10-year intervals), mean QALY decreased and mean cost/QALY increased for older patients, but despite lower HRQoL compared with healthy matched patients, the cost per hospital survivor and lifetime cost-utility remained reasonably low regardless of age, disease severity, or type or duration of mechanical ventilation.

The cost-effectiveness of protocolized sepsis care has been examined in 2 studies of comparable design, reaching similar conclusions. In a single-center study from Boston, Talmor and colleagues[35] compared 79 patients who presented to the emergency department in septic shock with 59 control patients. The analysis was performed from the perspective of the health care system using a lifetime horizon, and incremental cost/QALY gained (ICER) was the primary end point. Mortality was 20.3% in the protocol-treated group versus 29.4% in the control group (P not significant). The integrated sepsis protocol increased cost by $8800/patient, due largely to increased ICU LOS. However, the expenditure was found to be cost-effective, with an incremental cost of $11,274 per life-year saved and $16,309 per QALY gained. By contrast, Suarez and colleagues[17] evaluated the cost-effectiveness of the protocol derived from the Surviving Sepsis Campaign guidelines[36] in a cohort of 1465 patients from 59 medical-surgical ICUs located throughout Spain. Comparison was made with 854 patients treated for severe sepsis/septic shock before protocol implementation. The health care system perspective was used. The primary outcome was ICER. There was lower mortality (39.7% vs 44.0%, P<.05) for the protocol-treated patients. Mean costs were €1736 higher (95% CI 114–3356) for protocol-treated patients, largely from increased LOS. Mean life-years gained was 0.54 years higher for the protocol-treated group (95% CI 0.02–1.05 years). The adjusted ICER of the protocol was €4435. Sensitivity analysis showed protocol-based care to be cost-effective in 96.5% of bootstrap replications.

Other Examples Relevant to the ICU

Translating evidence into practice often relies on the adoption of a "bundle" of interventions rather than a single treatment; a prime example is the Surviving Sepsis

Box 4
Selected cost-effectiveness analyses of relevance to surgical critical care practice

Antibiotic Prophylaxis of Surgery for Closed Fractures
Slobogean et al,[42] 2010   Comparison of single- and multiple-dose prophylaxis
Time horizons of 90 days and 1 year
Base-case analysis, sensitivity analysis, probabilistic. Monte Carlo sensitivity analysis
Single-dose prophylaxis slightly more cost-effective, $2576 versus $2596 for an average gain of 272 QALD

Critical Care Interventions
Etchells et al,[43] 2012   Systematic literature review identified 5 comparative economic analyses that reported 7 comparisons of adequate methodological quality, 4 of which were cost-effective: Pharmacist-led medication reconciliation; chlorhexidine for "vascular catheter site care"; implementation of "Keystone ICU Initiative"[45] to prevent CLABSI; counting to detect retained surgical foreign bodies. The 3 interventions that were "economically unattractive" were bar-coded surgical sponges compared with standard counting, use of erythropoietin for critically ill patients to avoid transfusion, and related adverse events

Screening for MRSA
Olchanski et al,[45] 2011   Decision analysis with multivariable sensitivity analysis. PCR-based versus culture-based screening in several ICU populations: "High risk," ICU, previous MRSA colonization/infection. Screening resulted in cost savings of $12,158–$76,644/month compared with no screening. Same-day PCR-based screening of high-risk patients resulted in fewer infections and the lowest total cost. Sensitivity analysis showed that the results are sensitive to hospital size, test turnaround time, transmission rate, prevalence rate, and rate of conversion of colonization to infection

TBI Care
Whitmore et al,[46] 2012   Decision analytical model of 3 strategies for treating a patient with severe TBI: (1) Aggressive care (including invasive ICP monitoring and decompressive craniectomy); (2) Routine care, in which Brain Trauma Foundation guidelines are not followed; and (3) Comfort care, consisting of only 1 day of critical care, followed by floor care. Glasgow Outcome Scale Scores were converted to QALYs based on estimates of longevity and QoL from the literature. Societal perspective. Monte Carlo sensitivity analysis used for patients aged 20, 40, 60, and 80 years. Aggressive care yielded an additional 1.7 QALYs; although the cost-effectiveness of aggressive care diminished with advancing age, it was significant at all ages. Aggressive care was significantly less costly up to age 80, whereas comfort care was associated with poorer outcomes and higher costs up to age 80

Trauma Triage
Mohan et al,[47] 2012   Comparison of ICERs for current practice with interventions targeting attitudes toward transferring patients to trauma centers (decisional threshold) and ability to identify patients who should be transferred (perceptual sensitivity). Societal perspective. Markov analysis (decision model). Monte Carlo sensitivity analysis. The ICER of an intervention to change perceptual sensitivity was $62,799/QALY, compared with current practice, whereas the ICER of an intervention to change the decisional threshold was $104,795/QALY. Findings were most sensitive to the relative cost of hospitalizing patients with

		moderate-to-severe injuries and their RR of dying at nontrauma centers. There was 62% likelihood that intervention to change perceptual sensitivity (improve adherence to CPGs for trauma triage) was the more cost-effective alternative, even at a modest cost to intervene
Ventilator Bundle Mollar et al,[41] 2012		CER of use of a "ventilator bundle" versus standard care in 2 models for prevention of VAP, for patients ventilated for more than 48 h: One for the prevention of VAP per se; another for the prevention of death. Perspective of third-party payor, thus societal costs and direct medical costs were not considered. The cost per episode of VAP prevented was €4451, and €31,792 per death prevented. The ICER analysis showed that the ventilator bundle was more cost-effective for VAP prevention in 99.9% of cases, and 42.6% of cases was dominant (ie, had both better outcomes and lower cost). The ventilator was more cost-effective for prevention of death in 85.9% of cases, with both lower cost and better outcome (dominance) in 31.6% of cases

Abbreviations: CER, cost-effectiveness ratio; CI, confidence interval; CLABSI, central line–associated bloodstream infection; CPG, clinical practice guideline; ICER, incremental cost-effectiveness ratio; ICP, intracranial pressure; ICU, intensive care unit; MRSA, methicillin-resistant *Staphylococcus aureus;* PCR, polymerase chain reaction; QALD, quality-adjusted life-days; QALY, quality-adjusted life-years; QoL, quality of life; RR, relative risk; TBI, traumatic brain injury.

Campaign treatment guidelines.[36] Hence, it can be asked whether some of the bundled interventions are cost-effective. Two such care bundles include early goal-directed therapy (EGDT) for sepsis (which is itself incorporated into the Surviving Sepsis Campaign guidelines), and a 24-hour intensivist presence model for ICU staffing. Huang and colleagues[37] examined the cost-effectiveness of EGDT from both the hospital and societal perspectives. Use of EGDT had a nearly 100% probability of being cost-effective at a value of less than $20,000 per QALY. On the other hand, the cost-effectiveness of different models of ICU attending coverage remains poorly defined. For example, a 24-hour intensivist coverage model for the ICU is believed to be cost-saving from the perspective of the hospital, because the intensivist's continuous presence can improve outcomes, enhance patient throughput and the efficient use of resources, and focus efforts on prevention,[38] but cost-effectiveness from the societal perspective has not been demonstrated definitively. The savings associated with implementation of the 24-hour intensivist model derive largely from an anticipated reduction in ICU and hospital LOS, which cannot be assured (see the sepsis protocol data above). This conundrum illustrates the need to be explicit about perspective and sensitivity analyses when conducting CEAs.

Surprisingly, some of the bundled interventions for prevention of hospital-acquired infection, which are advocated by many, have not been evaluated either for effectiveness or cost-effectiveness. One such example is the Institute for Healthcare Improvement's "ventilator bundle."[39] In a recent systematic review of studies evaluating bundled interventions for prevention of VAP, the investigators found only weak evidence in support. More importantly, no rigorous evaluations of the cost-effectiveness of ventilator bundles for avoiding VAP were identified[40] (one has been published subsequently [Box 4]),[41] but the cost-effectiveness demonstrated was examined only from the perspective of the third-party payor. As additional bundled strategies are promoted as quality improvement initiatives and measures for reimbursement, rigorous assessment of cost-effectiveness will be essential. Given that health care resources are limited, reflexive adoption of some tactics may result in the diversion of resources that prove ultimately to be more cost-effective.

Several other ICU-related therapies have been subjected to cost-effectiveness analysis (see **Box 4**)[42–47] and have been found to be cost-effective. However, it should be noted that one therapy of recent interest, off-label administration of recombinant human Factor VIIa (rFVIIa) as rescue therapy for patients with hemorrhage who require massive transfusion,[48] was found to be not cost-effective. Among 353 patients with substantive bleeding at Royal Perth Hospital, Australia, 81 received rFVIIa. The total CPLY gained was $1,148,000, and the ICER was $736,000, greater than the usual acceptable cost-effective limit of $100,000 per life-year. The ICER increased with increasing severity of illness and transfusion requirement. Note that this analysis did not address specifically the use of rFVIIa for trauma.

A Cautionary Tale

The recent example of the introduction and subsequent withdrawal, 10 years later, of drotrecogin alfa (activated) (DAA) therapy for severe sepsis, should serve as a cautionary tale. Angus and colleagues[49] incorporated both real-time data from a clinical trial and modeling in a CEA of the therapy, specifically the incremental health care cost associated with 1 death averted at 28 days as a result of treatment with DAA. To determine cost, the investigators needed not only to establish the costs of DAA but also to account for the cost of the continued care and further health care resource consumption attendant thereto for survivors. Angus and colleagues[49] estimated that DAA cost society $160,000 per life saved. In determining the reference case, which required estimating the life expectancy of sepsis survivors and HRQoL, the cost of DAA was $48,000/QALY. The ICER improved to $27,000/QALY when the estimated risk of short-term death increased, and worsened to the point of cost-ineffectiveness (>$100,000/QALY) if the survivors were expected to live fewer than 5 years.

Of course, a therapy cannot be found to be cost-effective if ultimately the therapy is not effective.[19] Although a single Class I trial[50] and ample Class II and III data[51–55] implied that DAA was effective, other randomized trials were not supportive.[56,57] The ensuing heated controversy led to the recent failed trial of DAA for patients in septic shock,[19] leading to its withdrawal from the market.[20]

SUMMARY

The rapid growth in health care expenditure has engendered careful scrutiny of the practice of medicine with regard not only to effectiveness but also to efficiency. This shift necessitates that physicians understand the effectiveness of their interventions and the cost at which this effectiveness is obtained. Cost-effectiveness and cost-utility analyses have become crucial evaluative tools in medicine. Explicit articulation of comparative cost-effectiveness facilitates the allocation of limited resources. As physicians and policy-makers encounter CEA in the literature, they must evaluate such studies as they would any clinical study: with caution, skepticism, and attention to the methods used.[58]

REFERENCES

1. Value. Dictionary.com. Dictionary.com unabridged. Random House, Inc. Available at: http://dictionary.reference.com/browse/value. Accessed June 03, 2012.
2. Alexander JA, Hearld LR. Methods and metrics challenges of delivery-system research. Implement Sci 2012;7:15.

3. Huang IC, Wen PS, Revicki DA, et al. Quality of life measurement for children with life-threatening conditions: limitations and a new framework. Child Indic Res 2011;4:145–60.
4. Singer SJ, Burgers J, Friedberg M, et al. Defining and measuring integrated patient care: promoting the next frontier in health care delivery. Med Care Res Rev 2011;68:112–27.
5. Dodson TB. Outcomes research and the challenge of evidence-based surgery. Oral Maxillofac Surg Clin North Am 2010;22:1–4.
6. Andres PL, Haley SM, Ni PS. Is patient-reported function reliable for monitoring postacute outcomes? Am J Phys Med Rehabil 2003;82:614–21.
7. Werner RM, Greenfield S, Fung C, et al. Measuring quality of care in patients with multiple clinical conditions: summary of a conference conducted by the Society of General Internal Medicine. J Gen Intern Med 2007;22:1206–11.
8. Semel ME, Lipsitz SR, Funk LM, et al. Rates and patterns of death after surgery in the United States, 1996 and 2006. Surgery 2012;151:171–82.
9. Barie PS, Hydo LJ, Fischer E. Comparison of APACHE II and III scoring systems for mortality prediction in critical surgical illness. Arch Surg 1995;130:77–82.
10. Barie PS, Hydo LJ, Fischer E. Development of multiple organ dysfunction syndrome in critically ill patients with perforated viscus. Predictive value of APACHE severity scoring. Arch Surg 1996;131:37–43.
11. Barie PS, Hydo LJ, Eachempati SR. Longitudinal outcomes of intra-abdominal infection complicated by critical illness. Surg Infect (Larchmt) 2004;5:365–73.
12. Barie PS, Hydo LJ, Shou J, et al. Decreasing magnitude of multiple organ dysfunction syndrome despite increasingly severe critical surgical illness: a 17-year longitudinal study. J Trauma 2008;65:1227–35.
13. Glance LG, Osler TM, Mukamel DB, et al. Outcomes of adult trauma patients admitted to trauma centers in Pennsylvania, 2000-2009. Arch Surg 2012;147:732–7.
14. Cook DA, Duke G, Hart GK, et al. Review of the application of risk-adjusted charts to analyze mortality outcomes in critical care. Crit Care Resusc 2008; 10:239–51.
15. Shiramizo SC, Marra AR, Durão MS, et al. Decreasing mortality in severe sepsis and septic shock patients by implementing a sepsis bundle in a hospital setting. PLoS One 2011;6:e26790.
16. McKinley BA, Moore LJ, Sucher JF, et al. Computer protocol facilitates evidence-based care of sepsis in the surgical intensive care unit. J Trauma 2011;70: 1153–66.
17. Suarez D, Ferrer R, Artigas A, et al, Edusepsis Study Group. Cost-effectiveness of the Surviving Sepsis Campaign protocol for severe sepsis: a prospective nation-wide study in Spain. Intensive Care Med 2011;37:444–52.
18. Levy MM, Dellinger RP, Townsend SR, et al, Surviving Sepsis Campaign. The Surviving Sepsis Campaign: results of an international guideline-based performance improvement program targeting severe sepsis. Crit Care Med 2010;38: 367–74.
19. Ranieri VM, Thompson BT, Barie PS, et al, PROWESS-SHOCK Study Group. Drotrecogin alfa (activated) in adults with septic shock. N Engl J Med 2012;366: 2055–64.
20. Barie PS. The last Xigris® survivor. Surg Infect (Larchmt) 2011;12:423–5.
21. Available at: http://info.worldbank.org/etools/docs/library/48475/m2s5bowling.pdf. Accessed August 15, 2012.
22. Institute of Medicine. To err is human: building a safer health system. Washington, DC: National Academies Press; 1999.

23. McGlynn EA, Asch SM, Adams J, et al. The quality of health care delivered to adults in the United States. N Engl J Med 2003;348:2635–45.
24. Schwartz K, Vilquin JT. Building the translational highway: toward new partnerships between academia and the private sector. Nat Med 2003;9:493–5.
25. Price KF. Pricing Medicare's diagnosis-related groups: charges versus estimated costs. Health Care Financ Rev 1989. Available at: http://findarticles.com/p/articles/mi_m0795/is_n1_v11/ai_9338473. Accessed September 10, 2012.
26. Kahn JM, Rubenfeld GD, Rohrbach J, et al. Cost savings attributable to reductions in intensive care unit length of stay for mechanically ventilated patients. Med Care 2008;46:1226–33.
27. Dasta JF, McLaughlin TP, Mody SH, et al. Daily cost of an intensive care unit day: the contribution of mechanical ventilation. Crit Care Med 2005;33:1266–71.
28. Weinstein MC, Siegel JE, Gold MR, et al. Recommendations of the panel on cost-effectiveness in health and medicine. JAMA 1996;276:1253–8.
29. Shorr AF, Susla GM, Kollef MH. Linezolid for the treatment of ventilator-associated pneumonia: a cost-effective alternative to vancomycin. Crit Care Med 2004;32:137–43.
30. Shorr AF, Zilberberg MD, Kollef MH. Cost-effectiveness analysis of a silver-coated endotracheal tube to reduce the incidence of ventilator-associated pneumonia. Infect Control Hosp Epidemiol 2009;30:759–63.
31. Zilberberg MD, Kothari S, Shorr AF. Cost-effectiveness of micafungin as an alternative to fluconazole empiric treatment of suspected ICU-acquired candidemia among patients with sepsis: a model simulation. Crit Care 2009;13:R94.
32. Vainiola T, Roine RP, Pettila V, et al. Effect of health-related quality-of-life instrument and quality-adjusted life-year calculation method on the number of life years gained in the critical care setting. Value Health 2011;14:1130–4.
33. Edbrooke DL, Minelli C, Mills GH, et al. Implications of ICU triage decisions on patient mortality: a cost-effectiveness analysis. Crit Care 2011;15:R56.
34. Linko R, Suojaranta-Yilnen R, Karisson S, et al, FINNALI study investigators. One-year mortality, quality of life and predicted life-time cost-utility in critically ill patients with acute respiratory failure. Crit Care 2010;14:R60.
35. Talmor D, Greenberg D, Howell MD, et al. The costs and cost-effectiveness of an integrated sepsis treatment protocol. Crit Care Med 2008;36:1168–74.
36. Dellinger RP, Levy MM, Carlet JM, et al, International Surviving Sepsis Campaign Guidelines Committee; American Association of Critical-Care Nurses; American College of Chest Physicians; American College of Emergency Physicians; Canadian Critical Care Society; European Society of Clinical Microbiology and Infectious Diseases; European Society of Intensive Care Medicine; European Respiratory Society; International Sepsis Forum; Japanese Association for Acute Medicine; Japanese Society of Intensive Care Medicine; Society of Critical Care Medicine; Society of Hospital Medicine; Surgical Infection Society; World Federation of Societies of Intensive and Critical Care Medicine. Surviving Sepsis Campaign: international guidelines for management of severe sepsis and septic shock: 2008 [Erratum in: Crit Care Med 2008;36:1394–6.]. Crit Care Med 2008;36:296–327.
37. Huang DT, Clermont G, Dremsizov TT, et al, ProCESS Investigators. Implementation of early goal-directed therapy for severe sepsis and septic shock: a decision analysis. Crit Care Med 2007;35:2090–100.
38. Pronovost PJ, Needham DM, Waters H, et al. Intensive care unit physician staffing: financial modeling of the Leapfrog standard. Crit Care Med 2004;32:1247–53.

39. Institute for Healthcare Improvement. Available at: http://www.ihi.org. Accessed June 21, 2012.

40. Zilberberg MD, Shorr AF, Kollef MH. Implementing quality improvements in the intensive care unit: ventilator bundle as an example. Crit Care Med 2009;37: 305–9.

41. Mollar AH, Hansen L, Jensen MS, et al. A cost-effectiveness analysis of reducing ventilator-associated pneumonia at a Danish ICU with ventilator bundle. J Med Econ 2012;15:285–92.

42. Slobogean GP, O'Brien PJ, Brauer CA. Single-dose versus multiple-dose antibiotic prophylaxis for the surgical treatment of closed fractures. Acta Orthop 2010;81:256–62.

43. Etchells E, Koo M, Daneman N, et al. Comparative economic analyses of patient safety improvement strategies in acute care: a systematic review. BMJ Qual Saf 2012;21:448–56.

44. Waters HR, Korn R Jr, Colantuoni E, et al. The business case for quality: economic analysis of the Michigan Keystone Patient Safety Program in ICUs. Am J Med Qual 2011;26:333–9.

45. Olchanski N, Mathews C, Fusfeld L, et al. Assessment of test characteristics on the clinical and cost impacts of methicillin-resistant *Staphylococcus aureus* screening programs in US hospitals. Infect Control Hosp Epidemiol 2011;32: 250–7.

46. Whitmore RG, Thawant JP, Grady MS, et al. Is aggressive treatment of traumatic brain injury cost-effective? J Neurosurg 2012;116:1106–13.

47. Mohan D, Barnato AE, Rosengart ME, et al. Optimal approach to improving trauma care triage: a cost-effectiveness analysis. Am J Manag Care 2012;18: e91–100.

48. Ho KM, Litton E. Cost-effectiveness of using recombinant activated factor VII as an off-label rescue treatment for critical bleeding requiring massive transfusion. Transfusion 2012;52:1696–702.

49. Angus DC, Linde-Zwirble WT, Clermont G, et al. Cost-effectiveness of drotrecogin alfa (activated) in the treatment of severe sepsis. Crit Care Med 2003;31:1–11.

50. Bernard GR, Vincent JL, Laterre PF, et al, Recombinant human protein C Worldwide Evaluation in Severe Sepsis (PROWESS) study group. Efficacy and safety of recombinant human activated protein C for severe sepsis. N Engl J Med 2001; 344:699–709.

51. Vincent JL, Bernard GR, Beale R, et al. Drotrecogin alfa (activated) treatment in severe sepsis from the global open-label trial ENHANCE: further evidence for survival and safety and implications for early treatment. Crit Care Med 2005;33: 2266–77.

52. Barie PS. Current role of activated protein C therapy for severe sepsis and septic shock. Curr Infect Dis Rep 2008;10:368–76.

53. Barie PS, Hydo LJ, Shou J, et al. Efficacy of therapy with recombinant human activated protein C of critically ill surgical patients with infection complicated by septic shock and multiple organ dysfunction syndrome. Surg Infect (Larchmt) 2011;12:443–9.

54. Payon D, Sablotzki A, Barie PS, et al. International integrated database for the evaluation of severe sepsis and drotrecogin alfa (activated) therapy: analysis of efficacy and safety data in a large surgical cohort. Surgery 2007;141:548–61.

55. Casserly B, Gerlach H, Phillips GS, et al. Evaluating the use of recombinant human activated protein C in adult severe sepsis: results of the Surviving Sepsis Campaign. Crit Care Med 2012;40:1417–26.

56. Abraham E, Laterre PF, Garg R, et al, Administration of Drotrecogin Alfa (Activated) in Early Stage Severe Sepsis (ADDRESS) study group. Drotrecogin alfa (activated) for adults with severe sepsis and a low risk of death. N Engl J Med 2005;353:1332–41.

57. Nadel S, Goldstein B, Williams MD, et al, REsearching severe Sepsis and Organ dysfunction in children: A gLobal perspective (RESOLVE) study group. Drotrecogin alfa (activated) in children with severe sepsis: a multicentre phase III randomised controlled trial. Lancet 2007;369(9564):836–43.

58. Weinstein MC, Skinner JA. Comparative effectiveness and healthcare spending—implications for reform. N Engl J Med 2010;362:1845–6.

Mechanical Ventilation

Mollie M. James, DO, MPH*, Greg J. Beilman, MD

KEYWORDS

- Mechanical ventilation • Respiratory failure • ARDS • Algorithm

KEY POINTS

- The goal of therapy in patients with acute respiratory distress syndrome should be to opti-mize oxygenation while minimizing the risk of ventilator-induced lung injury and providing adequate ventilation.
- Appropriate use of ventilation modes and strategies, positive-end expiratory pressure levels, and recruitment maneuvers can improve oxygen delivery.
- Salvage therapies, such as prone positioning, inhaled epoprostenol and nitric oxide, and high-frequency oscillatory ventilation, have a well-established role in supportive manage-ment and are associated with improved oxygenation but not survival.

INTRODUCTION

Respiratory failure can be broadly defined as the inability of the lungs to provide adequate oxygenation or ventilation to support the organism's systemic metabolic functions. Symptoms of respiratory failure are distressing for patients and can lead to rapid clinical decompensation without appropriate and timely intervention. The authors' goal is to familiarize the reader about the most current supportive therapies available for respiratory failure and provide an algorithm (**Fig. 1**) for implementing these interventions in clinical practice.

BACKGROUND

Respiratory failure requiring mechanical ventilation (MV) makes up a significant portion of health care costs. Nearly 30% of intensive care unit (ICU) admissions in the United States are for MV. The rate of MV is 2.8 per 1000, accounting for 700 000 episodes annually. Treatment costs for this diagnosis in 2005 was $34 257 per patient, with an average stay of 14 days. This expense accounts for $27 billion annually. Respiratory failure actually accounts for 12% of all hospital costs and 7%

Division of Critical Care and Acute Care Surgery, Department of Surgery, University of Minnesota, 420 Delaware St SE, MMC 11, Minneapolis, MN 55455, USA
* Corresponding author.
E-mail address: mmjames@umn.edu

Surg Clin N Am 92 (2012) 1463–1474
http://dx.doi.org/10.1016/j.suc.2012.08.003
0039-6109/12/$ – see front matter © 2012 Elsevier Inc. All rights reserved.
surgical.theclinics.com

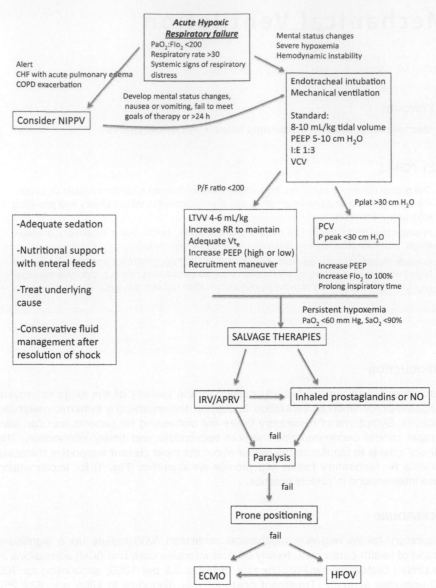

Fig. 1. The algorithm for ventilator management of ARDS. CHF, congestive heart failure; COPD, chronic obstructive pulmonary disease; ECMO, extracorporeal membrane oxygenation; FIo₂, fraction of inspired oxygen; HFOV, high-frequency oscillatory ventilation; I:E, inspiratory/expiratory ratio; IRV/APRV, inverse ratio ventilation/airway pressure release ventilation; LTVV, low tidal volume ventilation; NIPPV, noninvasive positive-pressure ventilation; NO, nitric oxide; PCV, pressure control ventilation; PEEP, positive end-expiratory pressure; P/F, PaO_2:FiO_2; Pplat, airway plateau pressures; RR, respiratory rate; SaO_2, saturation of arterial oxygen; VCV, volume control ventilation; Vte, minute ventilation.

of all hospital days. More than 50% of these expenditures involve patients older than 65 years.[1]

The incidence of acute lung injury (ALI) is nearly 80 per 100 000 person-years, with a mortality rate up to 40% for hospitalized patients.[2] Fifty-nine percent of patients with ALI present to community-based hospitals. Despite an increasing fund of knowledge regarding support for patients with acute respiratory distress syndrome (ARDS), survival remains minimally impacted. The first report of ARDS included a mortality risk of 58%, a number that declined through 1993.[3] Since 1994, the mortality remains stable at approximately 30%.[4] Heterogeneity in disease process results in varied mortality in subgroup populations (ie, younger patients do better than older patients); nonpulmonary sources leading to ARDS have better outcomes when compared with pulmonary-based ARDS, and trauma patients do better than most other groups.[2]

ALI and ARDS are both on the spectrum of the most severe form of respiratory failure. ALI is defined as a Pao_2/fraction of inspired oxygen (Fio_2) ratio of 300-200, whereas the more severe form, or ARDS, is defined as a Pao_2:Fio_2 ratio less than 200. To meet the complete definition, patients must be hypoxemic with new pulmonary infiltrates on chest radiograph, have a normal pulmonary capillary wedge pressure (to exclude left heart failure as a cause), and a predisposing condition associated with ARDS. The list of predisposing conditions is extensive but includes bacteremia, sepsis, pancreatitis, pneumonia, and trauma.

The pathophysiologic hallmark of ARDS is extensive inflammation and loss of capillary permeability in the lung tissue initiated by either a direct pulmonary insult (aspiration, exposure, infection) or an indirect process (pancreatitis, bacteremia, septic shock). This results in difficulty transporting oxygen from the alveoli into the bloodstream. The lungs lose compliance, becoming stiff and inelastic, which further limits gas exchange. MV to improve oxygenation and provide support can lead to ventilator-induced lung injury (VILI).[5] Injury to the lung parenchyma is in part caused by repeated opening and closing of alveoli causing injury of the tissue, with the volume and pressure used to ventilate the stiff lung resulting in an increased inflammatory cascade.[6] Long-term effects of this process can lead to pulmonary fibrosis.

Acute Support of Pulmonary Function

Noninvasive positive-pressure ventilation

Noninvasive positive-pressure ventilation (NIPPV) is used as a first-line therapy with increasing frequency for patients with respiratory failure. This therapy provides bilevel positive-pressure ventilation through a facemask. Because it is less invasive than endotracheal intubation, it is usually better tolerated and may require less sedation. NIPPV may be associated with lower rates of ventilator-associated pneumonia (VAP) because of the lack of a foreign body in the upper airway. NIPPV can improve oxygenation by increasing mean airway pressure with the resulting recruitment of alveoli, thus reducing the work of breathing. Ventilation is improved because of a higher effective tidal volume, which improves minute ventilation while lowering the work of breathing.[7]

Indications include hypoxemic respiratory failure caused by congestive heart failure and hypercapnic failure caused by exacerbations of chronic obstructive pulmonary disease (COPD).[7] Attempts to expand the indication to other disease processes, such as ARDS, pneumonia, and postoperative respiratory failure, produce varied results. Criteria for NIPPV include awake, alert patients who can tolerate the therapy. One must set defined treatment goals and proceed to intubation if those goals are not met within the predetermined timeframe. NIPPV is avoided in patients with any of the following contraindications: mental status change caused by traumatic brain injury, stroke, or seizure; active hemorrhage; hemodynamic instability; cardiac issues, such as arrhythmia or active ischemia; gastrointestinal (GI) issues that could lead to aspiration, such as nausea and vomiting, ileus, and recent GI surgery; facial trauma; secretions; and more than 2 organs with acute failure.[7]

NIPPV in ARDS NIPPV in ARDS has demonstrated some clinical success. Antonelli and colleagues[8] evaluated 147 patients admitted to the ICU with new-onset hypoxemic respiratory failure that were not endotracheally intubated. NIPPV advantages included avoiding intubation in 54%, lowering VAP rates (2% vs 20%, $P<.001$), reducing mortality (6% vs 53%, $P<.001$), and shortening MV duration. Factors leading to failure of NIPPV and intubation were older age, Simplified Acute Physiology Score II greater than 34, higher levels of positive end-respiratory pressure (PEEP), and a Pao_2:- Fio_2 ratio less than 175 after 1 hour of therapy.

NIPPV after extubation A frequent maneuver in our ICU is the attempt to prevent reintubation in recently extubated patients with NIPPV. Esteban and colleagues[9] addressed this clinical question and reported in a 2004 *New England Journal of Medicine*. This study evaluated 221 patients who failed extubation and were subsequently randomized to receive either standard therapy or NIPPV. The study was stopped after interim analysis because patients placed on NIPPV had higher mortality (25% vs 14%, relative risk [RR] 1.78 $P = .048$). Reintubation rates were the same in both groups, but the median time to intubation was longer when NIPPV was used (12 vs 2 hours 30 minutes, $P = .02$). A post hoc analysis of patients with COPD who were assigned to NIPPV showed a nonstatistical reduction in the rates of reintubation. This study suggests that NIPPV should not be used as a bridge to prevent reintubation.

Noninvasive weaning Contrary to the previously mentioned use of NIPPV after failure of extubation, this modality can be applied immediately after extubation to be used as another form of weaning. Candidates for this approach include patients with COPD who are clinically improving and otherwise stable but failing pressure support trials. A meta-analysis by Burns and colleagues[10] evaluated the results of 12 trials using NIPPV in this manner and found significantly reduced mortality (RR 0.55, confidence interval [CI] 95% 0.38–0.79, $P = .001$), lower rates of VAP (RR 0.29, CI 95% 0.38–0.79, $P = .001$), and shorter length of ICU (-6.27 days) and hospital stay (-7.19 days). Other factors were shorter duration of ventilation and shorter duration of invasive ventilation. Fewer tracheotomies were performed, and there was no increase in reintubation or arrhythmia. The benefits were most prominent in studies with patients with COPD.

Modes of MV

If patients have respiratory failure refractory to NIPPV or have a contraindication to NIPPV, they are endotracheally intubated. MV is directed to improve oxygenation and ventilation, reduce respiratory muscle effort, and recruit alveoli. Once MV is initiated, the physician must be aware of the complications of therapy. VILI can lead to long-term fibrosis of the parenchyma.[11] VAP rates can be as high as 25%, with the risk increasing with the duration of MV.[12] Patients often require sedation for anxiety or agitation, which is associated with delirium. Dyssynchrony with the ventilator may require heavy sedation or neuromuscular blockade. Positive-pressure ventilation is intimately tied to hemodynamic effects, including reduction in preload, reduction in afterload, increased stroke volume, and increased pulmonary artery pressures.[7,13] Finally, as with any invasive treatment, one must have a plan for the discontinuation of therapy and goals of treatment.

When supporting patients with respiratory failure, several modes of MV are available. If patients initiate each supported breath, it is called an assist-control mode. There are 2 options for this support: volume control and pressure control. In volume-controlled ventilation, the ventilator is set to deliver the same tidal volume with each breath. Most providers are familiar with the volume-control mode, and it is relatively straightforward to use. The inspiratory pressure is an uncontrolled variable in this mode of ventilation. As lung compliance drops, patients can develop high peak airway pressures.

Pressure-Controlled Ventilation (PCV)

Pressure-controlled ventilation (PCV) requires setting the inspiratory pressure and time while allowing a variation in the tidal volume. The ventilator delivers a breath to the preset pressure and then gradually reduces this pressure over the duration of the breath. This mode is helpful when the peak airway pressures are elevated and can also be effective for refractory hypoxemia and patient dyssynchrony. The inspiratory time can be lengthened, increasing the mean airway pressure and improving alveolar recruitment. Because the tidal volume is variable in this mode, it is important to monitor the tidal volume and minute ventilation to ensure patients adequately eliminate carbon dioxide.[5]

The aforementioned modes of ventilation follow the physiologic inspiratory/expiratory ratio of roughly 1:3. Either increasing or decreasing the inspiratory time can manipulate this ratio. In patients with COPD, decreasing the inspiratory time extends the expiratory phase to provide better ventilation that is necessary with air trapping. Conversely, when ventilating patients with hypoxemia, an initial strategy may include prolonging the inspiratory time, thus increasing the mean airway pressure and improving recruitment of alveoli.[5]

Airway Pressure Release Ventilation (APRV)

Airway pressure release ventilation (APRV) is a mode of inverse ratio ventilation that allows for an increase of the mean airway pressure without significantly increasing the peak airway pressure. The parameters of APRV include a T_{high} and T_{low} and P_{high} and P_{low}. T_{high} is the time in seconds during which patients are delivered the set positive pressure (P_{high}), whereas T_{low} is the time of exhalation, or breath release, and P_{low} is the baseline airway pressure. Increasing the mean airway pressure improves recruitment while potentially limiting volutrauma and barotrauma.

The ability for patients to spontaneously breathe during APRV is one advantage of this mode of ventilation. During P_{high}, patients can inspire and recruit dependent areas of the lung with lower transpleural pressure, avoiding the high airway pressure necessary in conventional modes. Because spontaneous breathing is more comfortable, the need for sedation and paralytics may be lower. Hemodynamics are dependent on the activity of spontaneous breathing: contraction of the diaphragm improves venous return and augments cardiac function. Small studies evaluating APRV have demonstrated improved hemodynamics compared with other modes of ventilation.[13]

Ventilator Strategies for ARDS

There are 3 hierarchical goals of ventilator support for patients with hypoxemic respiratory failure. These goals include adequate oxygenation, prevention of VILI, and adequate (not normal) ventilation. Achieving a normal P_{CO_2} is not one of the goals of supporting patients in this clinical setting.

Low tidal volume ventilation
One of the most influential studies on the treatment of ARDS was published in 2000 in the *New England Journal of Medicine*. The National Institutes of Health ARDS network

study evaluated low tidal volume ventilation (LTVV) compared with standard ventilation in patients with ALI or ARDS. The trial enrolled 861 patients before it was stopped early because of the survival benefit in the treatment arm. The treatment strategy included reducing tidal volume to 6 mL/kg predicted body weight with the aim of reducing plateau pressures to less than 30 cm H_2O. If plateau pressures were still high, the tidal volume was gradually reduced to 4 mL/kg in attempts to reduce plateau pressures to less than 30 cm H_2O. Conversely, if patients' plateau pressures were less than 25 cm H_2O, the tidal volume could be incrementally increased to 8 mL/kg PBW (predicted body weight). Inclusion criteria required a Pao_2:Fio_2 ratio less than 300, bilateral pulmonary infiltrates, and no evidence of elevated left atrial pressure. The LTVV strategy was instituted within 36 hours of onset of MV.[14] Results demonstrated that patients were ventilated differently: the mean tidal volume was 6 mL/kg versus 11.8 (P<.001), and the plateau pressures were 25 versus 33 cm H_2O (P<.001). End points included reduced mortality at 28 days; 31.0% versus 39.8% (P = .007) and more days without MV within the first 28 days (12 vs 10, P = .007).[14]

The LTVV strategy reduces VILI but also reduces minute ventilation. A consequence of this hypoventilation is hypercapnia leading to a respiratory acidosis, which highlights the principle of permissive hypercapnia. The level of Pco_2 is allowed to increase until the pH is less than 7.15, at which time a sodium bicarbonate infusion can be administered to prevent further reduction in pH. Hypercapnia in the setting of acute lung injury or ARDS is an expected consequence of the LTVV strategy and should not be aggressively corrected.

Recruitment maneuvers

Recruitment maneuvers (RM) are a group of strategies used to increase the mean airway pressure and open collapsed alveoli. Opening the alveoli improves ventilation capability and oxygenation. The lung tissue may be protected by opening alveoli that are collapsed or shear open and closed because of juxtaposed injured tissue. Strategies to recruit lung parenchyma include a prolonged inspiration at 30 to 50 cm H_2O for 30 to 40 seconds, a sigh breath with a high tidal volume, high pressures during PCV, or incrementally increasing PEEP. Most physicians using these strategies have noted temporary improvement in oxygenation with these maneuvers. Adverse effects associated with RM include hypotension caused by increased intrathoracic pressure (12%), transient desaturation (8%), and arrhythmia (1%). There is no overall mortality benefit with RM, but they may transiently improve oxygenation for patients with severe hypoxemia.[5] Most evidence suggests that a higher level of PEEP is required after a recruitment maneuver to keep the lung open.[15]

PEEP

PEEP is the pressure in the airway present during exhalation, which is a ventilator parameter that can be adjusted to increase recruitment of alveoli in ARDS. By increasing PEEP, oxygenation can be improved by stenting alveoli open. Studies have not demonstrated a survival advantage when PEEP levels are increased in ARDS. A study published in the 2004 New England Journal of Medicine compared high-PEEP to low-PEEP strategies in 549 patients. The low-PEEP group was ventilated with 8.3 cm H_2O, whereas the high-PEEP group had an average of 13.2 (P<.001). There was no difference between the groups in days free of ventilation in the first 28 days (14.5 vs 13.8) or mortality (24.9% vs 27.5%).[16]

Fluid management strategies

Management of fluid status is a frequent topic of debate among intensivists with critical care dogma dictating most clinical decisions. A 2006 article from the New England Journal of Medicine left us with data to guide therapy. The investigators randomized

1000 patients to a conservative versus liberal fluid strategy for the first 7 days after initiation of MV for ALI. The conservative group received a significantly higher cumulative furosemide dose. At 7 days, the conservative group had a fluid balance of −136 mL, compared with +6992 mL. Central venous pressure was 7 mm Hg in the conservative arm compared with 11 mm Hg in the liberal arm.[17] The primary end point was 60-day mortality, which was the same in both groups (25.5% vs 28.4%, P = .30). The conservative fluid strategy group had significantly more ventilator-free days (14.6 vs 12.1 P<.001) and days not spent in the ICU (13.4 vs 11.2) without a significant increase in shock, nonpulmonary organ dysfunction, or renal failure leading to dialysis. Thus, once shock has resolved, patients will have improved oxygenation but no difference in mortality, with a conservative fluid management strategy.[17]

Corticosteroids

Corticosteroids have been studied for treatment of ARDS for decades with conflicting results. A 2006 *New England Journal of Medicine* article did not support the routine use of steroids in patients with ARDS. Patients with ARDS (n = 180) were randomized to receive intravenous methylprednisolone (2 mg/kg bolus followed by 0.5 mg/kg every 6 hours for 7 days, then tapered) or standard therapy beginning day 7 after MV was initiated. The primary end point, 60-day mortality, was the same in both groups. The treatment group had fewer ventilator-free days within 28 days (6.8 vs 11.2, P<.001). There was a higher rate of death in patients who were started on steroids after 13 days of disease (35% vs 8%, P = .02). There was also a significant increase in myopathy and neuropathy in the patients receiving steroids (0 vs 9 patients, P = .001).[18]

One year later, Meduri and colleagues[19] reported conflicting results. They showed a clear clinical benefit in a single-institution study using a protocolized administration of corticosteroids in patients with early severe ARDS. Ninety-one patients were randomized to receive methylprednisolone infusion at 1 mg/kg/d (2:1, 63 patients in the treatment arm and 28 control patients) starting at the time of diagnosis of ARDS. Results demonstrated higher rates of extubation at 7 days (53.9% vs 25.0%, P = .01), reduced duration of MV (P = .002), improved ICU length of stay (P = .007), and improved ICU mortality (20.6% vs 42.9%, P = .03). Patients in the treatment arm also had lower infectious complications (P = .002). Important aspects of the protocol were emphasized: avoidance of neuromuscular blockade, avoidance of etomidate, and continuous infusion of the methylprednisolone to minimize fluctuations in glucose.

Additional negative evidence regarding corticosteroids in the ICU is found in the corticosteroid therapy of septic shock (CORTICUS) trial, which failed to show benefit of hydrocortisone treatment in patients with septic shock.[20] The use of corticosteroids for ARDS is likely another controversy that will continue. The authors do not currently use corticosteroids in treatment of ALI or ARDS, unless patients have objectively been diagnosed with adrenal insufficiency.

Salvage therapies for ARDS

There are several salvage therapies available for improving oxygenation in patients with severe ARDS. These therapies include inhaled vasodilators, high-frequency oscillatory ventilation (HFOV), prone positioning, and extracorporeal life support. These strategies have all demonstrated significant improvement in oxygenation in studied patient populations. However, this improvement has not been associated with improvement in patient survival.

Inhaled vasodilators

Two inhaled vasodilators have been used clinically in ARDS but neither has demonstrated reduction in overall mortality. Administering medications via inhalant allows preferential vasodilation of the pulmonary vasculature in well-aerated areas of lung, which reduces ventilation-perfusion ratio (V/Q) mismatch to improve oxygenation. Using recruitment maneuvers and PEEP in combination with inhaled agents shows some clinical benefit.[21]

Inhaled nitric oxide (iNO) relaxes the pulmonary vasculature because of its role in endothelial-derived relaxing factor. It was first used in humans with ARDS in the 1990s. A 1998 study by Dellinger and colleagues[22] investigated the dose-dependent relationship on oxygenation and mortality (1.25–80.0 ppm) in 177 patients with primary pulmonary ARDS. In this well-designed study, the 5-ppm dose of iNO was associated with improved oxygenation and reduction in ventilatory support. In post hoc analysis, this treatment group was found to have a higher rate of survival and removal from MV at 28 days. Park and colleagues[21] evaluated the use of iNO, RM, or iNO plus RM. He found that, in the RM plus iNO arm, there was improvement of the Pao_2:Fio_2 ratio at 2, 12, and 24 hours (171 baseline, 203, 215, 254 mm Hg).

Inhaled prostacyclins act on the pulmonary vasculature by inducing smooth muscle relaxation. During acute events in the lung, the intrinsic production of prostaglandin may be disrupted, leading to pulmonary vasoconstriction, especially in the setting of hypoxemia. There is a paucity of data regarding this therapy, limited mostly to small studies and case reports. In 1993, a clinical report of inhaled prostacyclin in 3 patients was published. The mean pulmonary artery pressures were reduced, and the Pao_2:Fio_2 ratio improved from 120 to 173 mm Hg. The patients returned to the initial parameters once the drug was discontinued.[23] To better understand the patient populations who benefit from inhaled prostacyclins, Domenighetti and colleagues[24] evaluated 15 patients with ARDS; 6 with a primary pulmonary process and 9 with secondary ARDS. Results demonstrate that the Pao_2:Fio_2 ratio dropped in the primary ARDS group (146–135) and improved in the secondary ARDS group (161–171). This small series suggests that secondary ARDS may be more responsive to the use of inhaled prostacyclins in clinical practice.

Prone positioning

One of the options for improving oxygenation in patients with ARDS is prone positioning. In most studies, 60% to 70% of patients demonstrate improved oxygenation after prone positioning. Theories behind the physiologic effects of prone positioning include improving ventilation, perfusion matching, recruiting alveoli in the larger posterior area of the lung, improved postural drainage, and reducing the pressure of the heart on surrounding lung parenchyma (**Fig. 2**).

Early studies evaluating prone positioning demonstrated improved oxygenation without mortality benefit. Duration of prone positioning was generally short (6 hours)

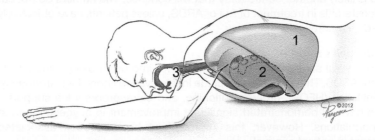

Fig. 2. The prone position has 3 theoretical benefits: (1) The dorsal aspect of the lung has a larger surface area for gas exchange and improves the ventilation: perfusion mismatch. (2) The weight of the heart is offloaded from surrounding lung tissue. (3) The airway is dependent in this position, facilitating postural drainage of secretions.

and patients included in the studies had ALI or ARDS, making the population hetero-geneous.[25–27] The Prone-Supine I was a study from Italy and Spain randomizing 295 patients to prone or supine positioning. The treatment arm showed improved in the Pao_2:Fio_2 ratio but no mortality benefit. A retrospective review found a reduction in mortality from 52% to 35% for the subset of patients who had a decrease in $Paco_2$ greater than 1 mm Hg after prone positioning.[27] The Prone-Supine II study expanded on these findings by increasing the duration of prone positioning to 20 hours daily. In the patients with severe ARDS, there was a nonsignificant trend toward lower mortality (37.8% vs 46.1%).[28]

Complications to be anticipated with prone positioning include endotracheal tube displacement or unintentional extubation, accidental removal of intravenous lines and other support tubes, and decubitus ulcer. During treatment, patients must be returned to the supine position intermittently for routine care. Lack of access to the anterior aspect of patients can be disastrous in the case of cardiac arrest. Pressure sores were reported in 36% of patients in the Prone-Supine I study and can compli-cate care, even with diligent attention to padding and monitoring for skin breakdown.[27]

HFOV

HFOV is a technology that originated in the neonatal ICU and has been applied to adults since the mid-1980s. Potential benefits of HFOV include a small tidal volume that limits alveolar overdistention and smaller variation of mean airway pressure that prevents recruitment and derecruitment of alveoli (atelectrauma). HFOV also creates a higher mean airway pressure, which promotes alveolar recruitment. The high-frequency ventilator vibrates to create a pulsation, as opposed to a full breath, which increases the mean airway pressure and creates an improved gas mixture in the alveoli.

In many settings, HFOV is used at the end of the algorithm for ARDS. Candidates for HFOV should be sedated and paralyzed to minimize patient factors of respiratory failure. Most patients treated with HFOV will have failed other strategies, such as inhaled agents, RM, and higher levels of PEEP. Patients should also be euvolemic; hypovolemia can lead to hypotension because of the increased intrathoracic pressure and diminished venous return.[29] Pneumothorax is another anticipated complication of treatment caused by the ventilation of noncompliant lung tissue.

The first randomized controlled trial evaluating the safety of HFOV versus conven-tional ventilation (CV) was reported in 2002 by Derdak and colleagues.[30] They random-ized 148 patients with severe ARDS to CV or HFOV. They found the mean airway pressure was significantly higher in the HFOV ($P = .0001$), suggesting the 2 groups had different respiratory mechanics. The mortality was reduced in the HFOV arm, 37% versus 52% ($P = .102$). The Pao_2:Fio_2 ratio improved over the first 16 hours but was not sustained ($P = .008$). This report was the first to demonstrate that HFOV was a safe alternative to CV in patients with severe ARDS.

Extracorporeal membrane oxygenation

Extracorporeal membrane oxygenation (ECMO), originally developed to support patients during cardiopulmonary bypass surgery, has been used over the last 4 decades to provide support for patients with severe, reversible respiratory failure. By providing gas exchange independent of the lungs, the need to push ventilation strategies that lead to VILI is reduced. The benefit of ECMO is complete rest of the lungs and ventilation with a low pressure until compliance recovers. Selecting patients who may benefit from this technology is key to its success. Potential patients must have reversible respiratory failure, failure of optimal medical management, or medical stabilization requiring high levels of support that would lead to additional lung injury. **Box 1** summarizes the indications and contraindications of ECMO. This therapy is becoming more widely available because of improved cannulation and support technology but continues to require significant resources.

The conventional ventilation or ECMO for severe audit respiratory failure (CESAR) trial from the United Kingdom is one of the largest studies focused on outcomes of ECMO for ARDS. The study randomized 180 patients to conventional management or referral to an ECMO center. The 6-month survival was higher in those treated at a referral center (63% vs 47%, RR 0.69, P = .03). In closely examining the data, only 75% of patients in the referral arm received ECMO. The data suggest that the benefit in treatment may be the algorithm of care leading to ECMO and not the intervention itself.[31] Recommendations now include transferring patients with severe ARDS to a center capable of ECMO. Another criticism of the study is that the ventilation management in the conventional treatment arm was not best available; only 70% of those patients received low tidal volume ventilation.

Improved survival in ARDS was also demonstrated in a 1997 study of 122 patients with severe ARDS treated with a clinical algorithm. The care protocol mandated ventilation with PCV, increased inspiratory times, RM, adequate PEEP, aggressive diuresis, and prone positioning. The patients who failed these interventions were then placed on ECMO. Forty-nine patients received ECMO and 73 patients were in the advanced treatment without ECMO (AT-sine). Overall survival for the 122 patients was 75%:89% in the AT-sine group and 55% in the ECMO group.[32]

Box 1
ECMO guidelines: patients who may be considered for ECMO support and contraindications to ECMO support

Consideration

Reversible cause of respiratory failure

Ability to anticoagulate patients

Failure of conventional ventilation strategies

Adults (aged 18–65 years)

Weight less than 175 kg

$Paco_2$ greater than 80

Pao_2:Fio_2 ratio less than 80

Contraindications

Aged older than 65 years

Weight greater than 175 kg

Chronic lung disease

High ventilation greater than 7 days

Intracranial hemorrhage

Moribund patients

Nonfatal comorbidities

SUMMARY

The treatment of respiratory failure requiring MV has advanced significantly over the last 20 years. Numerous studies reveal different strategies to guide therapeutic decisions. The goal of therapy in patients with ARDS should be to optimize oxygenation while minimizing risk of VILI and providing adequate ventilation. Protocols help apply interventions in a stepwise fashion to meet patients' physiologic demand and degree of critical illness. The result is a slight increase in overall survival. Appropriate use of ventilation modes and strategies, PEEP levels, and RM can improve oxygen delivery. Salvage therapies, such as prone positioning, inhaled epoprostenol and NO, and HFOV, have a well-established role in supportive management (see **Fig. 1**) and are associated with improved oxygenation but not survival. As our understanding of ECMO and its use in ARDS matures, this may become a more widely used salvage strategy with more widespread availability.

REFERENCES

1. Cooke CR. Economics of mechanical ventilation and respiratory failure. Crit Care Clin 2012;28(1):39–55, vi.
2. Rubenfeld GD, Caldwell E, Peabody E, et al. Incidence and outcomes of acute lung injury. N Engl J Med 2005;353(16):1685–93.
3. Raghavendran K, Napolitano LM. ALI and ARDS: challenges and advances. Crit Care Clin 2011;27(3):xiii–xxiv.
4. Phua J, Badia JR, Adhikari NK, et al. Has mortality from acute respiratory distress syndrome decreased over time?: a systematic review. Am J Respir Crit Care Med 2009;179(3):220–7.
5. Haas CF. Mechanical ventilation with lung protective strategies: what works? Crit Care Clin 2011;27(3):469–86.
6. Raghavendran K, Napolitano LM. Definition of ALI/ARDS. Crit Care Clin 2011; 27(3):429–37.
7. Barreiro TJ, Gemmel DJ. Noninvasive ventilation. Crit Care Clin 2007;23(2): 201–22, ix.
8. Antonelli M, Conti G, Esquinas A, et al. A multiple-center survey on the use in clinical practice of noninvasive ventilation as a first-line intervention for acute respiratory distress syndrome. Crit Care Med 2007;35(1):18–25.
9. Esteban A, Frutos-Vivar F, Ferguson ND, et al. Noninvasive positive-pressure ventilation for respiratory failure after extubation. N Engl J Med 2004;350(24): 2452–60.
10. Burns KE, Adhikari NK, Keenan SP, et al. Use of non-invasive ventilation to wean critically ill adults off invasive ventilation: meta-analysis and systematic review. BMJ 2009;338:b1574.
11. Blank R, Napolitano LM. Epidemiology of ARDS and ALI. Crit Care Clin 2011; 27(3):439–58.
12. American Thoracic Society, Infectious Diseases Society of America. Guidelines for the management of adults with hospital-acquired, ventilator-associated, and healthcare-associated pneumonia. Am J Respir Crit Care Med 2005;171(4): 388–416.
13. Habashi NM. Other approaches to open lung ventilation: airway pressure release ventilation. Crit Care Med 2005;33(Suppl 3):S228–40.
14. Ventilation with lower tidal volumes as compared with traditional tidal volumes for acute lung injury and the acute respiratory distress syndrome. The Acute Respiratory Distress Syndrome Network. N Engl J Med 2000;342(18):1301–8.

15. Marini JJ, Gattinoni L. Ventilatory management of acute respiratory distress syndrome: a consensus of two. Crit Care Med 2004;32(1):250–5.
16. Brower RG, Lanken PN, MacIntyre N, et al. Higher versus lower positive end-expiratory pressures in patients with the acute respiratory distress syndrome. N Engl J Med 2004;351(4):327–36.
17. Wiedemann HP, Wheeler AP, Bernard GR, et al. Comparison of two fluid-management strategies in acute lung injury. N Engl J Med 2006;354(24):2564–75.
18. Steinberg KP, Hudson LD, Goodman RB, et al. Efficacy and safety of corticosteroids for persistent acute respiratory distress syndrome. N Engl J Med 2006;354(16):1671–84.
19. Meduri GU, Golden E, Freire AX, et al. Methylprednisolone infusion in early severe ARDS: results of a randomized controlled trial. Chest 2007;131(4):954–63.
20. Sprung CL, Annane D, Keh D, et al. Hydrocortisone therapy for patients with septic shock. N Engl J Med 2008;358(2):111–24.
21. Park KJ, Lee YJ, Oh YJ, et al. Combined effects of inhaled nitric oxide and a recruitment maneuver in patients with acute respiratory distress syndrome. Yonsei Med J 2003;44(2):219–26.
22. Dellinger RP, Zimmerman JL, Taylor RW, et al. Effects of inhaled nitric oxide in patients with acute respiratory distress syndrome: results of a randomized phase II trial. Inhaled Nitric Oxide in ARDS Study Group. Crit Care Med 1998;26(1):15–23.
23. Walmrath D, Schneider T, Pilch J, et al. Aerosolised prostacyclin in adult respiratory distress syndrome. Lancet 1993;342(8877):961–2.
24. Domenighetti G, Stricker H, Waldispuehl B. Nebulized prostacyclin (PGI2) in acute respiratory distress syndrome: impact of primary (pulmonary injury) and secondary (extrapulmonary injury) disease on gas exchange response. Crit Care Med 2001;29(1):57–62.
25. Fernandez R, Trenchs X, Klamburg J, et al. Prone positioning in acute respiratory distress syndrome: a multicenter randomized clinical trial. Intensive Care Med 2008;34(8):1487–91.
26. Guerin C, Gaillard S, Lemasson S, et al. Effects of systematic prone positioning in hypoxemic acute respiratory failure: a randomized controlled trial. JAMA 2004;292(19):2379–87.
27. Gattinoni L, Tognoni G, Pesenti A, et al. Effect of prone positioning on the survival of patients with acute respiratory failure. N Engl J Med 2001;345(8):568–73.
28. Taccone P, Pesenti A, Latini R, et al. Prone positioning in patients with moderate and severe acute respiratory distress syndrome: a randomized controlled trial. JAMA 2009;302(18):1977–84.
29. Chan KP, Stewart TE, Mehta S. High-frequency oscillatory ventilation for adult patients with ARDS. Chest 2007;131(6):1907–16.
30. Derdak S, Mehta S, Stewart TE, et al. High-frequency oscillatory ventilation for acute respiratory distress syndrome in adults: a randomized, controlled trial. Am J Respir Crit Care Med 2002;166(6):801–8.
31. Peek GJ, Elbourne D, Mugford M, et al. Randomised controlled trial and parallel economic evaluation of conventional ventilatory support versus extracorporeal membrane oxygenation for severe adult respiratory failure (CESAR). Health Technol Assess 2010;14(35):1–46.
32. Lewandowski K, Rossaint R, Pappert D, et al. High survival rate in 122 ARDS patients managed according to a clinical algorithm including extracorporeal membrane oxygenation. Intensive Care Med 1997;23(8):819–35.

Removing the Critically Ill Patient from Mechanical Ventilation

Jeremy S. Juern, MD

KEYWORDS

- Respiration, artificial • Ventilator weaning • Tracheostomy • Sedation

KEY POINTS

- The goal sedation level is drowsy to calm and cooperative.
- Protocolized weaning results in less time on the ventilator.
- After the daily spontaneous breathing trial, the patient is either extubated or returned to a resting mode of ventilation.
- The most difficult airway is one in a patient with a halo vest—have a low threshold to perform tracheostomy in this group.
- A strategy of extubate to bilevel positive airway pressure is most appropriate in patients with chronic obstructive pulmonary disease.

INTRODUCTION

Mechanical ventilation is a life-saving intervention in a critically ill patient. Ever since the first ventilators were developed, physicians have been working on the best way to liberate patients from them. Efficient weaning from mechanical ventilation is important to decrease morbidity, mortality, and hospital length of stay (LOS). Weaning is a team effort involving nursing, pharmacy, and respiratory therapy. The physician is the leader of the team and must be actively involved in the process. In most cases, weaning is a straightforward endeavor. Occasionally weaning is more challenging and requires skill, experience, and intuition. The following is a practical, evidence-based approach to wean mechanical ventilation, with a focus on surgical patients.

SEDATION, ANALGESIA, AND SEDATION HOLIDAYS

Most patients who are intubated endotracheally need analgesia and sedation. The purpose of analgesia is to control pain. The purpose of sedation is to control anxiety, agitation, and delirium.

The author has nothing to disclose.
Division of Trauma and Critical Care, Department of Surgery, Medical College of Wisconsin, 9200 West Wisconsin Avenue, Milwaukee, WI 53226, USA
E-mail address: jjuern@mcw.edu

Analgesia

Fentanyl, hydromorphone, and morphine are common choices for analgesia. Fentanyl has an onset of 1–2 minutes and duration of 0.5–1 hour, which makes it easy to titrate. Morphine and hydromorphone have slightly longer time of onset (2–3 minutes) and longer duration of action (2–4 hours), making these drugs better for longer-term use. Any of these drugs can be used with intermittent dosing or a continuous infusion.[1]

Sedation

Anxiety comes from the noxious stimulation of the endotracheal tube, nasogastric tube, or orogastric tube. Further stimuli include being connected to monitors, blood draws, x-rays being performed, unusual sounds, disruption of sleep/wake cycle, lights being on, noise in general, and being turned. Agitation can also be secondary to base-line mental illness, traumatic brain injury, advanced age, and drugs used in the intensive care unit (ICU).

Choice of Sedation Agent

The ideal sedation agent will keep a patient calm and cooperative, has a short half-life, does not cause hypotension, and has a wide therapeutic window. No single agent is good for all situations. For short periods of intubation (<48 hours) intermittent- or continuous-infusion midazolam is an effective and inexpensive drug. For longer periods of intubation (>48 hours), a long-term and cost-effective agent such as lorazepam is ideal, given intermittently or as continuous infusion if needed. Another agent with a short half-life is propofol. This convenience comes with the increased cost and the risk of propofol infusion syndrome.[2] Defining the incidence of propofol infusion syndrome is difficult, but the risk definitely increases as the dose and number of days on propofol increases. Dexmedetomidine is an α_2 agonist that can provide sedation and analgesia. Dexmedetomidine may have an advantage over midazolam in that there is less time on the ventilator with the trade-off of more bradycardia.[3] If agitation from delirium is a component, then an antipsychotic, like haloperidol, can be used.[1]

Sedation Level

The goal is for the patient to be calm and cooperative. Multiple sedation scales have been developed; a commonly used scale is the Richmond Agitation-Sedation Scale (RASS). The RASS scale is reliable and reproducible and correlates with dose of sedation medicines.[4] The goal of RASS is 0 (alert and calm) or -1 (drowsy).

Sedation Holidays

Excess sedation must be avoided. It is well established that for patients on a continuous infusion of a sedative, and if the clinical situation allows, their sedation should be stopped at least once per day to evaluate their mental status and determine if they can undergo a weaning trial. This sedation holiday has been found to decrease the duration of mechanical ventilation and length of stay in the ICU.[5] A further study of 336 nonsurgical ICU patients found that a daily sedation interruption combined with a daily spontaneous breathing trial (SBT) resulted in decreased ventilator days, decreased ICU and hospital LOS, and improved 1-year survival.[6]

WEANING TRIALS
Is This Patient Ready for a Weaning Trial?

First, it should be determined why the patient was intubated and if that process is now over. Do they have a traumatic brain injury? Were they intoxicated when they came into the trauma bay? Do they have COPD? Is it a postoperative CABG that comes back intubated as a matter of protocol? Does the patient have pneumonia? The inciting process that caused respiratory failure should be resolved or improved before starting a weaning trial and working toward extubation.

What are Ventilator Criteria for Starting a Weaning Trial?

To start a weaning trial, the sedation should have worn off, and the patient should be awake, alert, and following commands. The patient should have adequate oxygenation (Partial pressure of oxygen >60 mm HG or oxygen saturation ≥92%) on minimal vent settings such as fraction of inspired oxygen ≤40% and Positive end-expiratory pressure (PEEP) ≤5. There should be no hemodynamic instability, signs of myocardial ischemia, or elevated intracranial pressure.

How Is a Weaning Trial Performed?

The most common way to perform a weaning trial is to perform an SBT. The patient is placed on a pressure support trial that provides no scheduled mechanical breaths. The ventilator will provide a continuous-positive airway pressure (CPAP) that is sufficient to overcome the resistance of the ventilator tubing and the endotracheal (ET) tube. Commonly accepted pressure support settings for a weaning trial are 5–8 cm H_2O. Some ventilators have built-in automatic tube compensation feature. The patient should be told about the weaning trial and given reassurance. Neither the fraction of inspired oxygen nor the PEEP is changed during a pressure support trial because they should have already been weaned down.

Another method of doing a weaning trial is a T-piece trial. A T-piece trial is one in which an oxygen tank is connected to a plastic T-piece at the end of the ET tube. It provides blow-by oxygen with minimal positive pressure to help overcome the resistance of the ET tube. Because of the pressure support setting on modern ventilators, T-piece weaning is used much less frequently in ICUs today.

What Parameters During an SBT Predict Successful Extubation?

The traditional parameters of a successful trial are:

- Vital capacity (VC) 12–15 mL/kg (840 mL–1050 mL in a 70-kg patient)
- Tidal volume (TV) ≥5–7 mL/kg (350 mL–490 mL in a 70-kg patient)
- Respiratory rate (RR) <25
- Maximum inspiratory pressure (also called negative inspiratory force) ≥20 cm H_2O.

All of these pulmonary numbers are based on predicted body weight, which is calculated from height. For example, a man who is 5 ft, 10 in tall has a predicted body weight of 68.5 kg. This ideal person has the same TV and vital capacity parameters as a man who is 5 ft, 10 in tall weighing 100 kg or 200 kg.

Rapid Shallow Breathing Index

An intubated patient who is tachypneic and takes shallow breaths during a weaning trial will continue to take shallow breaths once the ET tube is out, putting him or her at high risk for reintubation. The quantification of rapid and shallow breathing was first described in 1991 as the ratio of the respiratory frequency (f), divided by the tidal volume (V_T) in liters.[7] This ratio was subsequently called the *rapid shallow breathing index* (RSBI). For example, a patient taking 500 mL tidal volumes 20 times per minutes has an RSBI of 40 (20/0.5). An RSBI less than 100 had a sensitivity of 0.97 and specificity of 0.64 and was felt to be the best single predictor of successful weaning. In this original article, the RSBI protocol was performed with the patient disconnected from the ventilator, the patient breathing room air for 1 minute, and with measurements taken using a spirometer. The RSBI is rarely calculated this way today. Modern ventilators can calculate the RSBI over the time of a weaning trial with the patient still connected to the ventilator.

Subsequent research on the RSBI has been done in different patient populations, and its usefulness as a weaning parameter has been variable. In a study of 40 postoperative surgical patients on a pressure support of 5 cm H_2O, an RSBI of 65 had sensitivity of 0.9 and specificity of 0.8 for successful extubation.[8]

Summary of Parameters

Clinicians cannot always rely on any one number to indicate that a patient will be extubated successfully.[9] For example, consider a patient with a traumatic brain injury, an RSBI of 63 (f = 21, TV = 0.3) during a weaning trial, and a neurologic examination that shows they are not yet consistently following commands. Extubating at this time may result in the patient accumulating secretions, aspirating, and having subsequent reintubation. A patient like this may be better off with a tracheostomy and weaning them safely off the ventilator from there. Understanding everything that is going on with the patient is imperative to make the best decision about extubation.

PROTOCOL-DRIVEN WEANING FROM MECHANICAL VENTILATION

Traditionally, a physician writes an order for every single ventilator change. A synchronized intermittent mandatory ventilation wean involves gradually turning down the set rate of breaths until the patient is generating all of his or her own breaths. Then potentially a different physician is in charge of the analgesia and sedation regimen. This protocol may cause the patient to stay on mechanical ventilation longer because (1) the sedation level may be too deep for them to participate in a weaning trial and (2) when the patient is awake enough, the ventilator needs to be adjusted in a timely fashion to the appropriate setting so that weaning can take place.

Working together, physicians, nurses, respiratory therapists, and pharmacists developed protocols that allow weaning to happen without a specific directive from the physician. If a patient is deemed ready for a weaning trial, the protocol has the nurse lighten the sedation, and the respiratory therapist makes the vent changes to put the patient on an SBT. This coordination allows weaning trials to take place irrespective of physician workload in the ICU that day or even physician presence at the bedside.

The SBT is done typically once a day, usually in the morning. The typical length of time of the SBT is 30–120 minutes.[6] An SBT is considered a failure if the patient becomes tachypneic or hypoxemic or develops respiratory distress or an arrhythmia. In the event of failure, the patient is immediately returned to a resting mode of mechanical ventilation, such as assist/control or SIMV with a rate of 12–16. If the patient stays on the SBT and meets traditional weaning parameters and RSBI, a physician order is needed to extubate the patient. Most protocols call for the SBT to be done once a day, and if the procedure fails, it is not tried again until the next day. However, if for some reason other factors were not optimal at the time of the SBT (analgesia, sedation, delirium, fluid overload), it may be reasonable to try again later in the day after a period of rest and the other factors have been corrected.

Results of studies of protocol-driven weaning have been encouraging. One study involving medical ICU patients and trauma ICU patients showed the time on the ventilator was decreased by nearly half along with a decrease in VAP.[10] Another study in a multidisciplinary surgical ICU showed reduced use of mechanical ventilation, lower reintubation rates, and decreased ventilator-associated pneumonia.[11] Meta-analysis of 11 studies of protocolized weaning showed a 25% reduction in the total duration of mechanical ventilation for protocolized versus nonprotocolized weaning.[12] Overall, having a weaning protocol ensures that every patient who is eligible gets an SBT with extubation as early as possible.

ROLE OF TRACHEOSTOMY

The common indications for tracheostomy in a mechanically ventilated general surgery and trauma patient are prolonged mechanical ventilation/failure to wean (the most common reason), inability to protect airway (because of head injury or stroke), and inability to cough/handle secretions. The benefits of tracheostomy are less damage to the larynx, easier oral care, decreased work of breathing (less dead space), potentially less time spent in the ICU, and potentially decreased time spent on mechanical ventilation. Timing of tracheostomy has been controversial regarding early (around 7 days) versus late (≥10 days). One review and practice guideline showed no mortality difference between early and late tracheostomy. For trauma patients with head injuries, early tracheostomy decreased the days of mechanical ventilation and ICU LOS. For patients without head injuries there is less benefit regarding days of mechanical ventilations and ICU LOS.[13] Although are conflicting data, early tracheostomy does not seem to prevent ventilator-associated pneumonia.[14]

THE DIFFICULT-TO-WEAN PATIENT

It may be difficult to wean patients off the ventilator for a variety of reasons, including delirium and preexisting lung disease, such as COPD. One aspect of delirium in the ICU is agitation.[1] An agitated patient is commonly tachypneic; it is difficult to wean a tachypneic patient because their RSBI is high. The source of agitation, for example, inadequate analgesia, inadequate sedation, or delirium, must be controlled. The most common treatment for delirium is haloperidol (Haldol).[1] Caution is advised to watch for QT prolongation and extrapyramidal side effects from Haldol.

A patient may have decreased lung function because of COPD, which puts him or her at higher risk pneumonia. Treating pneumonia with appropriate antibiotics should result in improved lung function after a few days. A patient with COPD can be a challenge to mechanically ventilate. A general strategy is to avoid hyperinflation by keeping the minute volume ≤8 L/min, expiratory time ≥4 seconds, and a breathing rate of 8–12 breaths per minute.[15] These patients also have airway obstruction that will benefit from bronchodilators, typically albuterol and ipratropium combined, given via nebulizer or metered-dose inhaler. One study found significant improvement in airway obstruction without any change in heart rate or blood pressure.[16] Finally, COPD patients commonly have hypercapnia and subsequent chronic respiratory acidosis. They compensate for this condition with a chronic metabolic alkalosis, manifested by elevated bicarbonate. Increasing the ventilator respiratory rate to "blow them down" to a normal P_{CO_2} will result in excretion of that excess bicarbonate by the kidneys. Then, as the patient participates in subsequent SBTs, the hypercapnia will return, leading to an acute respiratory acidosis and difficulty weaning.

Once the problem is addressed in a difficult-to-wean patient, a careful wean can proceed. If progress is not being made, proceeding with tracheostomy is reasonable. With a tracheostomy, progressively longer periods are spent on pressure support followed by progressively longer periods on tracheostomy mask (humidified room air) trials until the patient is completely liberated from mechanical ventilation.

CONSIDERATIONS WHEN WEANING AND EXTUBATING
Is the Patient Going Back to the Operating Room Soon?

Consider the following scenario: The time is noon, the patient meets all criteria for extubation, but they are returning to the operating room the next morning. Should the patient be extubated? The answer is yes. If a patient meets all of the criteria for extubation and the only reason to keep them intubated is a return trip to the operating room they should still be extubated. A patient is always better off being able to cough out their own secretions rather than having them suctioned out.

Airway Swelling and Edema

Airway swelling and edema can contribute to postextubation stridor and subsequent reintubation. One way that has been proposed to predict the development of postextubation stridor is the cuff leak test. The cuff leak test is performed by thoroughly suctioning out the mouth and pharynx above the ET tube cuff. The air is let out of the cuff. There should be an audible sound as air flows around the ET tube. The tidal volumes will be lower on the ventilator, and this amount can be quantified. A further maneuver is to remove the circuit tubing from the ET tube, briefly occlude the end of the tube with a gloved hand, and again listen to see if the patient is moving air around the tube. If no air is moving around the tube, this may be a sign of airway edema. Unfortunately, the cuff leak test is not an accurate predictor of postextubation stridor.[17] But in high-risk patients, it may be most useful as an indicator to be more vigilant in monitoring the postextubation airway.[18]

The 2 common pharmacologic methods of decreasing airway swelling are epinephrine and corticosteroids. Aerosolized epinephrine has been studied primarily in pediatric critical care and it does help to treat laryngeal edema. There is no difference in the efficacy or safety profile between racemic epinephrine and the l-isomer of epinephrine.[19]

The role of corticosteroids to decrease airway swelling is less clear. A Cochrane review of 6 studies in adults found that corticosteroids were most useful when administered as multiple doses begun 12–24 hours before extubation as opposed to just a single dose closer to the time of extubation.[20] Several corticosteroid types and dosages were used in these studies. A reasonable approach is to use corticosteroids only in patients that are at high risk for airway swelling and postextubation stridor. An appropriate corticosteroid dose is methylprednisolone 20–40 mg intravenously every 4–6 hours for 12–24 hours before extubation.[21]

The Patient with the Difficult Airway

For every intubated patient in the ICU the physician in charge of the extubation should know the difficulty of the airway of the patient. This information must be known before extubation, not afterward when the airway is failing and the patient must be reintubated emergently. This information should be obtained by checking the emergency department or anesthesia record noting the Mallampati class, method of intubation (direct laryngoscopy, glidescope, fiberoptic, bougie use), and number of attempts, rather than relying on the nurses or the anesthesia providers to tell you about the difficult airway. If a difficult airway is discovered, a plan should be in place in case the patient needs to be reintubated emergently. Consider having intubation supplies in the room along with a bougie and cricothyroidotomy kit and an expert airway provider if appropriate.

The Patient in a Halo Vest

The most difficult airway is one in a patient in a halo vest because the cervical spine cannot be extended. In addition, if there is a spinal cord injury, the function of the diaphragm and accessory respiratory muscles may be impaired.

From an airway standpoint, first understand why the patient is in a halo vest. Look at the cervical spine images of the patient and understand the anatomy. If there is a spinal cord injury, know if muscles of respiration are affected. If they have had an operative fusion of the cervical spine, know if it was an anterior or posterior approach. Take into account other injuries, age, and comorbidities.

There must be a low threshold for performing a tracheostomy on a patient in a halo vest, because if extubation fails, it may be impossible to reintubate, resulting in death of the patient. Performing a tracheostomy and then weaning from the ventilator is the safe approach. If the patient had an anterior-approach cervical spine fusion with hardware, then waiting approximately 7 days to perform tracheostomy will result in a low risk of wound infection.[22] A percutaneous approach in this setting may be advantageous. It is better to have a living patient with a halo and a tracheostomy than to have a deceased patient and wishing that you would have done a tracheostomy.

WHAT IS THE ROLE OF NONINVASIVE MECHANICAL VENTILATION?

Noninvasive positive pressure ventilation (NPPV) is mechanical ventilation through a tight-fitting facemask. This mask makes it difficult or impossible for a patient to cough out secretions. The mode of mechanical ventilation can be CPAP ventilation or bilevel positive airway pressure (BPAP).

CPAP delivers one level of continuous positive pressure. BPAP has 2 settings: inspiratory positive airway pressure (IPAP) and expiratory positive airway pressure (EPAP). For either setting, the patient must be generating their own breaths. The IPAP is analogous to Pressure Support (PS) on a conventional ventilator, whereas EPAP is analogous to PEEP. A common initial setting for BPAP is "12 over 5," which means an IPAP of 12 cm H_2O with an EPAP of 5 cm H_2O. In BPAP, when a patient takes a breath, the machine will increase the pressure to the mask at the level of the IPAP. When the breath is finished, the pressure in the system will be at the EPAP level. For CPAP, the pressure is always at one level regardless of whether the patient is taking a breath.

Important contraindications to BPAP include cardiac arrest, respiratory arrest, inability to cooperate, inability to protect the airway, inability to clear secretions, recent facial surgery or facial trauma, or when prolonged duration of mechanical ventilation is anticipated. NPPV is most useful in patients with a COPD exacerbation or cardiogenic pulmonary edema. It may be useful in patients who are having a hard time after extubation. In this case, a short trial of NPPV can be attempted with careful monitoring of the arterial blood gas. If the patient does not show real improvement after 1–2 hours, they need to be intubated. A Cochrane review of NIPPV as a weaning strategy in adults with respiratory failure showed a positive effect on mortality and VAP rates. Caution is advised when interpreting these results because most patients had COPD and are not generalizable to all ICU patients.[23] A strategy of extubate to BPAP is fraught with danger and only has a chance at working in COPD patients.

BPAP IN GASTRIC BYPASS

Many patients undergoing gastric bypass surgery have diagnosed or undiagnosed sleep apnea and are at risk for postoperative respiratory failure. Can CPAP or BPAP be used after Roux-en-Y gastric bypass? Will the air pressure cause an anastamotic leak at the gastrojejunostomy? CPAP seems to be safe after Roux-en-Y gastric bypass, particularly for patients that were on it at home and use that same setting in the hospital.[24] There are case reports of BPAP causing anastamotic leaks,[25] probably because the BPAP has a higher pressure setting than CPAP. The lack of a pylorus means air can flow freely into the small bowel. CPAP and BPAP must be used judiciously in the postoperative gastric bypass patient, and it is always necessary to clear any intervention with the patient's surgeon.

SUMMARY

Patients must be weaned from mechanical ventilation as efficiently as possible. The most important component of weaning is the protocol-driven daily sedation holiday combined with an SBT. Oversedation must be avoided. Tracheostomy and noninvasive mechanical ventilation are important options to exercise at the right time. Understanding everything going on with the patient gives the best chance of an efficient wean from the ventilator.

REFERENCES

1. Jacobi J, Fraser G, Coursin D, et al. Clinical practice guidelines for the sustained use of sedatives and analgesics in the critically ill adult. Crit Care Med 2002;30: 119–41.
2. Diedrich DA, Brown DR. Propofol infusion syndrome in the ICU. J Intensive Care Med 2011;26(2):59–72.
3. Riker RR, Shehabi Y, Bokesch PM, et al. Dexmedetomidine vs midazolam for sedation of critically ill patients: a randomized trial. JAMA 2009;301(5):489–99.
4. Ely EW, Truman B, Shintani A, et al. Monitoring sedation status over time in ICU patients: reliability and validity of the Richmond agitation-sedation scale (RASS). JAMA 2003;289(22):2983–91.
5. Kress JP, Pohlman AS, O'Connor MF, et al. Daily interruption of sedative infusions in critically ill patients undergoing mechanical ventilation. N Engl J Med 2000;342: 1471–7.
6. Girard TD, Kress JP, Fuchs BD, et al. Efficacy and safety of a paired sedation and ventilator weaning protocol for mechanically ventilated patients in intensive care (awakening and breathing controlled trial):a randomized controlled trial. Lancet 2008;371:126–34.
7. Yang KL, Tobin MJ. A prospective study of indexes predicting the outcome of trials of weaning from mechanical ventilation. N Engl J Med 1991;324:1445–50.
8. Rivera L, Weissman C. Dynamic ventilatory characteristics during weaning in postoperative critically ill patients. Anesth Analg 1997;84:1250–5.
9. Meade M, Guyatt G, Cook D, et al. Predicting success in weaning from mechanical ventilation. Chest 2001;120:400S–24S.
10. Marelich GP, Murin S, Battistella F. Protocol weaning of mechanical ventilation in medical and surgical patients by respiratory care practitioners and nurses: effect on weaning time and incidence of ventilator-associated pneumonia. Chest 2000; 118:459–67.
11. Dries DJ, McGonigal MD, Malian MS, et al. Protocol-driven ventilator weaning reduces use of mechanical ventilation, rate of early reintubation, and ventilator-associated pneumonia. J Trauma 2004;56:943–52.
12. Blackwood B, Alderice F, Burns KE, et al. Protocolized versus non-protocolized weaning for reducing the duration of mechanical ventilation in critically ill adult patients. Cochrane Database Syst Rev 2010;(5):CD006904.

13. Holevar M, Dunham JC, Brautigan R, et al. Practice management guidelines of timing of tracheostomy: the EAST practice management guidelines work group. J Trauma 2009;67(4):870–4.
14. Terragni PP, Antonelli M, Fumagalli R, et al. Early vs late tracheostomy for prevention of pneumonia in mechanically ventilated adult ICU patients: a randomized controlled trial. JAMA 2010;303(15):1483–9.
15. Amato M. Acute respiratory failure in chronic obstructive pulmonary disease. In: Gabrielli A, Layon AJ, Yu M, editors. Critical care. $th edition. Philadelphia: Lippincot, Williams, and Wilkins; 2009. p. 2133–41.
16. Dhand R, Jubran A, Tobin MJ. Bronchodilator delivery by metered-dose inhaler in ventilator-supported patients. Am J Respir Crit Care Med 1995;151:1827–33.
17. Kriner EJ, Shafazand S, Colice GL. The endotracheal tube cuff-leak test as a predictor for postextubation stridor. Respir Care 2005;50(12):1632–8.
18. Deem S. Limited value of the cuff-leak test. Respir Care 2005;50(12):1617–8.
19. Nutman J, Brooks LJ, Deakins KM. Racemic versus l-epinephrine aerosol in the treatment of postextubation laryngeal edema: results form a prospective, randomized, double-blind study. Crit Care Med 1994;22:1591–4.
20. Khemani RG, Randolph A, Markovitz B. Corticosteroids for the prevention and treatment of post-extubation stridor in neonates, children and adults. Cochrane Database Syst Rev 2009;(3):CD001000.
21. Roberts RJ, Welch SM, Devlin JW. Corticosteroids for prevention of postextubation laryngeal edema in adults. Ann Pharmacother 2008;42:686–91.
22. O'Keefe T, Goldman RK, Mayberry JC, et al. Tracheostomy after anterior cervical spine fixation. J Trauma 2004;57:855–60.
23. Burns KE, Adhikari NK, Keenan SP, et al. Noninvasive positive pressure ventilation as a weaning strategy for intubated adults with respiratory failure. Cochrane Database Syst Rev 2010;(8):CD004127.
24. Ramirez A, Lalor PF, Szomstein S, et al. Continuous positive airway pressure in immediate postoperative period after laparoscopic roux-en-y gastric bypass: is it safe? Surg Obes Relat Dis 2009;5(5):544–6.
25. Vasquez TL, Hoddinott K. A potential complication of bi-level positive airway pressure after gastric bypass surgery. Obes Surg 2004;14:282–4.

Enteral Nutrition in the Critically Ill Patient

Panna A. Codner, MD

KEYWORDS

- Nutrition • Critical illness • Enteral nutrition • ICU

KEY POINTS

- Early enteral nutrition is the preferred route of nutrition for the critically ill patient.
- Enteral nutrition maintains the intestinal barrier to prevent bacterial translocation.
- Parenteral nutrition is beneficial in the small group of patients who are malnourished on arrival to the ICU or in patients in whom the intestinal tract is unable to be used for greater than a week.
- Attention to calories and blood sugar control may reduce complications in patients receiving parenteral nutrition.

INTRODUCTION

Clinical factors, such as premorbid nutritional status and severity of illness, determine the overall efficacy of nutritional support. Malnutrition may be defined as "a disorder of body composition in which macronutrient and/or micronutrient deficiencies occur when nutrient intake is less than required."[1] Malnutrition leads to reduced organ function, abnormal laboratory chemistry values, and poorer clinical outcome. For all hospitalized patients, the reported prevalence of malnutrition is as high as 50%. Although difficult to quantify, the incidence in intensive care unit (ICU) patients is closer to 5%. A malnourished patient is more likely to have infectious morbidity, a prolonged hospital stay, and increased mortality.[2] However, not all patients in the ICU need nutritional support, and disease and nutrition exhibit complex interactions. In critical illness, malnutrition results from abnormal nutrient processing and not starvation. Each individual patient should receive a nutritional formula specific to their disease process. Keeping this in mind, it is important to provide early nutritional support during critical illness. Approaches to nutritional support in the critically ill patient are detailed later in this article.

The author has nothing to disclose.
Division of Trauma and Critical Care, Department of Surgery, Medical College of Wisconsin, 9200 West Wisconsin Avenue, Milwaukee, WI 53226, USA
E-mail address: pcodner@mcw.edu

Surg Clin N Am 92 (2012) 1485–1501
http://dx.doi.org/10.1016/j.suc.2012.08.005
0039-6109/12/$ – see front matter © 2012 Published by Elsevier Inc.

METABOLIC RESPONSE TO INJURY

Injury and stress produce a constellation of signs and symptoms known as the "systemic inflammatory response syndrome" (SIRS), defined in 1992 by the American College of Chest Physicians and the Society of Critical Care Medicine.[3] Two or more of the following are required to diagnose SIRS:

- Body temperature of greater than 38°C or less than 36°C
- Heart rate greater than 90 beats per minute
- Respiratory rate greater than 20 breaths per minute or a $Paco_2$ level of less than 32 mm Hg
- Abnormal white blood cell count (>12,000/µL or <4000/µL or >10% bands)

Another important component of SIRS is a hypermetabolic response lasting up to 1 month after injury. Besides trauma, other etiologies associated with SIRS include ischemia, inflammation, infection, or a combination of these. SIRS is nonspecific and its pathophysiologic properties are independent of the inciting mechanism. The body's response to insult is inflammation and SIRS is considered a self-defense mechanism. The complex interactions between the various components of the inflammatory cascade and SIRS were summarized by Bone and coworkers[3] as a three-stage process:

- Stage I: For example, intestinal ischemia leads to local cytokine production, initiating an inflammatory response to promote wound healing and activation of the reticular endothelial system.
- Stage II: The local response is augmented by the release of small quantities of local cytokines, stimulating release of growth factor and recruitment of macrophages and platelets. This acute response is balanced by a reduction in proinflammatory mediators and release of endogenous antagonists.
- Stage III: The goal of stage II is homeostasis, and a significant systemic reaction occurs if this is not achieved. Dysregulated cytokine release leads to an overall destructive rather than protective environment, eventually resulting in end-organ dysfunction.

The progression from SIRS to organ dysfunction and multisystem organ failure (MSOF) is thought to result from a series of insults, with each additional insult provoking an exaggerated response. The key to preventing the multiple effects is timely identification of the cause of SIRS and appropriate resuscitation and therapy, including provision of adequate nutrition.

Hypermetabolism in critical illness is characterized by accelerated protein catabolism to supply energy and substrates for increased protein synthesis in visceral organs. Excessive protein breakdown in skeletal muscle leads to amino nitrogen production and an increase in urinary nitrogen excretion (with approximately 85% as urea) roughly proportional to the severity of injury. Nitrogen balance is determined by the net loss or gain of body protein and is a measure of the catabolic state of the patient. It is imperative to recognize that the accelerated proteolysis occurs even in noninjured extremities.

In addition to the spleen and heart, the liver uses the protein redistributed from skeletal muscle to synthesize structural, plasma, and acute-phase proteins. The amino acids arginine and glutamine comprise 50% to 75% of the amino acid nitrogen released from skeletal muscle. Both amino acids are important as glucose precursors and are central to the immune response. Glutamine is also important in acid-base homeostasis and is a precursor for glutathione.

GUT DISUSE

The gastrointestinal (GI) tract normally provides a barrier to invasion by pathologic microorganisms. The functional and structural integrity of the intestinal epithelium is affected by the intake and processing of nutrients and the route of delivery of these nutrients, such as enteral feeding. The GI tract is also home to one of the largest immune organs in the body, known as the gut-associated lymphoid tissue (GALT). This tissue contains 70% to 80% of all immunoglobulin-secreting cells.[4] The gut is responsible for 50% of the body's total immunoglobulin production, with the primary component for mucosal immunity and barrier integrity being IgA. Decreased gut use results in reduced mucosal mass (about 10%–15% in humans) and disruption of the intestinal mucosa.[5] When nutrients are not provided to the gut, there is shortening of the microvilli, the fingerlike projections in the intestinal wall that serve to increase the surface area for nutrient absorption, and the surface architecture of the small bowel mucosa is disrupted.[6,7] Animal studies have revealed reductions in villus height after only a few days of complete bowel rest. This effect is not prevented by the use of parenteral (intravenous) nutrition, but rather villus atrophy is commensurate with the duration of parenteral feeding.

The structural and functional changes occurring in the small intestine increase permeability. In addition, distinct metabolic changes occur during stress versus starvation, including increased caloric expenditure and metabolic rate, mobilization of carbohydrate and fat stores, protein breakdown, and loss of lean body mass.[8] The afferent limb of the stress response is the central nervous system, specifically activation of the hypothalamic-pituitary-adrenal axis and the autonomic nervous system. The effector response is mediated by the immune system (inflammatory cytokines, such as tumor necrosis factor [TNF]; interleukins [IL]-1 and -6; and the humeral response in the form of catecholamines, glucagon, insulin, cortisol, and growth hormone). Intestinal permeability is not increased as drastically in starvation alone as when the starvation is preceded by an injury.[9] Ammori and coworkers[10] reported that the increased gut permeability may be directly correlated to the severity of illness in patients with pancreatitis. In burn patients, the degree of gut permeability is inversely correlated to the percentage of goal calories provided by enteral nutrition (EN).[11]

BACTERIAL OVERGROWTH

During critical illness, the gut barrier hypothesis suggests that certain substances can cross the gut mucosal lining and initiate and amplify the SIRS response.[12] Decreased gut use leads to bacterial overgrowth and an increase in bacterial translocation. It has been demonstrated in animal models that intestinal IgA levels are inversely correlated with changes in intestinal permeability, degree of bacterial overgrowth, and translocation.[13] Bacterial overgrowth leads to a predominance of aerobic bacteria.[9] Reduced peristalsis (ileus) can also contribute to bacterial overgrowth. Bile salt secretions and secretory IgA (sIgA) levels are reduced, promoting bacterial adherence to the mucosa.[14] The phenomenon of bacterial translocation and increased gut permeability explains the approximately 30% of patients who are found clinically or at autopsy to suffer from severe sepsis and MSOF without an identifiable focus of infection.

It is not known whether the process of translocation involves live bacteria or such products as endotoxins.[15] After these products translocate across the bowel lumen, they enter the portal vein. An inflammatory cascade is initiated, including stimulation of Kupffer cells in the liver parenchyma. Moore and coworkers[15] failed to find bacteria or endotoxin in the portal blood of severely injured patients, including a subgroup developing MSOF. Although clinical trials of selective decontamination of the digestive tract resulted in reduced incidence of pneumonias, primary bacteremias, and other infectious complications by approximately 50%, they did not improve survival rates.[16] Another hypothesis is that gut-derived factors actually enter the mesenteric lymph rather than the portal bloodstream.[17] Support for this latter theory is obtained from indirect evidence in which hemorrhagic-shock–induced lung injury was prevented after division of mesenteric lymphatic ducts. The lung is the first organ exposed to mesenteric lymph and clinically is one of the first organs to fail in severely injured patients. In vitro studies of mesenteric lymph compared with portal vein plasma have revealed increased endothelial cell monolayer permeability, increased activation of neutrophils, and endothelial cell death. Proof of clinical translation is difficult to conclusively show and change in outcome is even harder but some translocation of bacteria or their products occurs in humans and provision of enteral nutrients may prevent this.

EFFECT OF NUTRITION DELIVERY METHOD ON GUT IMMUNE FUNCTION

Mucosal immunity is dependent on sIgA production. Although levels of sIgA diminish within 5 days of gut disuse whether or not parenteral nutrition (PN) is used,[14,18] lymphocyte populations are altered by an absence of EN. Normally, there is a balance between the proinflammatory arm and the anti-inflammatory arm of the immune system. The proinflammatory arm consists of differentiated T helper (Th) 1 lymphocytes and proinflammatory cytokines, such as IL-2, interferon gamma (IFN-γ), and TNF. Stimulation of naive cell differentiation into Th1 cells occurs by IL-12. The response of the proinflammatory arm of the immune system results in increased inflammation and is essential for host defense. This is counterbalanced by the anti-inflammatory response, consisting of IL-4-differentiated Th2 lymphocytes and secretion of additional IL-4, IL-6, and IL-10. The latter moderates Th1 response and is essential to prevent self-injury.[19] In addition, IL-4 stimulates IgA-positive B cells in Peyer patches; further differentiation of IgA-positive B cells produces sIgA-secreting plasma cells in the lamina propria.

Reduced gut use decreases IL-4 and IL-10 secretion and subsequent differentiation of naive lymphocytes into Th2 lymphocytes, eventually reducing sIgA levels.[20,21] In contrast, Th1 lymphocyte differentiation and production of IFN-β, TNF, and IL-2 are not affected by lack of EN.[22] This leads to an unbalanced ratio of Th1 to Th2 lymphocytes and upregulation of the proinflammatory arm of the immune system, possibly contributing to host injury.

EN not only affects differentiation of lymphocyte populations, but also expression of adhesion molecules important in homing of naive B cells to the intestinal lamina propria and GALT. Proper homing of B cells is mediated by the ligand MADCAM-1, whose expression is decreased with gut disuse.[20] Without an influx of B cells from the vascular space into the lamina propria, the intestinal Peyer patches atrophy. The decrease in IL-4 and IL-10 levels caused by intestinal disuse results in increased expression of the adhesion molecules ICAM-1 and E-selectin in the intestine and pulmonary microvasculature.[23] The latter plays a role in sequestration of polymorphonuclear neutrophils into the microvasculature, exacerbating organ injury.

GUT USE

The functional and structural integrity of the GI tract is positively affected by normal enteral feeding. The benefits of EN include maintenance of mucosal mass, cellular proliferation, production of brush border enzymes, and maintenance of villus height.[6,24] There is decreased intestinal epithelial cell permeability and small bowel blood flow is stimulated with provision of enteral nutrients.[25] A variety of endogenous agents, such as cholecystokinin, gastrin, bombesin, and bile salts, are produced. These agents have trophic effects on gut mucosa and can reverse the detrimental effects of PN on histologic and functional aspects of the intestinal tract. Cholecystokinin can partially restore the GALT system after use of PN.[26]

Enteral feeding encourages the proliferation of Th2 CD4+ helper T lymphocytes, which in turn stimulates the production and release of IgA-stimulating cytokines, such as IL-4, IL-5, IL-6, and IL-10.[27] Through a series of steps, IL-4 converts IgA-positive B cells in Peyer patches, whereas IL-10, IL-5, and IL-6 eventually promote differentiation of IgA-positive B cells into sIgA-secreting plasma cells in the lamina propria.[20]

Colonization resistance was first reported by van der Waaij[28] and describes a process in which the predominant anaerobic flora of the GI tract limits the overgrowth of potentially pathogenic (mostly aerobic) organisms. The normal gut environment contains more than 400 obligate species in a total concentration of 10^{11} to 10^{12} CFU/g of feces.[29,30] The concentration of aerobic flora is much lower, with aerobes accounting for less than 0.1% of the normal composition. Among the gram-negative bacilli in the bowel, $Escherichia$ $coli$ species are dominant. Secondary gram-negative bacilli other than E $coli$ are ingested daily with food, but these secondary gram-negative bacilli fail to colonize the bowel in the presence of successful E $coli$ populations in healthy volunteers.[31] Among the aerobic gram-positive cocci, the enterococci are dominant, whereas staphylococci or streptococci also populated the bowels of healthy volunteers at low concentrations ($<10^5$ CFU/g of feces).[32] Most endogenous infections are caused by aerobic flora, and provision of EN maintains the normal, predominant, anaerobic flora of the gut.[33]

Another important process is known as "oral tolerance." A small fraction of the food passing through the human adult intestinal tract consists of intact immunologic antigens.[34] Oral tolerance refers to hyporesponsiveness to these food antigens. The immune system is downregulated in its response to common antigens in food and in the commensal bacterial flora of the GI tract. An alternative pathway for CD4+ helper T-cell differentiation occurs to support this process. Special regulatory T cells (Th3 and Tr1) stimulated by enteral feeding help promote a balanced Th2-Th1 profile. Normal intestinal immunity is maintained by the large dietary and indigenous microbial antigenic loads.[34] The intestinal B-cell system is also stimulated by the antigenic constituents of food. Thus, continued EN supports a high concentration of IgA-secreting immunocytes and preserves the indigenous microbial flora in the gut, balancing the proinflammatory and anti-inflammatory arms and preventing an exaggerated inflammatory response.

Clinical investigations comparing EN with PN have shown that patients treated with EN demonstrate no apparent difference in mortality rate but that EN is associated with a significant reduction in infectious complications (relative risk [RR], 0.61; 95% confidence interval [CI], 0.44–0.84).[35] Early EN compared with delayed forms of nutrition also resulted in reduced mortality (RR, 0.52; 95% CI, 0.25–1.08) and fewer infectious complications (RR, 0.66; 95% CI, 0.36–1.22). Both of these findings approached but did not reach statistical significance.[35]

The site of EN delivery (gastric vs postpyloric) has also been studied. Postpyloric nutrition is associated with a decreased frequency of regurgitation and aspiration[36] and the incidence of ventilator-associated pneumonia was significantly reduced with this method.[37] Finally, EN is preferred to PN to avoid serious risk of catheter-induced sepsis in acute lung injury–acute respiratory distress syndrome.[38] In my ICU, a postpyloric nasojejunal feeding tube is placed within 72 hours of admission, preferably within 48 hours, and EN is initiated.

IMMUNONUTRITION

Immunonutrition refers to therapy in which a particular nutrient is administered to induce a specific metabolic function not usually associated with nutrition support.[39] These "immune-enhancing diets" are thought to modulate the immune system, facilitate wound healing, and reduce oxidative stress. When research first began in this area, nutrition was added as a therapeutic modality after control of the underlying disease process and restoration and stabilization of oxygen transport in patients who manifested severe malnutrition associated with organ dysfunction, nosocomial infections, and wound failure. Investigators believed that the postresuscitation phase consisted of a hypermetabolic pathologic state of persistent inflammation and suppression of immune function, eventually leading to MSOF and death. Enteral formulas containing supraphysiologic amounts of L-arginine, omega-3 fatty acids, L-glutamine, and antioxidants and vitamins have been developed and are discussed individually next. There is little direct evidence of the overall clinical efficacy of each of these immune compounds or their effects on hypermetabolism.

L-ARGININE

The amino acid L-arginine becomes an essential nutrient under stress conditions because the normal quantities endogenously produced to maintain muscle mass are insufficient because of increased protein turnover after injury. Arginine is required for stimulation and release of growth hormone, prolactin, insulin, and glucagon; plays a fundamental role in polyamine and nucleic acid synthesis; and is essential for growth but not viability of cells in vitro.[40] It is also a critical substrate for nitric oxide (NO) production,[41] which is mediated by a family of enzymes known as "nitric oxide synthases" (NOSs) that exist in constitutive and inducible isoforms.[42] NO is an important mediator of vascular dilation, protein synthesis in hepatocytes, and electron transport in hepatocyte mitochrondria.

Under normal circumstances and in some disease states, small quantities of NO are produced by the constitutive form of NOS (cNOS). This exerts a beneficial effect on tissue oxygenation and immune function.[43] Supplemental administration of arginine (which is then metabolized to NO by cNOS) is associated with increased lymphocyte and monocyte proliferation, enhanced T-cell production, activation of macrophages and natural killer cells, and increased phagocytosis. Manufacturers have noted the benefits of arginine and have added supraphysiologic concentrations to their immune-enhancing formulas. Unfortunately, this had led to excessive NO production mediated through the inducible isoform of NOS (iNOS) and can lead to excessive inflammation and vasodilatation. Inflammatory cytokines (eg, IL-1, TNF, and IFN-γ) mediate induction of iNOS.

Evidence concerning the effects of arginine administration on mortality is lacking. In critically ill patients with sepsis, arginine supplementation led to excessive mortality compared with an isonitrogenous control diet (23% vs 9.6%; $P = .03$).[44] In patients undergoing major cancer surgery, arginine supplementation has been associated with reduced length of stay.[40,45] The mechanism behind this is thought to be increased thymic and peripheral blood lymphocyte blastogenic responses to mitogens from arginine supplementation.

OMEGA-3 FATTY ACIDS

Polyunsaturated fatty acids (PUFAs) are a major component of cell membranes and consequently influence the structure and function of cellular membranes. Experimentally, dietary PUFAs reduce platelet aggregation, slow blood clotting, participate in cell surface enzyme activity, and limit the production of proinflammatory cytokines.[46] Synthesis of all PUFAs occurs in humans, except those in the omega-3 and omega-6 families.[47] Fish oil contains high concentrations of eicosapentaenoic acid, docosahexaenoic acid, and alpha-linolenic acid, which are naturally occurring omega-3 acids.[48] The omega-3 PUFAs alter the physiologic characteristics of cell membranes and compete with arachidonic acid for cyclooxygenase metabolism. In response to lipopolysaccharide stimulation, arachidonic acid metabolism results in formation of type 2 prostaglandins and type 4 leukotrienes. These substances promote immunosuppression and inflammation. In contrast, omega-3 PUFA are metabolized to type 3 prostaglandins and type 5 leukotrienes, which are less inflammatory and do not suppress immune function.[47,49] The North American diet contains very low levels of omega-3 PUFAs and n-3 PUFA can preferentially replace the n-6 PUFA, thus changing the physiologic characteristics of the cell membrane to stimuli, such as lipopolysaccharide.[39,50]

Gadek and colleagues[51] randomly assigned patients with acute lung injury–acute respiratory distress syndrome to either an experimental diet containing fish oils (eicosapentaenoic acid and docosahexaenoic acid) and antioxidants or a high-fat, low-carbohydrate control diet. Those receiving the experimental diet had higher plasma phospholipid fatty acid levels and fewer total cells and neutrophils recovered from bronchoalveolar lavage fluid. The experimental group also had fewer ventilator days, shorter ICU lengths of stay, fewer new organ failures, and a trend toward decreased mortality.[51] Unfortunately, it is difficult to attribute beneficial clinical outcomes solely to PUFAs when other nutrients, such as antioxidants, are also likely to exert a significant influence. In addition, the high-fat diet used for the control group may have been harmful.[52] This study and limited other studies do not clearly demonstrate the benefits of PUFAs.

L-GLUTAMINE

L-glutamine plays a central role in nucleotide synthesis and serves as an important fuel for rapidly dividing cells, such as lymphocytes and gut epithelial cells.[53] It is also important in endogenous synthesis of the antioxidant glutathione. Glutamine is considered a conditionally essential amino acid during stress and critical illness. Consumption may overcome endogenous production during these periods, and low circulating levels of glutamine have been associated with immune dysfunction and increased mortality.[54,55]

There is some debate whether the route of administration (parenteral vs enteral) affects the efficacy of glutamine. The gut and liver metabolize most enterally administered glutamine; therefore, it may not have a systemic effect. However, clinical studies have demonstrated that parenteral and enteral glutamine supplementation is beneficial in patients after bone marrow transplantation, multiple trauma, critical illness, or surgery.[56–58]

As a single agent, glutamine supplementation has a broad spectrum of beneficial effects in humans. These include reducing infectious complications, acting as a trophic agent for the GI tract, and upregulating the immune system. Ziegler and colleagues[56] published the first major clinical study demonstrating a reduction in infectious complications and hospital length of stay in patients with bone marrow transplant supplemented with glutamine. Houdijk and coworkers[57] reported a nonsignificant reduction in the number of infections in trauma patients receiving a glutamine-supplemented enteral formula compared with those receiving a control formula (20 [57%] of 35 vs 26 [70%] of 37).

Other human studies have described the benefits of glutamine as a trophic substance for the GI tract, repairing damaged intestinal epithelial cell layers, and maintaining the barrier function of the GI tract.[59] In burn patients, improved immune cell function and a reduction in mortality with enteral glutamine have been demonstrated.[60,61]

ANTIOXIDANTS, VITAMINS, AND TRACE MINERALS

Increased levels of reactive oxygen species (ROS) are present during critical illness because of an imbalance between protective endogenous antioxidant mechanisms and ROS production. Examples of ROS include superoxide anion, hydroxyl radical, hydrogen peroxide, and hypochlorous acid. Oxidative stress plays a central role in the pathophysiology of SIRS and MSOF.[62] ROS cause cellular injury through numerous mechanisms, including destruction of cell and organelle membranes through peroxidation of fatty acids; hyaluronic acid and collagen degradation; damage to DNA and RNA; and damage to key enzymes, such as Na^+/K^+-ATPase.[62,63]

The endogenous antioxidant defense system consists of enzymes, such as superoxide dismutase, catalase, glutathione peroxidase, and glutathione reductase. All of these enzymes contain heavy metals, such as manganese, selenium, copper, or zinc, at their active sites. When this system is overwhelmed, ROS react with target molecules and cause cellular damage. The endogenous system is the first line of defense against ROS, but cells can also use water-soluble nonenzymatic antioxidants, such as selenium, zinc, or vitamin C, or lipid-soluble antioxidants, such as vitamin E and betacarotene.[64]

Selenium

Selenium is the most-studied single nutrient. It is an important cofactor for the enzyme glutathione and exerts beneficial effects on immune function.[65] Selenium deficiency has been associated with encephalopathy, progressive muscle weakness, myopathy, and cardiomyopathy.[65,66] A study of selenium supplements in patients with necrotizing pancreatitis suggested that they reduced mortality,[65] whereas in SIRS patients three separate selenium studies produced three different outcomes: one reported reduced mortality, one described a nonsignificant trend toward reduced mortality, and the final study reported no effect.[65] Considered together, these four studies displayed a trend of reduced mortality with selenium supplementation.[65]

Zinc

Zinc is an essential element for cell growth, immune function, and disease resistance. A component of the enzyme superoxide dismutase, zinc regulates the expression of metalloproteins and plays a role in cell replication, protein synthesis, gene expression, and immune cell function.[67] Zinc deficiency can inhibit immunologic development; modify the barrier functions of the skin, lungs, and GI tract; and alter the number and function of immune cells, such as neutrophils, monocytes, macrophages, T cells, and B cells, resulting in decreased resistance to infection.[67]

In critically ill head-injury patients on ventilators, zinc supplementation was associated with a nonsignificant reduction in mortality.[67]

Vitamin C

Linus Pauling demonstrated the link between vitamin C and immune function in the 1970s. White blood cells normally contain high concentrations of vitamin C. In patients with cancer who have undergone surgical trauma or are being treated for major infections, dietary requirements for vitamin C are increased.[68]

Two randomized trials were conducted with patients suffering from pressure ulcers. The first study reported a significant reduction in wound area in those receiving high doses of vitamin C, whereas the second revealed no benefit.[69,70] Vitamin C improved chemotaxis, exhibited bactericidal activity, and resulted in shorter illness in patients with diseases involving dysfunctional phagocytic cells.[71]

Vitamin E

Vitamin E is a lipid-soluble antioxidant shown in animal studies to enhance natural killer cell function, antibody production, macrophage phagocytosis, and resistance to pathogens.[68] There is evidence to support the role of vitamin E in reducing the risk of prostate cancer. Newer conflicting data suggest no risk reduction. Based on these findings, studies examining the incidence of prostate cancer with vitamin E supplementation alone or in combination with selenium are underway.[72]

Betacarotene

Carotenoids are naturally occurring pigmented compounds present in a variety of plants in the human diet. Their chemical structure facilitates neutralization of free radicals, making them important antioxidants.[68]

Betacarotene has been associated with cancer prevention,[73] the mechanism of which may be related to its antioxidant and immune-enhancing properties.[74] The immune enhancements include an increase in circulating lymphocytes and T-cell mediated immunity.[75] The strongest evidence for the beneficial role of carotenoids is in the incidence of lung cancer, with eight out of eight prospective studies demonstrating a protective effect.[76]

PARENTERAL NUTRITION

In patients who cannot tolerate adequate EN, total PN (TPN) is an important source of calories and nutrients. Enteral feeding is always preferable, but there are patients in whom the intestinal tract cannot be used or that must be frequently returned to the operating room. TPN is also appropriate for patients who are malnourished before injury.[77] The main advantage to TPN is that full nutritional requirements may be met within 12 to 24 hours.

Patient Selection

In critically ill patients with a wide variety of disease processes (including pancreatitis, trauma, burns, and those on mechanical ventilation with an intact GI tract) TPN should never be selected over EN. The reduction of infections from the use of EN is consistent across almost all critical care patient populations.[78] In comparing standard therapy (no artificial nutritional support provided) with TPN, Braunschweig and colleagues[78] reported a significant reduction in infections with the former (RR, 0.77; 95% CI, 0.65–0.91). An even greater reduction in infectious complications was observed in well-nourished patients receiving standard therapy than with TPN. Trends toward reduced overall complications[78] and hospital length of stay[79] have also been described.

The one patient population in which TPN use reduces infectious morbidity, overall major complications, and mortality in comparison with standard therapy[79] is patients with protein-calorie malnutrition defined by a greater than 10% to 15% weight loss or low body mass index. TPN has greater efficacy in these patients and can favorably affect their outcome compared with standard therapy. The prevalence of this population in ICUs is low, ranging from 8.3% to 12.6%.[80]

Timing of TPN

The timing of TPN initiation is based on the underlying nutritional status of the patient. In critically ill patients without premorbid malnutrition (>10%–15% weight loss), it is reasonable to wait 7 to 10 days before starting TPN if oral intake is not possible.[81] An even longer waiting period of 10 to 14 days has been advocated. If TPN is not initiated after 14 days, mortality is increased in patients on standard therapy (dextrose solution) who are not yet eating.[82]

In malnourished patients TPN is superior to standard therapy in the first 7 to 10 days when the enteral route is not available, but should not be started unless it is anticipated that it will be continued for more than 7 to 10 days. Short-term TPN (<7 days) is not effective and does not favorably impact outcome.

Lipid Content

Recent investigations have demonstrated an increase in infectious complications with the use of TPN in surgically stressed patients.[80] This is contrary to findings from earlier studies that reported either a marginal benefit for patients receiving TPN or no difference.[83] One difference between the earlier and later studies is that patients in the more recent studies received a formulation in which 20% to 30% of the nonprotein calories were in the form of an intravenous fat emulsion (IVFE), compared with little or no intravenous lipid in the earlier studies.

IVFE is a widely used source of essential fatty acids. The long-term effects of withholding lipids in TPN are unknown. To prevent essential fatty acid deficiency at least 5% of total calories must be provided as a lipid emulsion. The consequences of not providing sufficient lipid are not observed until after the first 10 days of hospitalization.[84]

Lipid infusions have been associated with immune modulation and dysfunction in surgical patients receiving perioperative TPN.[85] Long-chain fats can cause immune suppression, promote dysfunction of the reticuloendothelial system, promote formation of prostanoids and leukotrienes, generate ROS, and negatively alter cell membrane composition.[85] Battistella and colleagues reported that IVFE in the early postinjury period increased infectious complications (pneumonia and catheter-related sepsis); prolonged pulmonary failure; and increased ICU and hospital length of stay.[86] One criticism of this study is that the no-lipid group did not have the missing calories replaced with additional carbohydrates and was underfed compared with the group receiving the lipid formulation.

Although IVFE is associated with a significant increase in infections in critically ill patients, lipid-free TPN is probably best reserved for short-term use (<10 days). In my ICU, IVFE is administered on Mondays and Thursdays with TPN.

Hyperglycemia

Most (50%–75%) of the total calories in the TPN admixture come from glucose (dextrose). In contrast, enteral formulas contain 40% to 55% carbohydrate. Parenteral nutrition leads to more frequent episodes of hyperglycemia. Hyperglycemia has been identified as the cause of increased complications during TPN and the reason for its reduced efficacy. Other studies noted that patients who developed infections had higher serum glucose values than their noninfected cohorts, but these values were still below those expected to increase the risk of infection (serum glucose >220 mg/dL).[87] A wide variety of factors play a role in the dysfunction resulting from hyperglycemia including impaired neutrophil chemotaxis and phagocytosis, less effective wound healing caused by glycosylation of immunoglobulins, complement cascade dysfunction, and promotion of inflammation.[88] Parenteral nutrition has also been shown to increase the endogenous production of glucose and decrease glucose oxidation.[78]

Van den Berghe and coworkers[89] demonstrated that compared with conventional treatment (target range for blood glucose concentration 10–11.1 mmol/L), achievement of tight glycemic control (4.4–6.1 mmol glucose/L) was associated with a lower incidence of sepsis (P = .003), a trend toward reduced ventilator days, and significant reductions in ICU length of stay (P <.04) and hospital mortality (P = .01).

More recent studies have compared this intensive regimen with a more conventional treatment goal of keeping target blood sugar levels at 10 mmol or less per liter. A blood glucose target of less than or equal to 10 mmol/L resulted in lower mortality than a target of 4.5 to 6 mmol/L.[90] Further studies are necessary to determine the optimum window for glycemic control with the use of TPN. In my surgical ICU population, blood sugar is maintained between 5 and 7.2 mmol/L (90–130 mg/dL) except in patients with total pancreatectomy.

PERMISSIVE UNDERFEEDING

When first considered, the concept of permissive underfeeding in critical illness (total caloric provision set at approximately 20 kcal/kg/d of actual or ideal body weight) may seem counterintuitive. Classical nutritional teaching emphasizes the provision of sufficient nutrients to meet tissue demands. Full nutrient support promotes growth and protein synthesis but may also stimulate pathologic processes, such as bacterial virulence, autoimmune disease, cytokine production, and inflammation, which are also dependent on nutrient supply. Permissive underfeeding is a strategy based on the concept that short-term dietary restriction minimizes pathologic processes while limiting organ dysfunction.[91]

Numerous studies have revealed that unrestricted nutrient intake optimizes growth in animals but shortens longevity. In normal and immunosuppressed animals, increased longevity was achieved when they were given protein-calorie restricted diets. The mechanism of this longevity is a delay in the onset of disease.[92,93] In humans, several studies have indicated a relationship between excessive calorie intake and increased rates of insulin resistance, infectious morbidity, and mortality.

When given PN in excess of 35 kcal/kg actual bodyweight, hyperglycemia (blood glucose concentration >200 mg/dL) occurred in greater than 50% of nondiabetic patients.[94] Another study compared a high-dose carbohydrate group (77% of total calories and 42.4 kcal/kg/d, on average) with lower doses of carbohydrates (60.6% of total calories and 34.3 kcal/kg/d, on average) and found more episodes of sepsis and higher mortality in the former group (both P <.05).[95] The higher carbohydrate formula in this study contained less protein, but this was not statistically significant. Most hypocaloric feeding is achieved by reducing the amount of carbohydrate or lipid.

Permissive underfeeding has been applied to EN. A recent study by Rice and coworkers[96] hypothesized that trophic feeding would result in shorter duration of mechanical ventilation and better GI tolerance. The study population included patients within 48 hours of acute lung injury and less than 72 hours of mechanical ventilation who were able to receive EN. The study group received 25% of their calculated caloric goal compared with 80% within 6 hours of randomization and demonstrated no improvement in ventilator-free days (14.9 vs 15 days, difference −0.1 [CI, −1.4 to 1.2]) or infectious complications but was associated with less GI intolerance.

Results of these and other studies suggest the detrimental mechanism of excess caloric consumption is a cycle of insulin resistance and subsequent hyperglycemia at lower rates of energy intake. Some degree of malnutrition may be protective and increase insulin sensitivity. Standard calorie intake in patients with sepsis may increase morbidity and mortality and permissive underfeeding may be beneficial, particularly in patients with sepsis.

SUPPLEMENTAL TPN

Supplemental TPN refers to the addition of TPN for patients receiving insufficient enteral feeding. When comparing EN with TPN-supplemented EN, there was no difference in morbidity or mortality, ICU length of stay, duration of mechanical ventilation, or incidence of respiratory infection.[97] Herndon and coworkers[98] reported a statistically significant increase in mortality in patients receiving supplemental TPN because of a greater depression of T-cell helper-suppressor ratios. In addition, supplemental TPN doubled the cost of nutritional support.[97]

However, low-dose enteral feeding or trophic feeds are beneficial in patients receiving TPN. A small amount of enteral support during TPN might attenuate gut atrophy and improve host defenses, limiting bacterial translocation.[99] This combination feeding may be tapered off when the patient tolerates more than 80% of protein and calorie needs by the intestinal tract. With combination feeding, it is still important not to overfeed the patient.

HOW I DO IT

In my surgical critical care population, I place a small-bore nasojejunal feeding tube into the postpyloric position and start tube feeds within 48 hours of admission to the ICU. The goal tube feed rate is achieved within 12 to 24 hours of placement. There are times when the feeding tube is unable to pass postpylorically and a potential delay in starting nutrition results. This is usually in a multiply injured trauma patient, and I elect to feed into the stomach taking other precautions, such as head of bed elevation. I do not spend the extra resources to send the patient to fluoroscopy for placement. If the patient is undergoing surgery, I ask the operating team to place a postpyloric nasojejunal tube. In the patient with an open abdomen whose bowel is in continuity, I start trophic feeds at 10 to 20 mL/h for the numerous benefits. A recent multi-institutional study by Burlew and coworkers[100] showed for patients without a bowel injury, EN in the open abdomen is associated with increased fascial closure rates ($P<.01$), decreased complications ($P = .02$), and decreased mortality ($P = .01$). It is recommended that EN should be initiated in these patients after resuscitation is completed. In patients with bowel injuries and an open abdomen, EN did not seem to impact outcomes (fascial closure [$P = .2$], complication rate [$P = .19$], or mortality [$P = .69$]). When the intestinal route is unavailable or the patient is not tolerating EN, I begin TPN only if I anticipate using it for more than 7 days. I always reevaluate the feasibility of enteral feeding on a daily basis. For all patients except total pancreatectomy patients, I monitor blood sugars and aim to keep levels lower than 130 mg/dL.

SUMMARY

The stress response to injury involves hypermetabolism, impaired protein synthesis, and a catabolic state. This leads to a metabolic derangement that requires appropriate nutritional support to counteract loss of body protein, improve the metabolic and immunologic responses, and improve overall morbidity and mortality. Optimizing nutritional therapy is based on fully understanding the premorbid nutritional status of the patient and the pathophysiology of the underlying critical illness.

The stress response may be modulated by provision of specific nutrients. It is possible that individual nutritional formulas could be tailored to the patient and disease. The enteral route is preferred in most circumstances, but there are specific situations in which TPN is necessary and may be beneficial, if attention is paid to hyperglycemia and total calorie intake.

REFERENCES

1. Cerra FB, Benitez MR, Blackburn GL, et al. Applied nutrition in ICU patients: a consensus statement of the American College of Chest Physicians. Chest 1997;111:769.
2. Bistrian BR, Blackburn GL, Hallowell E, et al. Protein status of general surgical patients. JAMA 1974;230:858.
3. Bone RC, Balk RA, Cerra FB. Definitions for sepsis and organ failure and guidelines for the use of innovative therapies in sepsis. The ACCP/SCCM Consensus Conference Committee. American College of Chest Physicians/Society of Critical Care Medicine. Chest 1992;101:1644–55.
4. Langkamp-Henken B, Glezer JA, Kudsk KA. Immunologic structure and function of the gastrointestinal track. Nutr Clin Pract 1992;7:100–8.
5. van der Hulst RR, van Kreel BK, von Meyenfeldt MF, et al. Glutamine and the preservation of gut integrity. Lancet 1993;29:1363–5.
6. Groos S, Hunefeld G, Luciano L. Parenteral versus enteral nutrition: morphological changes in human adult mucosa. J Submicrosc Cytol Pathol 1996;28:61–74.
7. Deitch EA, Winterton J, Li M, et al. The gut as portal of entry for bacteria: role of protein malnutrition. Ann Surg 1987;205:681–92.
8. Cerra FB. Hypermetabolism, organ failure, and metabolic support. Surgery 1987;101:1.
9. Kudsk KA. Importance of enteral feeding in maintaining gut integrity. Tech Gastrointest Endosc 2001;3:2–8.
10. Ammori BJ, Leeder PC, King RF, et al. Early increase in intestinal permeability in patients with severe acute pancreatitis: correlation with endotoxemia, organ failure, and mortality. J Gastrointest Surg 1999;3:252–62.
11. Ziegler TR, Smith RJ, O'Dwyer ST, et al. Increased intestinal permeability associated with infection in burn patients. Arch Surg 1988;123:1313–9.
12. Wilmore DW, Smith RJ, O'Dwyer ST, et al. The gut: a central organ after surgical stress. Surgery 1988;104:917–23.
13. Haskel Y, Xu D, Xu D, et al. Elemental diet-induced bacterial tranlocation can be hormonally modulated. Ann Surg 1993;217:634–42.
14. King BK, Li J, Kudsk KA. A temporal study of TPN-induced changes in gut-associated lymphoid tissue and mucosal immunity. Arch Surg 1997;132:1303–9.
15. Moore FA, Moore EE, Poggetti R, et al. Gut bacterial translocation via the portal vein: a clinical perspective with major torso trauma. J Trauma Acute Care Surg 1991;31:629–36.
16. Reidy JJ, Ramsey G. Clinical trials of selective decontamination of the digestive tract: a review. Crit Care Med 1990;18:1449–56.
17. Deitch EA. Role of the gut lymphatic system in multiple organ failure. Curr Opin Crit Care 2001;7(2):92–8.
18. Li J, Kudsk KA, Hamidian M, et al. Bombesin affects mucosal immunity and gut-associated lymphoid tissue in intravenously fed mice. Arch Surg 1995;130:1164–9.
19. Elson CO. The immunology of inflammatory bowel disease. In: Kirsner JB, editor. Inflammatory bowel disease. Philadelphia: WB Saunders; 2000. p. 208–39.

20. Kudsk KA. Current aspects of mucosal immunology and its influence by nutrition. Am J Surg 2002;183:390–8.
21. Hermsen JL, Gomez FE, Maeshima Y, et al. Decreased enteral stimulation alters mucosal immune chemokines. JPEN J Parenter Enteral Nutr 2008;32(1):36–44.
22. Wu Y, Kudsk KA, DeWitt RC, et al. Route and type of nutrition influence IgA-mediating intestinal cytokine. Ann Surg 1999;229:662–7.
23. Fukatsu K, Lundberg AH, Hanna MK, et al. Increased expression of intestinal P-selectin and pulmonary E-selectin during intravenous total parenteral nutrition. Arch Surg 2000;135:1177–82.
24. Groos S, Reale E, Hünefeld G, et al. Changes in epithelial cell turnover and extracellular matrix in human small intestine after TPN. J Surg Res 2003; 109(2):74–85.
25. Niinikoski H, Stoll B, Guan X, et al. Onset of small intestinal atrophy is associated with reduced intestinal blood flow in TPN-fed neonatal piglets. J Nutr 2004; 134(6):1467–74.
26. Dobbins WO. Gut immunophysiology: a gastroenterologist's view with emphasis on pathophysiology. Am J Phys 1982;242:1–8.
27. Lebman DA, Coffman RL. Cytokines in the mucosal immune system. In: Strober W, Mestecky J, Lamm ME, et al, editors. Handbook of mucosal immunology. San Diego (CA): Academic; 1994. p. 243–9.
28. van Der Waaij. Colonization resistance of the digestive tract-mechanism and clinical consequences. Food 1987;31(5–6):507–17.
29. Vollard EJ, Clasener HA. Colonization resistance. Antimicrobial Agents Chemother 1994;38(3):409–14.
30. Moore WE, Holdeman LV. Human fecal flora: the normal fecal flora of 20 Japanese-Hawaiians. Appl Microbiol 1974;27:961–79.
31. Murray BE, Mathewson HL, Dupont CD, et al. Emergence of resistant fecal *Escherichia coli* in travelers not taking prophylaxtic antimicrobial agents. Antimicrobial Agents Chemother 1990;34:515–8.
32. Vollard EJ, Clasener HA, Janssen AJ, et al. Influence of cefotaxime on microbial colonization resistance in healthy volunteers. J Antimicrob Chemother 1990;26:117–23.
33. Fink MP. Why the GI tract if pivotal in trauma, sepsis, and MOF. J Crit Illn 1991;6: 253–69.
34. Brandtzaeg PE. Current understanding of gastrointestinal immunoregulation and its relation to food allergy. Ann N Y Acad Sci 2002;964:13–45.
35. Heyland DK, Dhaliwal R, Drover JW, et al. Clinical practice guidelines for nutrition support in the adult critically ill patient. JPEN J Parenter Enteral Nutr 2003; 27(5):355–73.
36. Heyland DK, Drover JW, MacDonald S, et al. Effect of postpyloric feeding on gastroesophageal regurgitation and pulmonary microaspiration: results of a randomized controlled trial. Crit Care Med 2001;29:1495–501.
37. Heyland DK, Drover JD, Dhaliwal R, et al. Optimizing the benefits and minimizing the risks of enteral nutrition in the critically ill: role of small bowel feeding. JPEN J Parenter Enteral Nutr 2002;26:S51–7.
38. Ware LB, Matthay MA. The acute respiratory distress syndrome. N Engl J Med 2000;342(18):1134–349.
39. Cerra FB. Nutrient modulation of inflammatory and immune function. Am J Surg 1991;161:230–4.
40. Barbul A. Arginine and immune function. Nutrition 1990;6:53–9.
41. Evoy D, Lieberman MD, Fahey TH, et al. Immunonutrition: the role of arginine. Nutrition 1998;14:611–7.

42. Salzman AL. Nitric oxide in the gut. New Horiz 1995;3:33–45.
43. Muscara MN, Wallace JL. Nitric oxide: therapeutic potential of nitric oxide donors and inhibitors. Am J Phys 1999;276:G1313–6.
44. Dent DL, Heyland DK, Levy H, et al. Immunonutrition may increase mortality in critically ill patients with pneumonia: results of a randomized trial. Crit Care Med 2003;30:A17.
45. Reynolds JV, Thom AK, Zhang SM, et al. Arginine, protein calorie malnutrition and cancer. J Surg Res 1988;45:513–22.
46. Alexander JW. Immunoenhancement via enteral nutrition. Arch Surg 1993;128: 1242–5.
47. Alexander JW. Immunonutrition: the role of omega-3 fatty acids. Nutrition 1998; 14:627–33.
48. Schloerb PR. Immune-enhancing diets: products, components, and their rationales. JPEN J Parenter Enteral Nutr 2001;25(Suppl 2):S3–7.
49. Wachtler PH, Axel Hilger R, Konig W, et al. Influence of a pre-operative enteral supplement on functional activities of peripheral leukocytes from patients with major surgery. Clin Nutr 1995;14:275–82.
50. Kinsella J, Lokesh B, Boughton S, et al. Dietary PUFA and eicosanoids: potential effects on the modulation of inflammatory and immune cells: an overview. Nutrition 1990;6:24–5.
51. Gadek JE, DeMichele SJ, Karlstad MD, et al. Effect of enteral feeding with eicosapentaenoic acid, gamma-linolenic acid, and antioxidants in patients with acute respiratory distress syndrome. Enteral Nutrition in ARDS study group. Crit Care Med 1999;27:1409–20.
52. Garrel D, Razi M, Lariviere F, et al. Improved clinical status and length of care with low-fat nutrition support in burn patients. JPEN J Parenter Enteral Nutr 1995;19:482–91.
53. Manhart N, Vierlinger K, Spittler A, et al. Oral feeding with glutamine prevents lymphocyte and glutathione depletion of Peyer's patches in endotoxemic mice. Ann Surg 2000;234(1):92–7.
54. Oehler R, Pusch E, Dungel P, et al. Glutamine depletion impairs cellular stress response in human leucocytes. Br J Nutr 2002;87:S17–21.
55. Roth E, Funovics J, Muhlbacher F, et al. Metabolic disorders in severe abdominal sepsis: glutamine deficiency in skeletal muscle. Clin Nutr 1982;1:25–41.
56. Ziegler TR, Young LS, Benfell K, et al. Clinical and metabolic efficacy of glutamine-supplemented parenteral nutrition after bone marrow transplantation. Ann Intern Med 1992;116:821–8.
57. Houdijk APJ, Rijnsburger ER, Jansen J, et al. Randomised trial of glutamine-enriched enteral nutrition on infectious morbidity in patients with multiple trauma. Lancet 1998;352:772–6.
58. Griffiths RD, Jones C, Palmer TE. Six-moth outcome of critically ill patients given glutamine-supplemented parenteral nutrition. Nutrition 1997;13:295–302.
59. Wilmore DW, Shabert JK. Role of glutamine in immunologic responses. Nutrition 1998;14:618–26.
60. Ogle CK, Ogle JD, Mao JX, et al. Effect on glutamine on phagocytosis and bacterial killing by normal and pediatric burn patient neutrophils. JPEN J Parenter Enteral Nutr 1994;18:128–33.
61. Garrel F, Nedelec B, Samson L, et al. Decreased mortality and infectious morbidity in adult burn patients given enteral glutamine supplementation: a prospective, controlled, randomized clinical trial. Crit Care Med 2003;31(10): 2444–9.

62. Heyland DK, Dhaliwal R, Suchner U, et al. Antioxidants nutrients: a systematic review of trace elements and vitamins in the critically ill patient. Intensive Care Med 2005;31:327–37.

63. Lovat R, Preiser JC. Antioxidant therapy in intensive care. Curr Opin Crit Care 2003;9:266–70.

64. Tanswell AK, Freeman BA. Antioxidant therapy in critical care medicine. New Horiz 1995;3:330–41.

65. Heyland DK, Dhaliwal RD, Suchner MD. Immunonutrition. In: Rolandelli RH, Bankhead R, Boullata JI, editors. Clinical nutrition: enteral and tube feeding. 4th edition. Philadelphia: Elsevier Saunders; 2005. p. 224–42.

66. Marcus RW. Myopathy and cardiomyopathy associated with selenium deficiency: case report, literature review, and hypothesis. Maryland Med J 1993;42:669–74.

67. Prasad AS. Zinc, infection, and immune function. In: Calder PC, Field CJ, Gill HS, editors. Nutrition and immune function. 1st edition. New York: CABI Publishing; 2002. p. 193–207.

68. Hughes DA. Antioxidant vitamins and immune functions. In: Calder PC, Field CJ, Gill HS, editors. Nutrition and immune function. 1st edition. New York: CABI Publishing; 2002. p. 171–91.

69. Taylor TV, Rimmer S, Day B, et al. Ascorbic acid supplementation in the treatment of pressure-sores. Lancet 1974;2:544–6.

70. ter Riet G, Kessels AG, Knipschild PG. Randomized clinical trial of ascorbic acid in the treatment of pressure ulcers. J Clin Epidemiol 1995;48:1453–60.

71. Anderson R. Effects of ascorbate on normal and abnormal leucocyte functions. Int J Vitam Nutr Res Suppl 1982;23:23–34.

72. Klein EA, Thompson IM, Lippman SM, et al. SELECT: the next prostate cancer prevention trial. Selenium and Vitamin E Cancer Prevention Trial. J Urol 2001; 166:1311–5.

73. Peto R, Doll R, Buckley JD, et al. Can dietary beta-carotene materially reduce human cancer rates? Nature 1981;290:201–8.

74. Block G, Patterson B, Subar A. Fruit, vegetable, and cancer prevention: a review of the epidemiological evidence. Nutr Cancer 1992;18:1–29.

75. Alexander M, Newmark H, Miller RG. Oral beta-carotene can increase the number of OKT4+ cells in human blood. Immunol Lett 1985;9:221–4.

76. Ziegler RG, Mayne ST, Swanson CA. Nutrition and lung cancer. Cancer Causes Control 1996;7:157–77.

77. Van Way CW III. Nutritional support in the injured patient. Surg Clin North Am 1991;71:537–48.

78. Braunschweig CL, Levy P, Sheean PM, et al. Enteral compared with parenteral nutrition: a meta-analysis. Am J Clin Nutr 2001;74:534–42.

79. Heyland DK, MacDonald S, Keefe L, et al. Total parenteral nutrition in the critically ill patient: a meta-analysis. JAMA 1998;280:2013–9.

80. Veterans Affairs Total Parenteral Nutrition Cooperative Study Group: perioperative total parenteral nutrition in surgical patients. N Engl J Med 1991;325:525–32.

81. Klein S, Kinney J, Jeejeebhoy K, et al. Nutrition support in clinical practice: review of published data and recommendations for future research directions. National Institutes of Health, American Society for Parenteral and Enteral Nutrition, and American Society for Clinical Nutrition. JPEN J Parenter Enteral Nutr 1997;27: 133–56.

82. Sandstrom R, Drott C, Hyltander A, et al. The effect of postoperative intravenous feeding (TPN) on outcome following major surgery evaluated in a randomized study. Ann Surg 1993;217:185–95.

83. Heatley RV, Williams RH, Lewis MH. Pre-operative intravenous feeding: a controlled trial. Postgrad Med J 1979;55:541.
84. Koretz RL, Lipman TO, Klein S. AGA technical review on parenteral nutrition. Gastroenterology 2001;121:970–1001.
85. Kinsella JE, Lokesh B. Dietary lipids, eicosanoids, and the immune system. Crit Care Med 1990;18:S94.
86. Basttistella FD, Widergren JT, Anderson JT, et al. A prospective, randomized trial of intravenous fat emulsion administration in trauma victims requiring total parenteral nutrition. J Trauma Acute Care Surg 1997;43:52–60.
87. Kudsk KA, Laulederkind A, Hanna MK. Most infectious complications in parenterally fed trauma patients are not due to elevated blood glucose levels. JPEN J Parenter Enteral Nutr 2001;25(4):174–9.
88. Moore FA, Feliciano DV, Andrassy RJ, et al. Early enteral feeding, compared with parenteral, reduces postoperative septic complications: the results of a meta-analysis. Ann Surg 1992;216:172–3.
89. Van den Berghe G, Wouters P, Weekers F, et al. Intensive insulin therapy in critically ill patients. N Engl J Med 2001;345:1359–67.
90. NICE-SUGAR study investigators, Finfer S, Chittock DR, Su SY, et al. Intensive versus conventional glucose control in critically ill patients. N Engl J Med 2009;360(13):1283–97.
91. Zaloga GP, Roberts P. Permissive underfeeding. New Horiz 1994;2(2):257–63.
92. Nolen GA. Effect of various restricted dietary regimens on the growth, health and longevity of albino rats. J Nutr 1972;102:1477–94.
93. Berg BN, Simms HS. Nutrition and longevity in the rat. III. Food restriction beyond 800 days. J Nutr 1961;74:23–32.
94. Rosmarin DK, Wardlaw GM, Mirtallo J. Hyperglycemia associated with high, continuous infusion rates of total parenteral nutrition dextrose. Nutr Clin Pract 1996;11:151–6.
95. Vo NM, Waycaster M, Acuff RV, et al. Effects of postoperative carbohydrate overfeeding. Am Surg 1987;53:632–5.
96. Rice TW, Wheeler AP, Thompson BT, et al. Initial trophic vs full enteral feeding in patients with acute lung injury. The EDEN randomized trial. JAMA 2012;307(8): 795–803.
97. Bauer P, Charpentier C, Bouchet C, et al. Parenteral with enteral nutrition in the critically ill. Intensive Care Med 2000;26:893–900.
98. Herndon DN, Barrow RE, Stein M, et al. Increased mortality with intravenous supplemental feeding in severely burned patients. J Burn Care Rehabil 1989; 10:309–13.
99. Sax HC, Illig KA, Ryan CK, et al. Low-dose enteral feeding is beneficial during total parenteral nutrition. Am J Surg 1996;171:587–90, 100.
100. Burlew C, Moore E, Cuschieri J, et al. Who should we feed? A Western Trauma Association multi-institutional study of enteral nutrition in the open abdomen after injury. J Trauma Acute Care Surg 2012. in press.

Renal Management in the Critically Ill Patient

Kenneth S. Waxman, MD*, Galen Holmes, MD

KEYWORDS

- Renal function • Acute kidney injury • Prerenal azotemia • Peritoneal dialysis

KEY POINTS

- Alterations in renal function are common in surgical patients, where multiple factors affect the clinical picture and outcomes are influenced by prompt diagnosis and protective management strategies.
- Recent studies suggest that acute kidney injury occurs in up to two-thirds of intensive care unit patients and that increasing severity of acute kidney injury is associated with increasing mortality.
- Urinalysis with microscopy is a useful tool in determining the cause of acute kidney injury.
- Distinguishing between prerenal azotemia and acute tubular necrosis, two of the most common causes of acute kidney injury, can be complicated by a confusing clinical picture.

INTRODUCTION

Alterations in renal function are common in surgical patients, where multiple factors affect the clinical picture and outcomes are influenced by prompt diagnosis and protective management strategies. This is particularly true in critically ill patients.

ACUTE KIDNEY INJURY

Acute kidney injury (AKI) is defined by a decline in renal filtration marked by acute decrease in glomerular filtration rate (GFR). Although serum creatinine (S_{Cr}) is not a perfect marker for GFR, it is frequently used as a surrogate to estimate GFR. The true incidence of AKI and acute renal failure has been difficult to define, given the broad and various definitions used to quantify and study altered renal function. Recent introduction of consensus definitions, such as RIFLE criteria and Acute Kidney Injury Network (AKIN) staging, has allowed a more clear analysis of the impact of this problem. Recent studies suggest that AKI occurs in up to two-thirds of intensive care unit (ICU) patients and that increasing severity of AKI is associated with

Ventura County Health Care Agency, 2323 Knoll Drive, Ventura, CA 93003, USA
* Corresponding author.
E-mail address: kenneth.waxman@ventura.org

Surg Clin N Am 92 (2012) 1503–1518
http://dx.doi.org/10.1016/j.suc.2012.08.012
0039-6109/12/$ – see front matter © 2012 Elsevier Inc. All rights reserved.

surgical.theclinics.com

increasing mortality.[1] It is clear that AKI is associated with increased morbidity, such as increased hospital length of stay and cost of care,[2] and has been linked to other in-hospital complications, such as increased difficulty weaning from mechanical ventilation.[3] Preoperative risk factors for development of AKI include older age, emergent surgery, hepatic disease, obesity, high-risk surgery, and vascular disease in chronic obstructive pulmonary disease.[4] Although the incidence of AKI seems to be rising, overall outcomes are gradually improving.[5,6]

DEFINITION

The RIFLE criteria (**Table 1**), defined in 2004 by the Acute Dialysis Quality Initiative Group,[7] quantifies the severity of AKI. Studies by Hoste and colleagues[8] and Osterman and Chang[9] found that mortality progressively increased with increasing RIFLE severity, and that patients in all of the RIFLE classifications had higher mortality than those in the ICU without AKI.

In 2005, the AKIN formulated consensus diagnostic criteria for AKI. The consensus states "an abrupt (within 48 hours) reduction in kidney function is currently defined as an absolute increase in S_{Cr} of either ≥ 0.3 mg/dL or a percentage increase of $\geq 50\%$ (1.5-fold from baseline) or a reduction in urine output (documented oliguria of <0.5 mL/kg/hr for >6 hrs)." These criteria can only be applied in the face of adequate fluid hydration.[10] This AKIN staging system (**Table 2**), arguably more inclusive than the RIFLE criteria, simplifies the definition of AKI for researchers and AKIN correlates with outcomes. Chertow and colleagues[2] found that an acute absolute change in creatinine greater than or equal to 0.3 was associated with increased mortality, length of stay, and cost of care. Barrantes and colleagues[11] found that patients meeting this definition of AKI were three times as likely to die during hospitalization.

In 2007, Coca and colleagues[12] published a review and meta-analysis of eight studies that suggest that even smaller elevations in S_{Cr} than recommended in RIFLE and AKIN (on the order of 10%–24%) are associated with a twofold risk of short-term death in several clinical settings and hypothesize that the lack of successful interventions in the treatment of AKI may be in part caused by delay in diagnosis caused by the lag-time of S_{Cr}. They suggest that implementing a new, more sensitive definition of AKI may improve the success of proposed interventions.

Table 1
RIFLE criteria

	Serum Creatinine Criteria	Urine Output Criteria
Risk	Increased 1.5–2× baseline	<0.5 mL/kg/h for 6 h
Injury	Increased 2–3× baseline	<0.5 mL/kg/h for 12 h
Failure	Increased >3× baseline or Serum creatine >4 mg/dL with acute rise ≥ 0.5 mg/dL	<0.3 mL/kg/h for 24 h or Anuria for 12 h
Loss	Persistent renal failure for >4 wk	
End-stage renal disease	Persistent renal failure for >3 mo	

Data from Bellomo R, Ronco C, Kellum J, et al. Acute renal failure: definitions, outcome measures, animal models, fluid therapy and information technology needs. The Second International Consensus Conference of the Acute Dialysis Quality Initiative (ADOQI) Group. Crit Care 2004;8:R204–12.

Table 2		
Acute Kidney Injury Network staging system		
Stage	**Serum Creatinine Criteria**	**Urine Output Criteria**
I	Absolute increase ≥0.3 mg/dL or Increased 1.5–2× baseline	<0.5 mL/kg/h for 6 h
II	Increased 2–3× baseline	<0.5 mL/kg/h for 12 h
III	Increased >3× baseline or	<0.3 mL/kg/h for 24 h or
	Serum creatine ≥4 mg/dL with absolute increase ≥0.5 mg/dL	Anuria for 12 h
	or Need for renal replacement therapy	

Data from Mehta R, Kellum J, Shah S, et al. Acute Kidney Injury Network (AKIN): report of an initiative to improve outcomes in acute kidney injury. Crit Care 2007;11:R31.

DIAGNOSTIC APPROACH

Historical keys include the temporal nature of symptoms, comorbidities, and identification of potentially nephrotoxic medications. It is important to identify signs and symptoms suggestive of obstruction. Although the physical examination in the intensive care patient with AKI is frequently fraught with conflicting clinical findings and is of limited accuracy,[13] ascertaining clues to the patient's hemodynamics and volume status is valuable.

Urinalysis with microscopy is a useful tool in determining the cause of AKI. Presence of casts or other cells can suggest or confirm a diagnosis. Red cell casts suggest glomerulonephritis or vasculitis, whereas white cell casts may raise the possibility of interstitial nephritis or pyelonephritis. "Muddy brown" casts and renal tubular epithelial cells are pathognomonic for acute tubular necrosis (ATN) and differentiate ATN from prerenal azotemia, which has normal sediment or occasional hyaline casts.[14] Dark hemepositive urine without red blood cells on microscopy is diagnostic of rhabdomyolysis.

Distinguishing between prerenal azotemia and ATN, two of the most common causes of AKI, can be complicated by a confusing clinical picture. Aside from analysis of urine sediment, response to fluid repletion is frequently used in this distinction. Return to baseline of renal function in 24 to 72 hours after fluid repletion suggests a prerenal cause. Urine chemistries can also aid in the diagnosis. The fractional excretion of sodium (FENa) measures the ratio of the sodium excreted to the sodium filtered by the formula:

$$FENa = (urine\ sodium \times S_{Cr})/(serum\ sodium \times urine\ creatinine) \times 100$$

Prerenal azotemia is indicated by FENa less than 1%, whereas FENa greater than 1% suggests ATN. However, FENa may be spuriously low in patients with severe sepsis, heart failure, or cirrhosis despite the presence of ATN.[15] The FENa may be falsely elevated in patients on diuretics, with glucosuria, or with preexisting renal insufficiency. In the case of diuretic use, the fractional excretion of urea (FEurea) can accurately distinguish between prerenal azotemia and ATN by the following formula:

$$FEurea = (urine\ urea\ nitrogen \times S_{Cr})/(blood\text{-}urea\text{-}nitrogen \times urine\ creatinine) \times 100$$

Prerenal azotemia is indicated by a FEurea less than 35% and ATN by a value greater than 50%.[16] Although of variable utility, other serum and urinary measures can be used in aggregate to distinguish ATN from prerenal azotemia.[17–20] These tests are summarized in **Table 3**, in order of general usefulness.

Serologic tests, such as antinuclear antibody, hepatitis B surface antigen, and anti-glomerular basement membrane antibody, are useful for distinguishing the cause of glomerular diseases. Creatinine phosphokinase level can indicate rhabdomyolysis.

Blood-urea-nitrogen (BUN) levels reflect the balance between urea production, metabolism, and excretion and frequently rise as renal function declines. Numerous nonrenal sources of BUN exist, including dietary protein intake, parenteral hyperalimentation therapy, catabolism of endogenous proteins, corticosteroid administration, and upper gastrointestinal bleeding. However, a recent study by Beier and colleagues[21] suggests that elevation of BUN is predictive of long-term mortality, independent of normal creatinine.

BIOMARKERS

Most clinicians rely on changes in S_{Cr} and BUN as indicators of renal function because they are accessible and well established. However, S_{Cr} level is influenced by nonrenal factors, such as age, gender, race, body weight, muscle mass, protein intake, and drugs, and changes in this laboratory value tend to lag behind actual alterations in GFR. BUN is influenced by nutritional intake and the degree of catabolism, independently of renal function. For these reasons, alternatives to S_{Cr} and BUN serve as more specific markers, earlier indicators, and better prognostic tools for kidney injury. Belcher and colleagues[22] highlight one of the most promising of these markers, interleukin (IL)-18. A proinflammatory cytokine thought to be released by injured proximal renal tubules,[23] IL-18 is a mediator and biomarker of AKI and can be reliably measured in the urine. The authors cite research that identifies IL-18 as an early indicator of AKI, as a tool for distinguishing prerenal azotemia and hepatorenal syndrome from ATN, and as a prognostic tool to predict mortality and viability of renal transplant.[22] Belcher and colleagues[22] also discuss neutrophil gelatinase-associated lipocalin, an acute-phase reactant indicative of inflammatory injury, which is upregulated and released by proximal renal tubular cells within a few hours of tubular damage. Like IL-18, studies suggest that neutrophil gelatinase-associated lipocalin can be used as an early indicator,[24] in the differential diagnosis, and as a prognostic tool for AKI.[25] Kidney injury molecule 1 is a type 1 cell membrane glycoprotein only expressed by proximal tubular cells in response to injury. It is detectable in urine and has been shown to discriminate ATN from other causes of AKI and is also used as a prognostic tool, because it predicts outcomes.[22]

Table 3
Diagnostic indices distinguishing prerenal azotemia from acute tubular necrosis

Measurement	Prerenal Azotemia	Acute Tubular Necrosis
Urinalysis	Normal or hyaline casts	Muddy brown casts
Response to fluid repletion	Within 24–72 h	No response
FENa	<1%	>1%
FEurea	<35%	>50%
BUN/creatinine ratio	20	10
Urine sodium (mEq/L)	<20	>30
Urine osmolality (mOsm/L)	>350	300

Abbreviations: BUN, blood-urea-nitrogen; FENa, fractional excretion of sodium; FEurea, fractional excretion of urea.

Cystatin C is a cysteine protease inhibitor secreted by all nucleated cells and is freely filtered by the glomerulus. Although several studies suggest that serum cystatin C is better than S_{Cr} as a surrogate for GFR and thus better for the early detection of AKI,[26–29] another study suggests urinary cystatin C may be better.[30]

Liver-type fatty acid binding protein is an intracellular lipid chaperone found in the proximal renal tubules where it binds lipid peroxidation products thus mitigating tissue damage in ischemia-reperfusion injury. Although urinary levels may be affected by liver injury or systemic inflammation, they are largely determined by tubular injury.[31]

IMAGING

Imaging is an important part of the initial work-up in patients with AKI. The primary test of choice is ultrasound. Using ultrasound to determine kidney size and echogenicity, cortical thickness, and the presence or absence of hydronephrosis is convenient and noninvasive.[32] The presence of a thin rim of decreased echogenicity ("renal sweat") may surround the kidneys in patients with kidney injury.[33] Recent studies suggest that the use of color Doppler technology is useful in the diagnosis of AKI.[34] Measuring the resistivity index, an indicator of perfusion based on measurement of flow at the level of the arcuate or interlobar arteries, may help differentiate among prerenal azotemia (normal resistivity index), ATN (reduced resistivity index), and postrenal obstruction (elevated resistivity index). The authors also suggest that this value can be serially followed, because it normalizes with resolution of the renal insult. Another promising ultrasonographic technique for the diagnosis of AKI is contrast-enhanced ultrasound, which makes use of microbubble-based contrast agents to help quantify renal blood flow, which is thought to be decreased in AKI.[35] Ultrasound is critical for the diagnosis of hydronephosis in which it is more than 95% accurate in detecting dilation of the collecting systems and renal pelvis.[36,37] A postrenal obstructive cause of AKI is suggested when hydronephrosis is present bilaterally.[38] Assessing bladder volume with ultrasound is important in the case of bilateral hydronephrosis. A postvoid residual volume greater than 150 mL is suggestive of bladder-outlet obstruction[39] and if observed in the presence of a urinary catheter, catheter malfunction should be considered. If ultrasound is negative, computed tomography (CT) may be required to elucidate the cause of obstruction, such as obstructing stones or pelvic mass.

MEDICATION REVIEW

When evaluating cases of AKI, a thorough investigation of medications and ingestions is essential. Certain medications can elevate S_{Cr} levels without affecting GFR, leading to misdiagnosis of AKI. The drugs cimetidine and trimethoprim block tubular creatinine secretion,[40,41] whereas several drugs and substances interfere with the creatinine assay (Table 4). The drug tenofovir disoproxil fumarate, used in the treatment of HIV/AIDS, elevates S_{Cr} without affecting measured GFR by an undefined mechanism.[42]

Various medications and substances induce AKI by several mechanisms (Table 5). It is important to limit the use of nephrotoxic agents when possible, especially in combination. If AKI is present, medications should be appropriately dosed.

DIFFERENTIAL DIAGNOSIS
Prerenal Azotemia

Prerenal azotemia is one of the most common etiologies of AKI, caused by a decrease in renal perfusion. This can occur because of an absolute decrease in extracellular

| Table 4 |
| Nonrenal causes of elevated serum creatinine |

Interference with Creatinine Assay	Block Tubular Creatinine Secretion	Undefined
Acetone (found in DKA)	Cimetidine	Tenofovir
Cefoxitin	Trimethoprim	
Flucytosine		
Isopropol alcohol		
Methanol		
Methyldopa		

Abbreviation: DKA, diabetic ketoacidosis.
  Data from refs.[82–85]

fluid volume (ie, hemorrhage, gastrointestinal losses, burns); a decrease in the effective circulating volume (ie, heart failure, portal hypertension); or shifting volume out of the intravascular space (ie, third-spacing). Prerenal azotemia by definition is reversible if treated early with fluid resuscitation, improvement in underlying heart failure, or correction of the third-space defect. If untreated, poor perfusion leads to tissue ischemia and cell death, representing a progression to intrinsic renal disease. An important cause of prerenal azotemia is abdominal compartment syndrome. High intra-abdominal pressures (>20 mm Hg bladder pressure) result in the clinical triad of oliguria, dyspnea with high peak airway pressures hindering ventilation, and hypotension transiently responsive to fluid resuscitation. If detected early, medical management can be effective,[43] but as with all compartment syndromes, timely surgical decompression with a decompressive laparotomy is usually necessary.

Postrenal Azotemia

Postrenal azotemia occurs because of obstruction of urinary flow at any point in the urinary tract from the renal collecting system to the level of the urethra. Increased back-flow builds pressure and decreases filtration. This type of azotemia can be caused by prostatic disease; neurogenic bladder; obstruction of an in-dwelling urinary catheter; abdominal or pelvic tumors; adhesions from prior surgery or radiation; vesicoureteral reflux; ureteral or bladder stones; medications causing crystals or fibrosis; or myeloma light chains (in multiple myeloma). The obstruction must be corrected to resolve the azotemia. Complications of postrenal azotemia include urinary tract infection secondary to urinary stasis, hyperkalemia caused by impaired excretion, and rarely postobstructive diuresis marked by significant diuresis leading to hypotension.

Intrinsic Renal Disease

Intrinsic renal disease results from injury to the parenchyma of the kidney, including the glomeruli, the interstitium, and the renal tubules.

Glomeruli

Glomerular disease is classified as nephritic or nephrotic and can have an acute or insidious onset. Nephritic syndrome is characterized by hematuria, proteinuria, hypertension, and edema caused by pores in the glomeruli allowing leakage of red blood cells and protein into the urine. Etiologies include bacterial endocarditis, systemic lupus erythematosus, poststreptococcal glomerulonephritis, hepatitis B antigenemia, IgA nephropathy, and hepatorenal syndrome. The hallmark of nephrotic syndrome is marked proteinuria with minimal hematuria and anasarca. Frequently, the diagnosis of

Table 5
Medications associated with direct and indirect nephrotoxicity

Direct Nephrotoxicity					Indirect Nephrotoxicity		
ATN	Osmotic Nephrosis	Interstitial Nephritis	Glomerular Injury	Crystal deposition (intrarenal obstruction)	Decrease in Intrarenal Blood Flow	Retroperitoneal fibrosis (ureteral obstruction)	Volume Depletion
Iodinated contrast	Hypertonic solutions	NSAIDs	NSAIDs	Indinavir	Ergotamine		Diuretics (loop, mannitol, thiazide)
Aminoglycosides	IVIG	Beta-lactams	Zoledronate	Sulfadiazine	Sotalol		
Amphotericin B		Quinolones	Pamidronate	Sulfamethoxazole	Propranolol		
Pentamidine		Sulfonamides	Ticlopidine	Methotrexate	Bromocriptine		
Foscarnet		Phenytoin	Clopidogrel	High-dose acyclovir			
Cisplatinum		Allopurinol	Cyclosporine				
Acetaminophen		Thiazide and loop diuretics	Gemcitabine				
Cidofovir		Indinavir					
Adefovir		PPIs					
Tenofovir		Vancomycin					
Melphalan							
IVIG							
Hetastarch							
Mannitol							

Abbreviations: ATN, acute tubular necrosis; IVIG, intravenous immunoglobulin; NSAIDS, nonsteroidal inflammatory drugs; PPIs, proton pump inhibitors.
Data from Pannu N, Nadim MK. An overview of drug-induced acute kidney injury. Crit Care Med 2008;36(4):S216–23.

nephrotic syndrome requires renal biopsy. Causes include minimal change disease, focal segmental glomerulosclerosis, and membranous nephropathy.

Interstitium

There are many conditions affecting the renal interstitium including allergic; drug-induced; infectious (bacterial, viral, fungal, parasitic); autoimmune (systemic lupus erythematosus, Sjögren syndrome, Goodpasture syndrome); infiltrative (lymphoma, sarcoid); and idiopathic forms of disease. The most common cause of acute interstitial nephritis is drug-induced disease, which is thought to underlie 60% to 70% of cases.[44] Illicit drugs, penicillins, cephalosporins, sulfonamides, and nonsteroidal anti-inflammatory drugs are some of the most common offenders. Acute interstitial nephritis can cause fever, rash, eosinophilia, and eosinophiluria; however, none of these are reliably diagnostic. Kidney biopsy is the gold standard of diagnosis, but rarely needed. Timely discontinuation of the offending agent is usually effective treatment. The use of steroids in drug-induced acute interstitial nephritis is controversial, but a recent study suggests that early administration of steroids (within 2 weeks) may prevent long-term sequelae.[45] Hyperuricemia, hyperuricosuria, and hyperphosphatemia, seen in tumor lysis syndrome, can cause deposits of crystals in the renal interstitium and tubules, leading to AKI. Similarly, ingestion of oral sodium phosphate solutions in bowel preparations for colonoscopy has been recognized as a cause of AKI from crystal deposition.[46] Allupurinol and rasburicase have been used for the prevention and treatment of tumor lysis syndrome.[47]

Tubules

ATN was originally thought to be caused by a period of ischemia followed by reperfusion causing extensive necrosis. More recently investigators emphasize the role of endothelial dysfunction, systemic inflammatory mediators, and oxidative stress in causing AKI.[48] With this in mind, the term currently is more often used to describe a clinical situation with adequate renal perfusion to maintain tubular integrity but not enough to sustain glomerular filtration.[49] This is particularly true in the case of sepsis and shock of any cause. ATN is also caused by toxins, most commonly the aminoglycoside antibiotics. Other toxins causing ATN include platinum, antifungals, rhabdomyolysis, hemolysis, and radiographic contrast (see **Table 5**). Risk factors for ATN include volume contraction, age, and concomitant use of other nephrotoxins. Prevention of ATN is focused on achieving euvolemia while maintaining renal perfusion and avoiding further renal insults. Rhabdomyolysis is caused by massive breakdown of muscle, releasing myoglobin, which can result in ATN. Rhabdomyolysis can be precipitated by drugs (heroin, cocaine, statins, alcohol); multiple trauma; crush injuries; seizures; muscle compression; and extreme exertion. Contrast-induced nephropathy (CIN) is an acute decline in renal function seen after administration of intravenous radiographic contrast, specifically an increase in S_{Cr} of 25% above baseline or absolute increase of 0.5 mg/dL within 48 hours after administration of parenteral contrast. Although not well understood, it is likely the result of several factors. Transient hypotension caused by osmotic diuresis, vasoconstriction of glomerular vessels, and direct cytotoxic effect has been hypothesized.[50] CIN is the third most common cause of hospital-acquired renal injury and is most prevalent among those with underlying renal disease.[51] Nephrogenic systemic fibrosis is a recently diagnosed disease that occurs in patients with preexisting stage IV and V chronic kidney disease or acute renal failure that has been linked to intravenous administration of gadolinium-based contrast media for magnetic resonance imaging. Shortly after exposure to gadolinium (2–12 weeks) patients develop skin thickening and fibrosis, similar to scleroderma, and can have rapid progression to joint contractures and severe disability. Systemic involvement may occur, leading to cardiomyopathy, pulmonary fibrosis, pulmonary hypertension, diaphragmatic paralysis, and death. The pathophysiology of the disease still remains unclear, but recent studies have demonstrated gadolinium deposits in tissues of patients diagnosed with nephrogenic systemic fibrosis.[52] Currently, prevention of nephrogenic systemic fibrosis entails avoidance of gadolinium administration in this population. Several treatment options (steroids, intravenous immunoglobulin, UV light, renal transplant) have been studied and have some benefit, but the evidence is based on small case studies or case reports and requires further evaluation.

RENAL PROTECTIVE STRATEGIES
Prevention of CIN

It is generally accepted that low-volume nonionic low-osmolar or iso-osmolar contrast media are associated with a decreased incidence of CIN than the high-osmolar agents.[53] For this reason, the high-osmolar preparations should be avoided. Such agents are currently not commonly used in clinical practice. Volume expansion has been accepted as the primary prevention of CIN, although choice of fluid has been controversial. Several meta-analyses of isotonic sodium bicarbonate show benefit over isotonic saline. However, a recent randomized controlled trial (RCT) suggested no difference between the two fluids, both of which were beneficial in preventing CIN.[54] Although the evidence suggests that bicarbonate may be superior, adequate volume resuscitation with either fluid is acceptable. N-acetylcysteine is a free radical scavenger that has been shown to decrease the incidence of CIN compared with placebo[55] and saline alone.[56] However, several studies found no benefit to N-acetylcysteine in the prevention of CIN. Despite an unproved benefit, because it is safe and inexpensive, many experts recommend N-acetylcysteine for its possible benefit.[57]

Other Preventative Strategies

The most important priority in renal protection is to maintain renal perfusion. Fluid choice, specifically crystalloid or colloid, for this purpose has been controversial. The landmark SAFE study[58] compared saline and albumin and found no difference in survival or need for renal replacement therapy (RRT) between the two groups. However, in post hoc analysis, albumin was found to have increased mortality in traumatic brain injury and a trend to decreased mortality in septic shock.

The use of synthetic colloids for volume expansion has been cautioned because of numerous studies implicating an increased risk of renal dysfunction. This increased risk of AKI was confirmed by a recent systematic review of the use of hydroxyethyl starches in patients with sepsis[59] and suggests that its use should be avoided. When fluid resuscitation is administered in critically ill patients, the amount given is also an important decision. An observational study in patients with AKI reported increased mortality associated with a positive fluid balance[60] and an RCT in patients with acute lung injury reported fewer ventilator days with conservative fluid management, which did not increase the need for RRT.[61] Erythropoetin has some promising nonerythropoietic properties, including tissue protection and antiapoptotic effect in animal models of brain, heart, and kidney. Despite preclinical data showing protective effects in AKI, the EARLYARF RCT in humans did not show benefit in erythropoetin administration.[62] However, proponents of erythropoetin cite the use of poorly validated biomarkers, among other flaws in study design that may have been responsible for the apparent failure.[63] The use of diuretics, such as mannitol and furosemide, in the prevention and treatment of AKI is extensive but they have not been conclusively found to shorten the duration of AKI, reduce the need for RRT, or improve overall outcomes.[64] Although it is based on anecdotal studies performed in the early 1960s, the prophylactic use of mannitol, together with an adequate hydration policy, is standard practice in many vascular and cardiac surgical units. Mannitol is beneficial in preventing ATN in postrenal transplant patients[65] and in severe crush injury.[66] In a recent study, high-dose furosemide showed a protective effect on mortality in patients with acute lung injury but no significant effect after adjustment for post-AKI fluid balance, which when positive, was strongly associated with mortality.[67] Atrial natriuretic peptide seems to dilate afferent glomerular arterioles and constrict efferent glomerular arterioles and may selectively increase GFR. It also inhibits agents that vasoconstrict the glomerular blood flow. Although the most recent RCT shows promising results in reducing the need for dialysis in cardiac surgery patients,[68] previous studies did not show any benefit.[69,70] Further studies are needed before its use is recommended.

It has been shown that dopamine at low doses increases renal perfusion and GFR and for this reason, dopamine was evaluated for its role in renal protective strategies. Despite numerous studies on this subject, none have yielded evidence to support this use of dopamine, and some results suggest it may worsen renal perfusion.[71] Fenoldopam, a dopamine-1 receptor agonist used in hypertensive emergencies, increases renal blood flow at its lowest dose. Although it failed to show benefit in sepsis, it has shown promise in surgical patients and the critically ill. In a recent meta-analysis of 16 randomized trials it seems to reduce mortality and need for RRT.[72]

A promising study by Heemskerk and colleagues[73] reports a significant decrease in plasma creatinine after an infusion of alkaline phosphatase in intensive care patients with severe sepsis or septic shock. The authors propose that exogenous alkaline phosphatase attenuates production of nitric oxide, a systemic vasodilator that causes compensatory renal vasoconstriction, by inhibiting inducible nitric oxide synthase, an enzyme that catalyzes production of nitric oxide. Reduction in nitric oxide may protect renal function; however, larger trials are needed to determine the presence of morbidity or mortality benefit. Other agents evaluated for potential use in prevention of CIN or ATN include theophylline and prostaglandin E_1. Both have shown promising but conflicting results, requiring further study before their use is recommend.

TREATMENT
Nonrenal Care that Affects AKI

It is clear that hyperglycemia and hypoglycemia during the postoperative period or during critical illness correlate with adverse outcomes. A recent study in surgical ICU patients also suggests that the presence of hyperglycemia and hypoglycemia in the same patient is associated with higher mortality risk.[74] Several studies suggest that intensive insulin therapy is associated with decreased incidence of AKI and reduced need for RRT, and may be renoprotective in critically ill surgical patients.[75] However, the largest and most recent RCT comparing intensive insulin therapy with conventional glucose control found no difference in need for RRT.[76] Lung protective ventilation is a mainstay in the treatment of acute respiratory distress syndrome because of the ARDSnet trial, which also suggested that the low-volume ventilation also may be beneficial for the kidney. The damaging effects of high-volume and high-pressure ventilation have been increasingly reported[77] and validate the use of lower volumes.

Renal Replacement Therapy

Despite numerous clinical trials evaluating pharmacologic agents for use in treating AKI, RRT remains the mainstay in treatment. Approximately 4% of critically ill patients who develop AKI require RRT.[78] The goal of RRT in AKI is to support nonrenal organs while awaiting recovery of renal function. However, standardization of practice in regards to initiation, dose, and modality of RRT has not been established and remains controversial.

Timing of initiation of RRT

Generally accepted indications for initiation of dialysis include severe acidemia, severe hyperkalemia, ingestion of a dialyzable substance causing renal injury, volume overload, and clinically apparent signs of uremia. Evidence suggests a benefit to early initiation; however, each study has variable definitions of early and late and differing markers to trigger initiation, including BUN, oliguria, ICU admission, and S_{Cr}.[79] Continued studies are needed to further define optimal initiation.

Frequency and rate of RRT

When determining the appropriate dose of dialysis, wide variation in clinical practice exists. Numerous studies are available, but there are conflicting data on outcomes. The largest and only multicenter trial looking at outcomes related to amount of renal support was the Acute Renal Failure Trial Network Study.[80] This study, following customary practice, assigned hemodynamically stable patients to the intermittent hemodialysis (IHD) group and hemodynamically unstable patients to continuous renal replacement modalities. The intensive management strategy had IHD six times per week or continuous therapy at 35 mL/kg/h. The less intense management strategy had IHD three times per week or continuous therapy at 20 mL/kg/h. They found no significant difference between groups in 60-day survival or renal recovery.

Modalities for RRT

Peritoneal dialysis is a simple but limited method for clearance of solute and ultrafiltration. It offers hemodynamic stability but can compromise respiratory status because of the dialysate volume. Its role in the ICU is therefore limited. Ultrafiltration is a technique that allows rapid removal of volume without significant solute removal. This protects intravascular volume and causes less hypotension. This strategy is useful in treating volume-overloaded states. IHD is the most frequently used method for RRT in the United States. This method uses a semipermeable biocompatible synthetic membrane and an electrochemical gradient maintained by continuous dialysate flow to remove solute. The major benefit of IHD is rapid removal of solute. Volume removal is frequently limited by hypotension. Another frequent drawback is hypoxia during treatments. Continuous renal replacement therapies are commonly used for RRT internationally, but used less frequently in the United States. Continuous therapies use hemofiltration, a technique that, like ultrafiltration, removes volume, but also has equal removal of solute because of the high permeability of the membrane used. In this case, solute clearance is dependent on volume filtered and because the volume filtered is substantial, replacement fluid is infused continuously to avoid hemodynamic instability. Hemodiafiltration adds a dialysate flow to supplement hemofiltration clearance. It is unclear if this addition adds benefit to hemofiltration alone. Continuous venovenous hemofiltration and continuous venovenous hemodiafiltration are two frequently used methods of CRRT that have been compared with IHD. It was initially thought that these continuous methods were safer for hemodynamically unstable patients and more physiologic and thus better for the critically ill. However, studies to determine the optimal method of RRT have yielded contradictory results. In a recent meta-analysis of nine randomized trials, Bagshaw and colleagues[81] found no difference in mortality or renal recovery between continuous and intermittent modalities. They comment on numerous problems with study design and quality that may undermine the results. Other drawbacks to the continuous modalities are the higher cost and need for anticoagulation. Hybrid therapies exist and have not yet been evaluated by prospective randomized trials. The most common hybrid modality is slow low-efficiency dialysis. Slow low-efficiency dialysis is a technique that is based on the observation that slower flow and longer treatments of IHD improve the inherent hemodynamic instability. Slow low-efficiency dialysis is usually continued over 8 to 12 hours nightly, avoiding typical daytime interruptions (procedures, radiology, surgery) and allowing for daytime mobilization. Presently, many questions regarding the variables of RRT remain unanswered and current practice is based largely on clinician choice, available resources, and cost.

SUMMARY

AKI is common in the hospital setting and morbidity and mortality outcomes depend on early recognition and early intervention. Identifying patients at risk of AKI is critical in prevention, early identification, and appropriate treatment.

REFERENCES

1. Hoste E, Schurgers M. Epidemiology of acute kidney injury: how big is the problem? Crit Care Med 2008;36(4):S146–51.
2. Chertow GM, Burdick E, Honour M, et al. Acute kidney injury, mortality, length of stay, and costs in hospitalized patients. J Am Soc Nephrol 2005;16:3365–70.
3. Vieira JM, Castro I, Curvello-Neto A, et al. Effect of acute kidney injury on weaning from mechanical ventilation in critically ill patients. Crit Care Med 2007;35(1): 184–91.
4. Kheterpal S. Predictors of postoperative acute renal failure after noncardiac surgery in patients with previously normal renal function. Anesthesiology 2007; 17(6):892–902.
5. Waikar S, Curhan G, Wald R, et al. Declining mortality in patients with acute renal failure, 1988-2002. J Am Soc Nephrol 2006;17:1143–50.
6. Xue J, Daniels F, Star R, et al. Incidence and mortality in patients with acute renal failure in Medicare beneficiaries, 1992-2001. J Am Soc Nephrol 2006;17: 1135–42.
7. Bellomo R, Ronco C, Kellum J, et al. Acute renal failure: definitions, outcome measures, animal models, fluid therapy and information technology needs. The Second International Consensus Conference of the Acute Dialysis Quality Initiative (ADOQI) Group. Crit Care 2004;8:R204–12.
8. Hoste EA, Clermont G, Kersten A, et al. RIFLE criteria for acute kidney injury are associated with hospital mortality in critically ill patients: a cohort analysis. Crit Care 2006;10:R73.
9. Osterman M, Chang R. Acute kidney injury in the intensive care unit according to RIFLE. Crit Care Med 2007;35:1837–43.
10. Mehta R, Kellum J, Shah S, et al. Acute Kidney Injury Network (AKIN): report of an initiative to improve outcomes in acute kidney injury. Crit Care 2007;11:R31.
11. Barrantes F, Tian J, Vazquez R, et al. Acute kidney injury criteria predict outcomes of critically ill patients. Crit Care Med 2008;36(5):1397–403.
12. Coca SG, Peixoto AJ, Garg AX, et al. The prognostic importance of a small decrement in kidney function in hospitalized patients: a systematic review and meta-analysis. Am J Kidney Dis 2007;50(5):712–20.
13. Peixoto AJ. Birth, death, and resurrection of the physical exam: clinical and academic perspectives on bedside diagnosis. Yale J Biol Med 2001;74(4):221–8.

14. Crowley ST, Peixoto AJ. Acute kidney injury in the intensive care unit. Clin Chest Med 2009;30(1):29–43.
15. Steiner RW. Interpreting the fractional excretion of sodium. Am J Med 1984;77: 699.
16. Cavounis CP, Nisar S, Guro-Razuman S. Significance of fractional excretion of urea in the differential diagnosis of acute renal failure. Kidney Int 2002;62(6): 2223–9.
17. Miller TR, Anderson RJ, Linas SL, et al. Urinary diagnostic indices in acute renal failure: a prospective study. Ann Intern Med 1978;89(1):47.
18. Espinel CH, Gregory AW. Differential diagnosis of acute renal failure. Clin Nephrol 1980;13:73.
19. Esson ML, Shrier RW. Diagnosis and treatment of acute tubular necrosis. Ann Intern Med 2002;137:744.
20. Perazella MA, Coca SG, Kanbay M, et al. Diagnostic value of urine microscopy for differential diagnosis of acute kidney injury in hospitalized patients. Clin J Am Soc Nephrol 2008;3:1615.
21. Beier K, Eppanapally S, Bazick HS, et al. Elevation of blood urea nitrogen is predictive of long-term mortality in critically ill patients independent of "normal" creatinine. Crit Care Med 2011;39(2):305–13.
22. Belcher JM, Edelstein CL, Parikh CR. Clinical applications of biomarkers for acute kidney injury. Am J Kidney Dis 2011;57(6):930–40.
23. Parikh CR, Jani A, Melnikov VY, et al. Urinary interleukin-18 is a marker of human acute tubular necrosis. Am J Kidney Dis 2004;43(3):404–15.
24. Nickolas TL, O'Rouke MJ, Yang J, et al. Sensitivity and specificity of a single emergency department measurement of urinary neutrophil gelatinase-associated lipocalin for diagnosing acute kidney injury. Ann Intern Med 2008; 148(11):810–9.
25. Haase M, Bellomo R, Devarajan P, et al. Accuracy of neutrophil gelatinase-associated lipocalin (NGAL) in diagnosis and prognosis in acute kidney injury: a systematic review and meta-analysis. Am J Kidney Dis 2009;56(6):1012–24.
26. Herget-Rosenthal S, Marggraf G, Husing J, et al. Early detection of acute renal failure by serum cystatin C. Kidney Int 2004;66:1115–22.
27. Le Bricon T, Leblanc I, Benlakehal M, et al. Evaluation of renal function in intensive care: plasma cystatin C vs. creatinine and derived glomerular filtration rate estimates. Clin Chem Lab Med 2005;43:953–7.
28. Delanaye P, Lambermont B, Chapelle JP, et al. Plasmatic cystatin C for the estimation of glomerular filtration rate in intensive care units. Intensive Care Med 2004;30:980–3.
29. Villa P, Jimenez M, Soriano MC, et al. Serum cystatin C concentration as a marker of acute renal dysfunction in critically ill patients. Crit Care 2005;9:R139–43.
30. Koyner JL, Bennett MR, Worcester EM, et al. Urinary cystatin C as an early biomarker of acute kidney injury following adult cardiothoracic surgery. Kidney Int 2008;74:1059–69.
31. Portilla D, Dent C, Sugaya T, et al. Liver fatty acid-binding protein as a biomarker of acute kidney injury after cardiac surgery. Kidney Int 2008;73(4):465–72.
32. Ritchie WW, Vick CW, Glocheski SK, et al. Evaluation of azotemic patients: diagnostic yield of initial US examination. Radiology 1988;167:245 7.
33. Yassa NA, Peng M, Ralls PW. Perirenal lucency ("kidney sweat"): a new sign of renal failure. AJR Am J Roentgenol 1999;173:1075–7.
34. Capotondo L. The role of color Doppler in acute kidney injury. Arch Ital Urol Androl 2010;82(4):275–9.

35. Schneider A. Bench-to-bedside review: contrast enhanced ultrasonography. A promising technique to assess renal perfusion in the ICU. Crit Care 2011;15(3):157.
36. Lee JK, Baron RL, Melson GL, et al. Can real-time ultrasonography replace static B-scanning in the diagnosis of renal obstruction? Radiology 1981;139:161–5.
37. Ellenbogen PH, Schieble FW, Talner LB, et al. Sensitivity of gray scale US in detecting urinary tract obstruction. Am J Roentgenol 1978;130:731–3.
38. Stuck KJ, White GM, Granke DS, et al. Urinary obstruction in azotemic patients: detection by sonography. Am J Roentgenol 1987;149:1191–3.
39. Taal. Brenner and Rector's the kidney, 9th ed.
40. Rocci ML Jr, Vlasses PH, Ferguson RK. Creatinine serum concentrations and H2-receptor antagonists. Clin Nephrol 1984;22(4):214.
41. Berg KJ, Gjellestad A, Nordby G, et al. Renal effects of trimethoprim in ciclosporin- and azathioprine-treated kidney-allografted patients. Nephron 1989;53(3):218.
42. Vrouenraets SM, Fux CA, Wit FW, et al. Persistent decline in estimated but not measured glomerular filtration rate on tenofovir may reflect tubular rather than glomerular toxicity. AIDS 2011;25(17):2149–55.
43. Cheatham ML. Nonoperative management of intraabdominal hypertension and abdominal compartment syndrome. World J Surg 2009;33:1116–22.
44. Perazella MA, Markowitz GS. Drug-induced acute interstitial nephritis. Nat Rev Nephrol 2010;6(8):461–70.
45. Gonzalez E, Gutierrez E, Galeano C, et al. Early steroid treatment improves the recovery of renal function in patients with drug-induced acute interstitial nephritis. Kidney Int 2008;73(8):940–6.
46. Ehrenpreis ED, Parakkal D, Semer R, et al. Renal risks of sodium phosphate tablets for colonoscopy preparation: a review of adverse drug reactions reported to the US FOOD and Drug Administration. Colorectal Dis 2011;13(9):e270–5.
47. Malaguarnera G, Giordana M, Malaguarnera M. Rasburicase for the treatment of tumor lysis in hematological malignancies. Expert Rev Hematol 2012;5(1):27–38.
48. Lameire NH. The pathophysiology of acute renal failure. Crit Care Med 2005;21:197–210.
49. Kellum JA. Acute kidney injury. Crit Care Med 2008;36(4):S141–5.
50. Persson PB, Tepel M. Contrast medium-induced nephropathy: the pathophysiology. Kidney Int Suppl 2006;100:S8–10.
51. Nash K, Hafeez A, Hou S. Hospital-acquired renal insufficiency. Am J Kidney Dis 2002;39:930–6.
52. Nainani N, Panesar M. Nephrogenic systemic fibrosis. Am J Nephrol 2009;29:1–9.
53. Barret BJ, Carlisle EJ. Meta-analysis of the relative nephrotoxicity of high and low-osmolality iodinated contrast media. Radiology 1993;188:171–8.
54. Brar SS, Shen AY, Jorgensen MB, et al. Sodium bicarbonate vs. sodium chloride for the prevention of contrast medium-induced nephropathy in patients in patients undergoing coronary angiography: a randomized trial. JAMA 2008;300:1038–46.
55. Tepel M, van der Giet M, Schwarzfeld C, et al. Prevention of radiographic-contrast-agent-induced reductions in renal function by acetylcysteine. N Engl J Med 2000;343:180–4.
56. Kelly AM, Dwamena B, Cronin P, et al. Meta-analysis: effectiveness of drugs for preventing contrast-induced nephropathy. Ann Intern Med 2008;148:284–94.
57. Dennen P, Douglas IS, Anderson R. Acute kidney injury in the intensive care unit: an update and primer for the intensivist. Crit Care Med 2010;38(1):261–75.
58. Finfer S, Bellomo R, Boyce N, et al. A comparison of albumin and saline for fluid resuscitation in the intensive care unit. N Engl J Med 2004;350:2247–56.

59. Wiedermann CJ. Systematic review of randomized clinical trials on the use of hydroxyethyl starch for fluid management in sepsis. BMC Emerg Med 2008;8:1.
60. Payen D, de Pont AC, Sakr Y, et al. A positive fluid balance is associated with a worse outcome in patients with acute renal failure. Crit Care 2008;12:R74.
61. Wiedemann HP, Wheeler AP, Bernard GR, et al. Comparison of two fluid-management strategies in acute lung injury. N Engl J Med 2006;354:2564–75.
62. Endre ZH, Walker RJ, Pickering JW, et al. Early intervention with erythropoietin does not affect the outcome of acute kidney injury (the EARLYARF trial). Kidney Int 2010;77:1020–30.
63. Patel N, Collino M, Yaqoob M, et al. Erythropoietin in the intensive care unit: beyond treatment of anemia. Ann Intensive Care 2011;1:40.
64. Venkataram R, Kellum JA. The role of diuretic agents in the management of acute renal failure. Contrib Nephrol 2001;158–70.
65. van Valenberg PL, Hoitsma AJ, Tiggeler RG, et al. Mannitol as an indispensable constituent of an intraoperative hydration protocol for the prevention of acute renal failure after renal cadaveric transplantation. Transplantation 1987;44:784–8.
66. Better OS, Rubinstein I. Management of shock and acute renal failure in casualties suffering from the crush syndrome. Ren Fail 1997;19:647–53.
67. Grams ME, Estrella MM, Coresh J, et al. Fluid balance, diuretic use, and mortality in acute kidney injury. Clin J Am Soc Nephrol 2011;6(5):966–73.
68. Sward K, Valsson F, Odencrants P, et al. Recombinant human atrial natriuretic peptide in ischemic acute renal failure: a randomized placebo-controlled trial. Crit Care Med 2004;32:1310–5.
69. Lewis J, Salem MM, Chertow GM, et al. Atrial natriuretic factor in oliguric acute renal failure. Anaritide acute renal failure study group. Am J Kidney Dis 2000; 36:767–74.
70. Meyer M, Pfarr E, Schirmer G, et al. Therapeutic use of the natriuretic peptide ularitide in acute renal failure. Ren Fail 1999;21:85–100.
71. Lauschke A, Teichgraber UK, Frei U, et al. 'Low-dose' dopamine worsens renal perfusion in patients with acute renal failure. Kidney Int 2006;69:1669–74.
72. Landoni G, Biondi-Zoccai GG, Tumlin JA, et al. Beneficial impact of fenoldopam in critically ill patients with or at risk for acute renal failure: a meta-analysis of randomized clinical trials. Am J Kidney Dis 2007;49(1):56–68.
73. Heemskerk S, Masereeuw R, Moesker O, et al. Alkaline phosphatase treatment improves renal function in severe sepsis or septic shock patients. Crit Care Med 2009;37(2):417–23.
74. Chi A, Lissauer ME, Kirchoffner J, et al. Effect of glycemic state on hospital mortality in critically ill surgical patients. Am Surg 2011;77(11):1483–9.
75. Schetz M, Vanhorebeek I, Wouters PJ, et al. Tight blood glucose control is reno-protective in critically ill patients. J Am Soc Nephrol 2008;19:571–8.
76. Finfer S, Chittock DR, Su SY, et al. Intensive vs. conventional glucose control in critically ill patients. N Engl J Med 2009;360:1283–97.
77. Pierson DJ. Respiratory considerations in the patient with renal failure. Respir Care 2006;51(4):413–22.
78. Uchino S, Kellum JA, Bellomo R, et al. Acute renal failure in critically ill patients: a multinational, multicenter study. JAMA 2005;294:813–8.
79. Bagshaw SM, Uchino S, Bellomo R, et al. Timing of renal replacement therapy and clinical outcomes in critically ill patients with severe acute kidney injury. J Crit Care 2009;24:129–40.
80. Palevsky PM, Zhang JH, O'Connor TZ, et al. Intensity of renal support in critically ill patients with acute kidney injury. N Engl J Med 2008;359:7–20.

81. Bagshaw SM, Berthiaume LR, Delaney A, et al. Continuous versus intermittent renal replacement therapy for critically ill patients with acute kidney injury: a meta-analysis. Crit Care Med 2008;36(2):610–7.

82. Molitch ME, Rodman E, Hirsch CA, et al. Spurious serum creatinine elevations in ketoacidosis. Ann Intern Med 1980;93(2):280.

83. Saah AJ, Koch TR, Drusano GL. Cefoxitin falsely elevates creatinine levels. JAMA 1982;247(2):205.

84. Mitchell EK. Flucytosine and false elevation of serum creatinine level. Ann Intern Med 1984;101(2):278.

85. Herrington D, Drusano GL, Smalls U, et al. False elevation in serum creatinine levels. JAMA 1984;252(21):2962.

Common Complications in the Critically Ill Patient

Kathleen B. To, MD, Lena M. Napolitano, MD*

KEYWORDS

- Venous thromboembolism • Ventilator-associated pneumonia
- Central line-associated bloodstream infection • Urinary tract infection
- Surgical site infection

KEY POINTS

- Critically ill patients in intensive care units (ICUs) are subject to many complications associated with the advanced therapy required for treatment of their serious illnesses.
- Many of these complications are health care-associated infections and are related to indwelling devices, including ventilator-associated pneumonia, central line-associated bloodstream infection, and catheter-associated urinary tract infection.
- Surgical site infection is also a common complication amongst surgical ICU patients.
- Venous thromboembolism, including deep venous thrombosis and pulmonary embolus, is another common complication in critically ill patients.
- All efforts should be undertaken to prevent these complications in surgical critical care, and national efforts are under way for each of these complications.

COMMON COMPLICATIONS IN THE CRITICALLY ILL PATIENT

Critically ill patients in intensive care units (ICUs) are subject to many complications associated with the advanced therapy required to treat their serious illnesses. Many complications are health care-associated infections (HAIs) related to indwelling devices. These complications include ventilator-associated pneumonia (VAP), central line-associated bloodstream infection (CLABSI), and catheter-associated urinary tract infection (CA-UTI). Surgical site infection (SSI) is also a common complication amongst surgical ICU (SICU) patients. Another common complication is venous thromboembolism (VTE), including deep venous thrombosis (DVT) and pulmonary embolus (PE). National efforts to prevent each of these complications are under

The authors have nothing to disclose.
Division of Acute Care Surgery [Trauma, Burns, Surgical Critical Care, Emergency Surgery], Department of Surgery, University of Michigan Health System, Ann Arbor, MI, USA
* Corresponding author. Room 1C340A-UH, University Hospital, 1500 East Medical Center Drive, Ann Arbor, MI 48109-5033.
E-mail address: lenan@umich.edu

Surg Clin N Am 92 (2012) 1519–1557
http://dx.doi.org/10.1016/j.suc.2012.08.018
0039-6109/12/$ – see front matter © 2012 Elsevier Inc. All rights reserved.

way. In this article, epidemiology, risk factors, diagnosis, treatment, and prevention of these complications in critically ill patients are discussed.

HAIS IN THE ICU

HAIs are a significant cause of morbidity and mortality in the United States, with 1.7 million reported in 2002, of which 417,946 (24.6%) were among adults and children in ICUs. The estimated deaths associated with HAIs in US hospitals were 98,987: of these, 35,967 were for pneumonia, 30,665 for bloodstream infections, 13,088 for urinary tract infections (UTIs), 8205 for SSIs, and 11,062 for infections of other sites.[1] National data regarding HAIs in US ICUs were initially reported by the Centers for Disease Control and Prevention (CDC) National Nosocomial Infections Surveillance (NNIS) system, and is currently reported by the National Healthcare Safety Network (NHSN). Similar to the NNIS system, NHSN facilities voluntarily report their HAI surveillance data for aggregation into a single national database, which provides national data regarding HAIs. The NHSN was established in 2005 to integrate and supersede 3 legacy surveillance systems at the CDC: the NNIS system, the Dialysis Surveillance Network, and the National Surveillance of Healthcare Workers. NHSN has both a patient safety and a healthcare personnel safety surveillance component. In the patient safety component, there is a device-associated module (**Fig. 1**). The device-associated module includes 4 separate options: CLABSI, VAP, CA-UTI, and dialysis incident (DI). DI is used only by chronic outpatient dialysis centers.

CLABSI
Epidemiology

ICU patients are at increased risk for CLABSI because 48% of ICU patients have indwelling central venous catheters (CVCs), accounting for 15 million central line

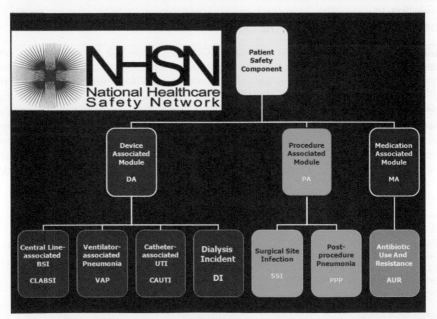

Fig. 1. The patient safety component of the NHSN of the CDC includes a device-associated module, including common HAIs in the ICU, including CLABSI, VAP, and CA-UTI.

days per year in US ICUs. CLABSIs are linked to mortality that ranges between 12% and 25% and result in increased ICU and hospital length of stay.

Risk Factors

The most significant risk factor for CLABSI is the presence of a CVC with duration of catheterization for more than 7 days.[2] Peripherally inserted CVCs (PICCs) are associated with a similar CLABSI rate compared with CVCs placed in the internal jugular or subclavian position.[3] PICCs are associated with an increased risk for upper extremity DVT.[4]

Diagnosis

The new CDC definition for CLABSI was published in 2008 (**Box 1**).[5] There are 3 potential routes of infection related to central lines: (1) extraluminal, from contiguous skin flora; (2) intraluminal, from contamination of the catheter hub and lumen or contamination of the infusate; and (3) hematogenous, from a distant unrelated site of infection (**Fig. 2**).

Treatment

Treatment principles for a CLABSI include removal of the infected device, and administration of empiric intravenous antimicrobials targeted against the likely causative bacterial pathogen and modified based on the final culture results. The Clinical Practice Guidelines for the Diagnosis and Management of Intravascular Catheter-Related Infection were updated in 2009. These guidelines review specific treatments based on pathogen identified, and whether complications (suppurative thrombophlebitis, endocarditis, osteomyelitis) are present (**Fig. 3**).[6] Significant changes have occurred in the microbiology of CLABSI in US hospitals (**Fig. 4**). Coagulase-negative staphylococci remain the most common CLABSI pathogen, but there has been a significant increase in *Candida* as causative pathogens and a significant reduction in *Staphylococcus*

Box 1
Laboratory-confirmed bloodstream infection (LCBI)

LCBI criteria 1 and 2 may be used for patients of any age, including patients ≤1 year of age.

LCBI must meet at least 1 of the following criteria:

1. Patient has a recognized pathogen cultured from 1 or more blood cultures

    and

    Organism cultured from blood is not related to an infection at another site.

2. Patient has at least 1 of the following signs or symptoms: fever (>38°C), chills, or hypotension

    and

    Signs and symptoms and positive laboratory results are not related to an infections at another site

    and

    Common skin contaminant (ie, diphtheroids [*Corynebacterium* spp], *Bacillus* [not *B anthracis*] spp, *Propionibacterium* spp, coagulase-negative staphylococci [including *Staphylococcus epidermidis*], viridians group streptococci [*Aerococcus* spp, *Micrococcus* spp]) cultured from 2 or more blood cultures drawn on separate occasions.

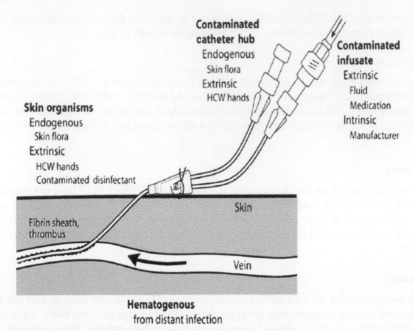

Fig. 2. Three potential routes of infection (CLABSI) related to central line use in critically ill patients.

aureus isolates (from 14.3% to 9.9% of all pathogens). Methicillin-resistant *S aureus* (MRSA) remains a common cause of CLABSI in US ICUs.

Prevention

Most CLABSI are preventable, and CLABSI prevention is important because the Center for Medicare and Medicaid Services (CMS) decided to disallow incremental payments associated with secondary conditions that it sees as preventable complications of medical care, including CLABSI, on October 1, 2008.[7] The state of Michigan Keystone Project, beginning in 2003, significantly reduced the incidence of CLABSIs (66% reduction) in 108 Michigan ICUs within 18 months, using 5 evidence-based procedures: hand washing; full-barrier precautions during CVC insertion; chlorhexidine skin preparation; avoidance of femoral site placement; and removal of unnecessary CVCs as soon as possible. This project was credited with saving 1500 lives and $200 million.[8] The Keystone Project implemented the Comprehensive Unit-Based Safety Program (CUSP), which has expanded to hospitals nationwide and to other settings beyond ICUs ("On the CUSP: Stop BSI"). This effort was funded in large part by the Agency for Healthcare Research and Quality as part of an action plan to reduce the incidence of HAIs.[9] A recent report by the CDC found that hospital ICUs decreased the number of CLABSI cases by more than half (58% reduction), from 43,000 in 2001 to 18,000 in 2009.[10] This decrease represents up to 6000 lives saved and $1.8 billion in cumulative excess health care costs saved since 2001.

What should we do to prevent CLABSIs? The Guidelines for Prevention of Intravascular Catheter-Related Infections[11,12] were recently updated in 2011, replacing the previous 2002 guidelines. Major areas of emphasis include (1) educating and training health care personnel who insert and maintain catheters; (2) using maximal sterile

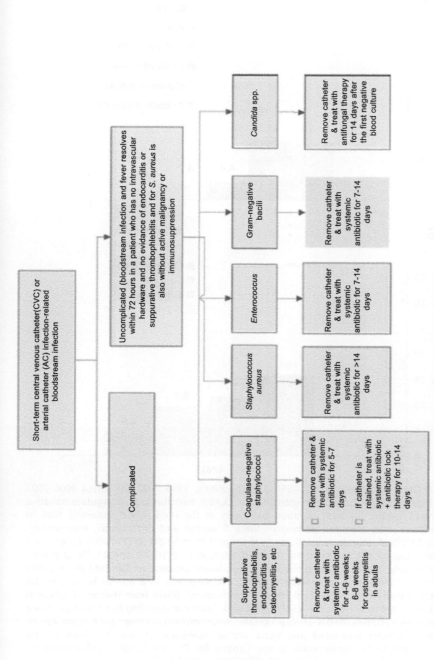

Fig. 3. Short-term CLABSI treatment includes removal of the CVC, adjustment of antimicrobial therapy based on the culture results, and variable duration of antimicrobial therapy based on the pathogen isolated and the clinical condition of the patient. (*From* Mermel LA, Allon M, Bouza E, et al. Clinical practice guidelines for the diagnosis and management of intravascular catheter-related infection: 2009 update by the Infectious Diseases Society of America. Clin Infect Dis 2009;49(1):1–45; with permission.)

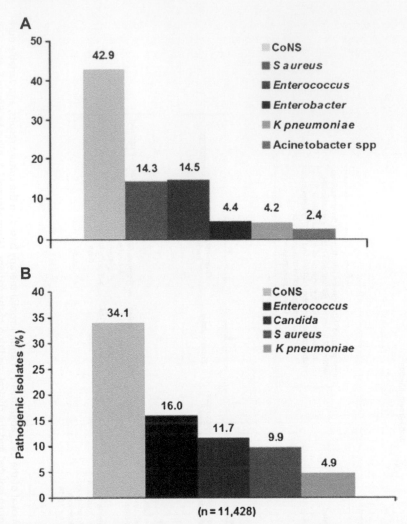

Fig. 4. Causative pathogens for CLABSI in US hospitals, 1986–2003 (*A*) versus 2006–2007 (*B*). Significant changes have been identified in CLABSI microbiology. Coagulase-negative *Staphylococci* remain the most common pathogen. In the NNIS report spanning 1986 to 2003, the next most common pathogens were *S aureus* and *Enterococci*, representing 14.3% and 14.5% of isolates, respectively. In the report from NHSN (2006–2007), *Enterococci* and *Candida* spp were the next most common, representing 16.0% and 11.7% of pathogens, respectively. These figures document a significant increase in *Candida* as causative pathogens for CLABSI and conversely, a significant reduction in *S aureus* isolates in the most recent period (from 14.3% to 9.9% of all pathogens). (*Data from* Hidron AI, Edwards JR, Patel J, et al. National Healthcare Safety Network Team Participating National Healthcare Safety Network Facilities. NHSN annual update: Antimicrobial-resistant pathogens associated with healthcare-associated infections: annual summary of data reported to the National Healthcare Safety Network at the Centers for Disease Control and Prevention, 2006–2007. Infect Control Hosp Epidemiol 2008;29:996–1011.)

barrier precautions (cap, mask, sterile gown, sterile gloves, sterile full-body drape) during CVC insertion; (3) using a greater than 0.5% chlorhexidine skin preparation with alcohol for antisepsis; and (4) avoiding routine replacement of CVCs as a strategy to prevent infection. The use of antiseptic-impregnated (chlorhexidine/silver sulfadia-zine) or antibiotic-impregnated (minocycline/rifampin) short-term CVCs[13] and chlorhexidine-impregnated sponge dressings[14] is recommended only if the CLABSI rate is not decreasing despite adherence to these initial strategies. These guidelines also emphasize performance improvement by documenting and reporting rates of compliance, with all components of the bundle as benchmarks for quality assurance and performance improvement. There has been a significant decline in ICU CLABSI rates in the United States (**Table 1**) related to prevention efforts.

VAP
Epidemiology

Hospital-acquired pneumonia (HAP) is the most common life-threatening HAI. Most are associated with mechanical ventilation (VAP), and associated with significant increases in length of ICU and hospital stay, mortality, and costs.[15] VAP is a potentially life-threatening complication in surgical critical care.[16] In a study of 554 critically ill trauma patients with VAP, patients with VAP alone had a case fatality rate of 12% versus a 26% case fatality rate in patients with concomitant bacteremia.[17] Reports from the NHSN document a recent decline in VAP rates related to the implementation of prevention strategies. However, the highest rates of VAP remain in SICUs, particularly in burn and trauma ICUs (**Table 2**).[18] VAP preventive strategies are therefore important to implement in all surgical patients.

Postoperative pneumonia incidence varies dependent on risk factors, ranging from an incidence of 1.5% to as high as 15.3% in high-risk groups. The 30-day postoperative mortality for all groups can be as high as 21%, dependent on the severity of illness, comorbidities, and causative pathogens.[19,20] In a study of 48,247 adults who underwent colectomy with data available in the American College of Surgeons National Surgical Quality Improvement Program (2005–2008), postoperative pneumonia was significantly more common in patients undergoing emergent versus elective surgery (11.1% vs 2.9%) and decreased in the overall cohort over time (4.60% in 2005 to 3.97% in 2008).[21]

Pathophysiology

Both HAP and VAP are caused by introducing bacteria into the sterile lower respiratory tract. The pathogenesis of the bacteria is exacerbated by impaired host defenses. This bacterial introduction occurs by 2 important mechanisms: (1) bacterial colonization of the aerodigestive tract and (2) aspiration of contaminated secretions into the lower airway.[22–25] Factors promoting the pathogenesis of VAP include the presence of invasive devices (endotracheal tube), medications altering gastric emptying and pH, and contaminated water, medications, and respiratory therapy equipment (**Fig. 5**).

VAP Clinical and Surveillance Definitions

Pneumonia is an acute infection of the pulmonary parenchyma. In 2005, the American Thoracic Society (ATS)/Infectious Diseases Society of America (IDSA) provided guidelines to further categorize pneumonia into HAP (pneumonia occurring >48 hours after hospital admission), VAP (pneumonia that develops 48 hours after endotracheal intubation), and health care-associated pneumonia (HCAP) (**Fig. 6**).[26] HCAP is pneumonia that occurs in a patient with health care contact as defined by 1 or more of the

Table 1
Decline in CLABSI rates per 1000 central line days in ICUs in the United States (NHSN)

Type of ICU	2004 Pooled Mean[a]	2006 Pooled Mean[b]	2007 Pooled Mean[c]	2008 Pooled Mean[d]	2009 Pooled Mean[e]	2010 Pooled Mean/50% Median[f]
Burn	7.0	6.8	5.6	5.5	5.3	3.5/2.2
Medical: major teaching	5.0	2.9	2.4	2.6	2.2	1.8/1.4
Medical: all other	–	–	–	1.9	1.6	1.3/0.7
Medical cardiac	3.5	2.8	2.1	2.0	1.7	1.3/0.9
Medical/surgical: major teaching	4.0	2.4	2.0	2.1	1.7	1.4/1.0
Medical/surgical: all other, ≤15 beds	3.2	2.2	1.5	1.5	1.4	1.1/0.0
Medical/surgical: all other, >15 beds	–	–	–	1.5	1.3	1.0/0.8
Neurologic	–	–	1.2	1.4	1.8	1.2/0.6
Neurosurgical	4.6	3.5	2.5	2.5	1.5	1.3/0.8
Pediatric cardiothoracic	–	–	–	3.3	2.5	2.1/1.7
Pediatric medical	–	–	1.0	1.3	2.6	1.9/1.9
Pediatric medical/surgical	6.6	5.3	2.9	3.0	2.2	1.8/1.4
Surgical: major teaching	4.6	2.7	2.3	2.3	1.8	1.4/1.0
Surgical: all other	–	–	–	–	–	1.0/0.6
Surgical cardiothoracic	2.7	1.6	1.4	1.4	1.2	0.9/0.6
Trauma	7.4	4.6	4.0	3.6	2.6	1.9/1.5

[a] NNIS System Report, data summary from January 1992 through June 2004, issued October 2004. Am J Infect Control 2004;32:470–485.

[b] Edwards JR, Peterson KD, Andrus ML, et al. National Healthcare Safety Network (NHSN) Report, data summary for 2006, issued June 2007. Am J Infect Control 2007;35:290–301.

[c] Edwards JR, Peterson KD, Andrus ML, et al. National Healthcare Safety Network (NHSN) Report, data summary for 2006 through 2007, issued November 2008. Am J Infect Control 2008;36:609–26.

[d] Edwards JR, Peterson KD, Mu Y, Banerjee S, Allen-Bridson K, Morrell G, Dudeck MA, Pollock DA, Horan TC. National Healthcare Safety Network (NHSN) report: data summary for 2006 through 2008, issued December 2009. Am J Infect Control 2009;37(10):783–805.

[e] Dudeck MA, Horan TC, Peterson KD, Allen-Bridson K, Morrell GC, Pollock DA, Edwards JR. National Healthcare Safety Network (NHSN) report, data summary for 2009, device-associated module. Am J Infect Control 2011;39(5):349–67.

[f] Dudeck MA, Horan TC, Peterson KD, Allen-Bridson K, Morrell G, Pollock DA, Edwards JR. National Healthcare Safety Network (NHSN) Report, data summary for 2010, device-associated module. Am J Infect Control 2011;39(10):798–816.

Table 2
Decline in VAP cases per 1000 ventilator days in ICUs in the United States. (Note higher VAP rates in surgical and neurosurgical ICUs and highest rates in burn and trauma ICUs.)

Type of ICU	2004 Pooled Mean[a]	2006 Pooled Mean[b]	2007 Pooled Mean[c]	2008 Pooled Mean[d]	2009 Pooled Mean[e]	2010 Pooled Mean/ 50% Median[f]
Burn	12.0	12.3	10.7	10.7	7.4	5.8/3.3
Medical: major teaching	4.9	3.1	2.5	2.4	1.9	1.4/1.0
Medical: all other	–	–	–	2.2	1.4	1.0/0.0
Medical carciac	4.4	2.8	2.5	2.1	1.5	1.3/0.0
Medical/surgical: major teaching	5.4	3.6	3.3	2.9	2.0	1.8/1.1
Medical/surgical: all other, ≤15 beds	5.1	2.7	2.3	2.2	1.4	1.2/0.0
Medical/surgical: all other, >15 beds	–	–	–	1.9	1.2	1.1/0.3
Neurologic	–	–	7.1	6.7	3.9	4.8/4.8
Neurosurgical	11.2	7.0	6.5	5.3	3.8	3.1/2.3
Pediatric cardiothoracic	–	–	–	0.6	0.7	0.7
Pediatric medical	–	–	–	2.3	0.9	1.1
Pediatric medical/surgical	2.9	2.5	2.1	1.8	1.1	1.2/0.0
Surgical: ma,or teaching	9.3	5.2	5.3	4.9	3.8	3.5/1.7
Surgical: all other	–	–	–	–	–	2.5/1.2
Surgical carciothoracic	7.2	5.7	4.7	3.9	2.1	1.6/0.4
Trauma	15.2	10.2	9.3	8.1	6.5	6.0/5.3

[a] NNIS System Report, data summary from January 1992 through June 2004, issued October 2004. Am J Infect Control 2004;32:470–485.
[b] Edwards JR, Peterson KD, Andrus ML, et al. NHSN Facilities. National Healthcare Safety Network (NHSN) Report, data summary for 2006, issued June 2007. Am J Infect Control 2007;35:290–301.
[c] Edwards JR, Peterson KD, Andrus ML, et al. National Healthcare Safety Network Facilities. National Healthcare Safety Network (NHSN) Report, data summary for 2006 through 2007, issued November 2008. Am J Infect Control 2008;36:609–26. Erratum in: Am J Infect Control 2009;37:425.
[d] Edwards JR, Peterson KD, Mu Y, Banerjee S, Allen-Bridson K, Morrell G, Dudeck MA, Pollock DA, Horan TC. National Healthcare Safety Network (NHSN) report: data summary for 2006 through 2008, issued December 2009. Am J Infect Control 2009;37(10):783–805.
[e] Dudeck MA, Horan TC, Peterson KD, Allen-Bridson K, Morrell GC, Pollock DA, Edwards JR. National Healthcare Safety Network (NHSN) report, data summary for 2009, device-associated module. Am J Infect Control 2011;39(5):349–67.
[f] Dudeck MA, Horan TC, Peterson KD, Allen-Bridson K, Morrell G, Pollock DA, Edwards JR. National Healthcare Safety Network (NHSN) Report, data summary for 2010, device-associated module. Am J Infect Control 2011;39(10):798–816.

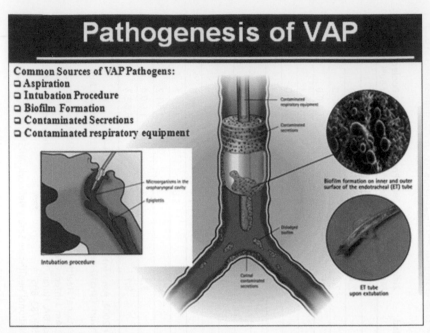

Fig. 5. Pathway of colonization of airway in VAP.

following criteria: a patient hospitalized for 2 days or more in an acute care facility within 90 days of infection; a patient residing in a nursing home or long-term care facility; a patient who has attended a hospital or hemodialysis center; a patient who has received intravenous antibiotic therapy, chemotherapy, or wound care within

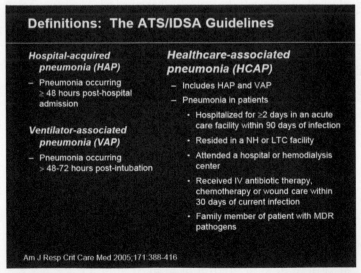

Fig. 6. ATS/IDSA Guideline: pneumonia definitions. (*Data from* American Thoracic Society. Guidelines for the management of adults with hospital-acquired, ventilator-associated, and healthcare-associated pneumonia. Am J Respir Crit Care Med 2005;171(4):388–416.)

30 days of the current infection; and any patient who is a family member of a patient with a multidrug-resistant (MDR) pathogen.

The CDC NHSN VAP definition for surveillance (last updated in 2002) uses a combination of radiologic, clinical, and laboratory criteria in patients who are ventilated for greater than 48 hours. Three components make up the current pneumonia (PNEU) definitions: an "X-ray" component (required), a "Signs and symptoms" component (required), and a "Laboratory" component (optional). Pneumonia is characterized into 3 types including clinically defined pneumonia (PNEU-1), common bacterial, fungal, or atypical pneumonia (PNEU-2), and pneumonia in immunocompromised patients (PNEU-3) (**Fig. 7**). The diagnosis requires new or progressive and persistent infiltrate/consolidation/cavitation on 2 or more serial chest radiographs. In addition, it must meet minimum criteria in 2 separate clinical categories (**Fig. 8**) and minimum criteria in laboratory categories (**Fig. 9**).

The CDC has recommended a significant change to VAP surveillance in the United States. A VAP Surveillance Definition Working Group was convened in September 2011 by the CDC's Division of Healthcare Quality Promotion in collaboration with the CDC Prevention Epicenters, the Critical Care Societies Collaborative (http://ccsconline.org), other professional societies, subject matter experts, and federal partners. There is currently no gold-standard, valid, reliable definition for VAP. Therefore, the Working Group pursued a different approach: development of a surveillance definition algorithm for detection of ventilator-associated events (VAEs). This algorithm detects a broad range of conditions or complications occurring in mechanically ventilated adult patients. The Working Group focused on definition criteria that use objective, clinical data expected to be readily available across the spectrum of mechanically ventilated patients. These criteria are less likely to be influenced by variability in resources, subjectivity, and clinical practices and are potentially amenable to electronic data capture. The proposed algorithm to detect VAEs in adult patients serves a surveillance function and is not designed for use in the clinical care of patients.[27]

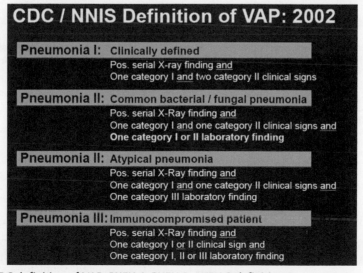

Fig. 7. CDC definition of VAP: PNEU-1, PNEU-2, PNEU-3 definitions.

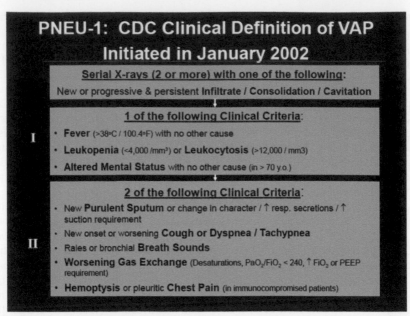

Fig. 8. CDC clinical definition of VAP for PNEU-1.

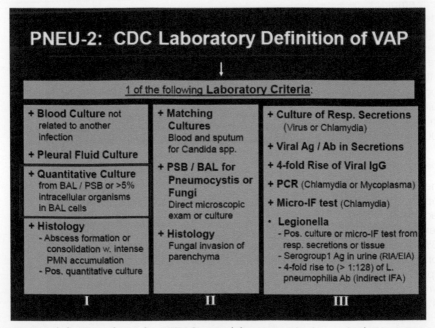

Fig. 9. CDC definition of VAP for PNEU-2 - one laboratory criteria required.

Diagnosis

The diagnosis of VAP is difficult because the clinical findings are nonspecific and the differential diagnosis can be broad.[28] When findings at autopsy are used as a reference, the combination of radiographic infiltrate plus 2 of 3 clinical features (fever >38°C, leukocytosis/leukopenia, purulent secretions) resulted in 69% sensitivity and 75% specificity for pneumonia.[29] Only 43% of patients with radiographic evidence of infiltrate were found to have VAP by postmortem examination.[30]

When VAP is suspected, we recommend diagnostic lower respiratory tract sampling for microscopic evaluation and quantitative culture, which can be performed with flexible bronchoscopy (bronchoalveolar lavage [BAL]) or without bronchoscopy (mini-BAL) with similar safety and diagnostic accuracy.[31] In patients with left lower lobe infiltrates and possible VAP, bronchoscopic BAL is preferred to obtain a sample from this area, because mini-BAL sampling catheters most commonly advance into the right lower lobe bronchus. Bronchoscopic sampling is not associated with improved mortality, or reduced duration of ventilation or ICU or hospital length of stay. However, it does influence antibiotic selection and de-escalation of antibiotics.[32]

Given the severity of VAP and the frequency of serious conditions that can mimic VAP, additional tests that provide further evidence for VAP are clearly warranted.[33] At present, no sensitive and specific biomarker is currently available to confirm a VAP diagnosis. C-reactive protein, procalcitonin, and soluble triggering receptor expressed on myeloid cells (sTREM-1, a member of the immunoglobulin superfamily whose expression on phagocytes is specifically upregulated by microbial products) have been evaluated as biomarkers for diagnosing VAP. Multiple studies have confirmed that C-reactive protein and procalcitonin have poor diagnostic value for VAP.[34–36] Additional studies have confirmed conflicting results for sTREM-1.[37–40]

Treatment

Early empiric broad-spectrum antimicrobial therapy for VAP should be initiated, ideally after obtaining lower respiratory tract quantitative cultures. An assessment of clinical response and cultures over the next 48 hours is imperative. If there is clinical improvement and culture results are negative, consider stopping antibiotics. If culture results are positive, consider de-escalating or narrowing the antibiotics based on sensitivities. If there is no clinical response, consider searching for other causes. If cultures are negative, assess for other pathogens, complications, or other sources of infection. If cultures are positive, adjust antibiotic therapy and search for other sources as well. An algorithm for diagnosis and treatment of pneumonia provided by the ATS/IDSA 2005 guidelines is shown in **Fig. 10**.

Specific Antibiotic Treatment

The initiation of early, appropriate empiric antibiotics to treat VAP significantly improves patient survival.[41] The microbiology of VAP has changed over the past decade (**Fig. 11**). For years (1992–1999), S aureus and Pseudomonas aeruginosa were the 2 leading causative pathogens for VAP, each representing approximately 18% of all isolates. Enterobacter spp and Klebsiella pneumoniae were less common, comprising 12% and 7% of VAP isolates, respectively.[42,43] The most recent NHSN report (2006–2007) for VAP confirms a significant change in VAP pathogens.[44] S aureus is now the leading VAP pathogen, representing 24.4% of all isolates, with 54.4% confirmed as MRSA, making MRSA the leading VAP pathogen. In the 2007 EPIC II point-prevalence study of infection in critically ill patients performed on May 8, 2007, MRSA infection in ICU patients was independently associated with an almost

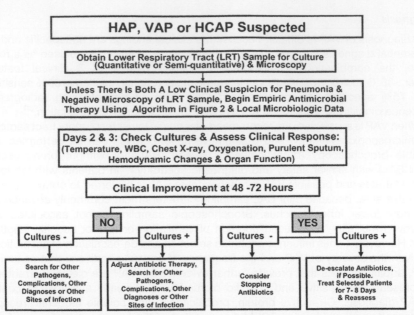

Fig. 10. Algorithm for diagnosis and treatment of suspected HAP, VAP, or HCAP. (*Reprinted with permission of* the American Thoracic Society. Copyright © 2012 American Thoracic Society. American Thoracic Society. Guidelines for the management of adults with hospital acquired, ventilator-associated, and healthcare-associated pneumonia. Am J Respir Crit Care Med 2005;171(4):388–416. Official journal of the American Thoracic Society. This document was published in 2005 and is currently in revision. Certain aspects of this document may be out of date and caution should be used when applying it to patient care.)

50% higher likelihood of hospital death compared with methicillin-sensitive *S aureus* (MSSA) infection, and the most common site of infection was the respiratory system.[45] *Pseudomonas aeruginosa* decreased from 18% to 16.3% and *Enterobacter* decreased from 12% to 8.4%. *Acinetobacter baumanii* is now the third most common VAP pathogen, comprising 8.4% of all VAP isolates. This MDR pathogen is difficult to eradicate, and is a significant issue for infection control. Empiric antibiotics for VAP should cover these potential causative pathogens, and knowledge of the local ICU antibiogram is important in antibiotic choice.[46]

Necrotizing pneumonias are an increasing problem and are associated with a higher mortality in our critically ill patients. Pathogens associated with necrotizing pneumonia include *Pseudomonas* and MRSA. Concurrent with the emergence of community-associated MRSA (CA-MRSA), there are increasing reports of community-acquired necrotizing pneumonia in young healthy patients, some after a viral prodrome and influenza infection.[47,48] In the most recent report from the CDC of 51 cases of *S aureus* community-acquired pneumonia, median age was 16 years and 44% had no underlying comorbidities. Influenza was confirmed in 33% of the cohort, and 91% of these patients died. MRSA was confirmed in 37 of the 51 patients and 48% died. Empiric coverage for MRSA pneumonia was provided in only 43% of these patients.[49]

Concomitant use of antibiotics that suppress toxin production is advocated for the treatment of severe and invasive CA-MRSA infections, including pneumonia. The rationale for their use in CA-MRSA pneumonia includes (1) the presumed role of the Panton-Valentine leukocidin (PVL) toxin, a staphylococcal toxin known to be associated with tissue necrosis,[50] and (2) the high morbidity and mortality observed.

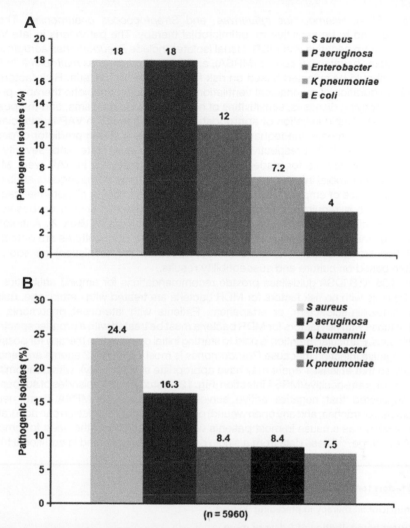

Fig. 11. Causative pathogens for VAP in US hospitals. (*A*)1992–1999 versus (*B*) 2006–2007 NHSN Report. *S aureus* increased from 18% to 24.4%. MRSA is now the leading causative pathogen, comprising 54.4% of all *S aureus* isolates. Note higher rate of *Acinetobacter* in 2006–2007. (*Data from* Hidron AI, Edwards JR, Patel J, et al. National Healthcare Safety Network Team Participating National Healthcare Safety Network Facilities. NHSN annual update: Antimicrobial-resistant pathogens associated with healthcare-associated infections: annual summary of data reported to the National Healthcare Safety Network at the Centers for Disease Control and Prevention, 2006–2007. Infect Control Hosp Epidemiol 2008;29:996–1011.)

Some therefore advocate treatment with agents that suppress toxin production (clindamycin, linezolid) and urge the avoidance of agents (ie, β-lactams) that can lead to increased production of PVL and other exotoxins in patients with MRSA pneumonia.[51]

The choice of antibiotic treatment in VAP depends on the microorganism isolated. These organisms differ based on duration of mechanical ventilation. Patients who develop VAP early (<4 days of mechanical ventilation) have different isolates than those who develop VAP later (>4 days).[22] The usual pathogens in early VAP are *S* aureus (MSSA), *Haemophilus influenzae*, and *Streptococcus pneumoniae*. These pathogens tend to be sensitive to antimicrobial therapy. The pathogens in late VAP tend to be gram negative and MDR. Usual isolates include *Pseudomonas aeruginosa*, *Acinetobacter baumanii*, *S aureus* (MRSA), and *Stenotrophomonas maltophilia*.[52] The antibiotic should be selected based on risk factors for MDR bacteria. Risk factors in addition to duration of mechanical ventilation include recent antibiotic therapy, presence of underlying diseases, sensitivities of hospital or ICU organisms, and the possibility of HCAP. Rapid initiation of appropriate antibiotic therapy in VAP is associated with improved outcome. Inadequate antibiotic therapy is a strong predictor of death in patients with VAP, irrespective of underlying disease state and severity of illness.[53–56] Risk factors for inadequate antimicrobial treatment in VAP were MDR bacteria, polymicrobial infection, and late-onset VAP.[57] To avoid inadequate antibiotic therapy, early use of empiric broad-spectrum antibiotics to cover all potential causative pathogens is required. Empiric antibiotics for pneumonia should be based on national guidelines and with consideration of local antibiograms (**Box 2**). Antibiotics are started when a clinical diagnosis is made immediately after cultures are obtained. Antibiotics are modified to a more narrow spectrum (de-escalation) as soon as possible based on culture and susceptibility results.

The 2005 ATS/IDSA guidelines provide recommendations for empiric antibiotics for VAP. Patients with no risk factors for MDR bacteria are treated with ceftriaxone, quinolones, ampicillin-sulbactam, or ertapenem. Patients with late-onset pneumonia (>5 days) or those with risk factors for MDR bacteria must be treated with a broader spectrum of antibiotics. Particular attention is paid to starting initial combination therapy for possible gram-negative infection (because *Pseudomonas* is most common, 2 agents are recommended so that at least 1 agent may have appropriate susceptibility), with concomitant coverage of gram-positive/MRSA infection (**Fig. 12**). A study of 924 episodes of suspected VAP suggested that negative active surveillance cultures for MRSA (from nares, oropharynx, or trachea, and any open wound) performed on ICU admission can accurately exclude MRSA as a cause in most patients with VAP, decreasing the need for empiric MRSA coverage.[58] These data from a single center must be validated in additional trials.

Box 2
Risk factors for MDR pathogens causing HAP, HCAP, and VAP

- Antimicrobial therapy in preceding 90 days
- Current hospitalization of 5 days or more
- High frequency of antibiotic resistance in the community or in the specific hospital unit
- Presence of risk factors for HCAP:

    Hospitalization for 2 days or more in the preceding 90 days

    Residence in a nursing home or extended care facility

    Home infusion therapy (including antibiotics)

    Chronic dialysis within 30 days

    Home wound care

    Family member with MDR pathogen
- Immunosuppressive disease or therapy

Data from American Thoracic Society. Guidelines for the management of adults with hospital-acquired, ventilator-associated, and health care-associated pneumonia. Am J Respir Crit Care Med 2005;171(4):388–416.

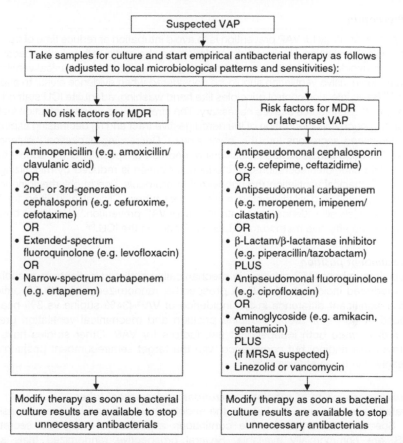

Fig. 12. Initial empiric antibiotic therapy for HAP, VAP, and HCAP with risk for MDR pathogens. (*Data from* American Thoracic Society. Guidelines for the management of adults with hospital-acquired, ventilator-associated, and healthcare-associated pneumonia. Am J Respir Crit Care Med 2005;171(4):388–416.)

Duration of Antibiotics for VAP

A landmark prospective, randomized multicenter trial compared 8 versus 15 days of antibiotic treatment of VAP in 401 patients in 51 ICUs.[59] No difference in 30-day mortality was identified (18.8% vs 17.2%) and no differences in ventilator-free days, organ failure-free days, length of ICU stay and 60-day mortality were identified. However, there was a higher recurrence of infection rate for nonfermenting gram-negative bacilli, including *Pseudomonas aeruginosa*. In addition, more MDR pathogens appeared in the 15-day treatment group (42% vs 62%, *P* = .038). Based on the results of this study, optimal duration of therapy for VAP should be 8 days, except in those isolates that are nonfermenting gram-negative bacilli, including *Pseudomonas aeruginosa* and *Acinetobacter* species, for which longer duration of antimicrobial therapy is recommended.

However, the duration of antimicrobial therapy for VAP caused by MRSA needs additional evaluation, because the studies that evaluated treatment duration included an insufficient number of MRSA-infected patients. Most clinicians provide a minimum of 14 days of therapy for MRSA pneumonia, and if there is concomitant bacteremia, more prolonged antibiotic therapy may be required. Duration of antimicrobial therapy should be assessed according to each patient's clinical course as well.

VAP Prevention

The foremost strategy for VAP prevention is to avoid intubation or reduce time of duration of mechanical ventilation. Noninvasive ventilation may be particularly valuable because it can lead to avoidance of intubation or shortening the duration of mechanical ventilation, therefore noninvasive ventilation should be considered when evidence exists to support its use.[60] Basic infection control principles like hand washing, adequate ICU staff education, and optimal resource use are necessary. The strategies to prevent infection include (1) reducing bacterial colonization of the aerodigestive tract and (2) decreasing aspiration of contaminated secretions into the lower airway. Decreasing aspiration incidence is achieved through semirecumbent positioning, and use of specialty endotracheal tubes that aspirate subglottic secretions. Bacterial colonization is reduced by minimizing the days on mechanical ventilation through weaning protocols, use of chlorhexidine in the posterior pharynx and silver-coated endotracheal tubes. Clinical guidelines for VAP prevention review all evidence-based strategies for VAP prevention.[61] Ventilator bundles are used as an effective method to reduce VAP rates in the ICU.[62]

Semirecumbent position

The semirecumbent (45°) position in mechanically ventilated patients is associated with a reduced incidence of VAP. A prospective randomized trial with 86 patients found a significant difference in the incidence of VAP (34% supine vs 3% head of the bead at 45°, $P = .003$).[63] Supine position and mechanical ventilation greater than 7 days were both independent risk factors for VAP. Other studies have not confirmed this finding, but compliance with the target semirecumbent position was not reached in these studies.[64,65]

Continuous aspiration of subglottic secretions endotracheal tubes

Aspirated secretions may pool above the endotracheal cuff and increase the risk for VAP. Specialty tubes that provide continuous aspiration of subglottic secretions (CASS) are commercially available. Several prospective randomized trials show a decreased VAP rate of VAP with CASS endotracheal tubes. A meta-analysis of 5 studies with 896 patients showed a reduction of VAP by nearly half (relative risk [RR] = 0.51), and delayed the onset of VAP by 6.8 days and reduced ICU length of stay by 3 days. Despite these beneficial outcomes, no improvement in mortality was identified. A study in cardiac surgical patients (n = 714) also confirmed a significant VAP reduction with use of the CASS tube.[66] The CASS tube is ideal for patients who are expected to require mechanical ventilation greater than 72 hours, but this may be difficult to predict.[67] Management of CASS tubes requires particular attention to detail for maintenance, frequent monitoring, and their use is associated with increased cost.[68]

Chlorhexidine gluconate

One strategy to reduce bacterial colonization of the aerodigestive tract is the use of oral chlorhexidine gluconate (0.12%). One trial in cardiac surgical patients documented a significant decrease in the incidence of nosocomial pneumonia and mortality.[69] A prospective, randomized, double-blind, placebo-controlled, multicenter trial also confirmed a significant reduction in VAP with use of chlorhexidine.[70] A meta-analysis of similar trials concluded that the use of chlorhexidine was associated with a 26% RR reduction in VAP.[71] In addition, it has also been shown that use of chlorhexidine in combination with protocol-driven weaning from mechanical ventilation reduces the incidence of VAP in SICU patients.[72] The addition of manual toothbrushing to chlorhexidine oral care does not help to prevent VAP.[73,74]

Silver-coated endotracheal tube
Another strategy to reduce bacterial colonization is the use of silver-coated endotracheal tubes. Silver prevents biofilm formation, delays airway colonization, has bactericidal activity, and reduces bacterial burden. The North American Silver-Coated Endotracheal Tube (NASCENT) randomized single-blind multicenter phase III trial enrolled 2003 patients expected to require mechanical ventilation for more than 24 hours. The primary outcome measure was VAP (defined as BAL >10^4 CFU/mL). Use of the silver-coated endotracheal tube was associated with a significant VAP reduction (4.8% vs 7.5%, RR 36%) and was associated with a significant delay in time to VAP.[75]

Spontaneous awakening and breathing trials
Prolonged mechanical ventilation is a risk factor for VAP, which increases by 1% to 3% with each day of mechanical ventilation.[76] The use of a weaning protocol, a sedation protocol, or both has been shown to reduce the duration of mechanical ventilation.[77] The Awakening and Breathing Controlled (ABC) trial enrolled 336 patients requiring mechanical ventilation at 4 tertiary care hospitals. The group was divided into an intervention group (n = 168), who received daily spontaneous awakening trials (SATs) and spontaneous breathing trials (SBTs), and a control group (n-168), who received sedation and usual care with SBTs. The study found a significant difference in 1-year mortality between the control and intervention group (58% vs 44%, *P* = .01). Routine use of SAT and SBT should be standard in all mechanically ventilated patients.

Selective decontamination
Selective decontamination of the digestive tract and oropharynx are strategies aimed at preventing colonization with virulent bacteria. The spectrum of studies includes oral administration of antibiotics via nasogastric tubes and intravenous administration for up to 4 days.[78] Several studies have shown modest benefit in pneumonia rate and mortality.[79,80] However, this modality has not been used widely in the United States because of significant concern about potential emergence of MDR bacteria.[81]

Tracheostomy
Previous studies have suggested that tracheostomy was superior to prolonged intubation for VAP prevention,[82] but 2 recent large, prospective, randomized clinical trials have found no difference in VAP or any other outcomes measures comparing early (6–8 days) versus late (13–15 days) tracheostomy in 419 patients[83] or comparing early (4 days) versus late (after 10 days) in 909 patients in the TracMan trial.[84] Thus, early tracheostomy should not be performed for VAP prevention, but may be considered for other reasons, such as patient comfort and airway protection, as in patients with severe traumatic brain injury.

CA-UTI
Epidemiology

UTIs are the most common HAI in acute care hospitals in the United States, and account for approximately 23% of nosocomial infections in the ICU; of these, 97% are CA-UTI.[85] Each year, there are more than 500,000 cases of CA-UTIs in the United States, accounting for 30% or more of HAIs.[86] Although not directly linked with mortality, CA-UTIs are associated with approximately 20% of hospital-acquired bacteremia, which in turn has a mortality of 10%.[87]

Risk Factors

The most important risk factors for the development of a CA-UTI are the presence and duration of a urinary catheter. The incidence of catheter-associated bacteriuria

(CA bacteriuria) is 3% to 8% per day of indwelling catheter.[88,89] Urinary catheters are used in 15% to 25% of all hospitalized patients, and 5% to 10% of nursing home residents. Often these catheters are placed for inappropriate indications and are not removed in a timely fashion. In 1 survey of US hospitals, more than 50% of physicians did not monitor which patients were catheterized and more than 75% did not monitor the durations or discontinuation of indwelling catheters.[90] This situation leads to increased risk for bacteriuria. Other risk factors include female gender, obesity, immunodeficiency, and length of stay in an ICU.[91]

Diagnosis

The CDC distinguishes between symptomatic UTI (SUTI) and asymptomatic bacteriuria (ASB) according to defined criteria listed in **Box 3** and **Table 3**.[92] Patients with SUTI have 1 or more of the following symptoms: fever, rigors, altered mental status, malaise, or lethargy with no other identified cause, flank pain, costovertebral angle tenderness, acute hematuria, pelvic discomfort, dysuria, urgency or frequency of urination, suprapubic pain or tenderness, or in the case of patients with spinal cord injury, increased spasticity, autonomic dysreflexia, or sense of unease. UTIs are considered CA-UTI if the patient has an indwelling urethral or suprapubic catheter, undergoes intermittent self-catheterization (ISC), or had removal within the last 48 hours or less of a urethral, suprapubic, or condom catheter. By contrast, catheter-associated ASB (CA-ASB) is defined as the presence of 10^5 cfu/mL or more of 1 or more bacterial species in a single catheter urine specimen in a patient without UTI symptoms. Pyuria is not a distinguishing factor between CA-UTI and CA-ASB, and should not be used as an indication for antimicrobial therapy.

Treatment

Patients with indwelling catheters should not undergo routine screening and treatment of ASB, with the exception of pregnant women and patients who undergo urologic procedures for which visible mucosal bleeding is anticipated. Women who have had short-term indwelling catheters with persistent CA-ASB for 48 hours or more after catheter removal may be considered for antimicrobial treatment; data are insufficient to make recommendations in men. Urine cultures should be obtained before initiating antimicrobial therapy for presumed CA-UTI and tailored to specific organisms based on culture results. For indwelling catheters present for 2 weeks or more, catheter replacement may hasten resolution of symptoms. If the catheter can be removed, then a midstream voided urine specimen should be obtained for urine culture before initiation of antimicrobial treatment. Length of treatment should be tailored to specific clinical scenarios. In women 65 years old or younger without upper urinary tract symptoms, a 3-day regimen should be sufficient. In patients who are not severely ill and have CA-UTI, 5 to 7 days of antimicrobial coverage is recommended for prompt resolution of symptoms; 10 to 14 days of treatment is recommended for patients with delayed resolution of symptoms.

Prevention

Effective from January 1, 2012, the Joint Commission's Board of Commissioners approved a new National Patient Safety Goal regarding CA-UTIs for hospitals in the United States (**Table 4**).[93,94] These goals reflect the guidelines set forth by the IDSA for the diagnosis, prevention, and treatment of CA-UTIs. As to be expected, the best prevention is limiting catheter use to only clear indications (**Box 4**), with prompt catheter removal as soon as it is no longer necessary. Condom catheters may be considered in men who have minimal postvoid residual volume, but there are insufficient data to suggest that these decrease UTI rates compared with indwelling catheters.

Box 3
Definitions of CA-UTI (SUTI and ASB) in adults under the NNIS system and the NHSN through December 2008

Catheter-associated SUTI must meet at least 1 of the following 2 criteria:

1. Criterion 1:

   a. Patient has had an indwelling urinary catheter within 7 days before the culture; and

   b. Patient has at least 1 of the following signs or symptoms with no other recognized cause: fever (temperature, >38°C), urgency, frequency, dysuria, or suprapubic tenderness; and

   c. Patient has a positive urine culture result (ie, $\geq 10^5$ microorganisms/mL of urine with no more than 2 species of microorganisms).

2. Criterion 2:

   a. Patient has had an indwelling urinary catheter within 7 days before the culture; and

   b. Patient has at least 2 of the following signs or symptoms with no other recognized cause: fever (temperature, >38°C), urgency, frequency, dysuria, or suprapubic tenderness; and

   c. Patient has at least 1 of the following:

      i. Positive dipstick result for leukocyte esterase or nitrate;

      ii. Pyuria (urine specimen with ≥ 10 WBCs/mm^3 or $3\geq$ WBCs/high-power field of unspun urine);

      iii. Organisms seen on Gram stain of unspun urine;

      iv. At least 2 urine cultures with repeated isolation of the same uropathogen (gram-negative bacteria or *Staphylococcus saprophyticus*) with $\geq 10^2$ colonies/mL in nonvoided specimens;

      v. Concentration of $\leq 10^5$ colonies/mL for a single uropathogen (gram-negative bacteria or *S saprophyticus*) in a patient being treated with an effective antimicrobial agent for a UTI;

      vi. Physician diagnosis of a UTI;

      vii. Physician institutes appropriate therapy for a UTI.

CA-ASB must meet the following criteria:

1. Patient has had an indwelling urinary catheter within 7 days before the culture; and

2. Patient has a positive urine culture result (ie, $\geq 10^5$ microorganisms/mL of urine with no more than 2 species of microorganisms); and

3. Patient has no fever (temperature, >38°C), urgency, frequency, dysuria, or suprapubic tenderness.

Abbreviation: WBC, white blood cell.

Data from Burton DC, Edwards JR, Srinivasan A, et al. Trends in catheter-associated urinary tract infections in adult ICUs-United States, 1990-2007. Infect Control Hosp Epidemiol 2011;32(8):748–56. PubMed PMID: 21768755.

ISC should be considered an alternative to indwelling catheters to reduce CA-UTI. There are fewer associated complications to ISC compared with indwelling Foley catheters, and some advantages include fewer instances of CA-ASB, pyelonephritis, epididymitis, periurethral abscess, urethral stricture, vesicoureteral reflux, hydronephrosis, bladder and renal calculi, bladder cancer, and autonomic dysreflexia. A recent Cochrane review of randomized and quasirandomized trials

Table 3	
Risk factors for development of CA-UTI, symptomatic versus asymptomatic	
SUTI	**Bacteriuria**
Prolonged catheterization[a]	Disconnection of drainage system[a]
Female sex[b]	Lower professional training of inserter[a]
Older age[b]	Placement of catheter outside the operating room[b]
Impaired immunity[b]	Incontinence[b]
	Diabetes
	Meatal colonization
	Renal dysfunction
	Orthopedic/neurology services

[a] Main modifiable risk factors.
[b] Also inform recommendations.
Available at: http://www.cdc.gov/HAI/pdfs/toolkits/CAUTItoolkit_3_10.pdf.

comparing indwelling Foley catheters versus ISC for surgical patients with short-term bladder drainage (defined as ≤14 days' duration) found that there were significantly more cases of CA-ASB in the indwelling Foley catheter group (RR, 2.90; 95% confidence interval, 1.44–5.84).[95]

Table 4	
Performance measures approved by the Joint Commission on Accreditation of Healthcare Organizations as a National Patient Safety Goal (NPSG) for 2012	
Requirement	**Level of Evidence**
EP2: Insert indwelling urinary catheters according to established evidence-based guidelines that address the following:	
Limiting use and duration to situations necessary for patient care	A-II
Using aseptic techniques for site preparation, equipment, and supplies	A-III
EP3: Manage indwelling urinary catheters according to established evidence-based guidelines that address the following:	
Securing catheters for unobstructed urine flow and drainage	A-III
Maintaining the sterility of the urine collection system	A-I
Replacing the urine collection system when required	B-III
Collecting urine samples	A-III
EP4: Measure and monitor CA-UTI prevention processes and outcomes in high-volume areas by doing the following:	
Selecting measures using evidence-based guidelines or best practices	A-II or B-II for all
Monitoring compliance with evidence-based guidelines or best practices	
Evaluating the effectiveness of prevention efforts	
Note: Surveillance may be targeted to areas with a high volume of patients using indwelling catheters. High-volume areas are identified through the hospital's risk assessment as required in IC.01.03.01, EP 2	B-III

NPSG.07.06.01: Implement evidence-based practices to prevent indwelling CAUTI.[a]
   Note: This NPSG is not applicable to pediatric populations. Research resulting in evidence-based practices was conducted with adults, and there is not consensus that these practices apply to children.
   [a] Evidence-based guidelines for CA-UTI are located at: Compendium of Strategies to Prevent Healthcare-Associated Infections in Acute Care Hospitals at, http://www.shea-online.org/about/compendium.cfm Guideline for Prevention of Catheter-associated Urinary Tract Infections, 2009 at http://www.cdc.gov/hicpac/cauti/001_cauti.html.
   Available at: http://www.jointcommission.org/assets/1/18/r3_report_issue_2_9_22_11_final.pdf.

Box 4

Examples of appropriate and inappropriate indications for indwelling urethral catheter use (Note: these indications are based primarily on expert consensus)

Examples of appropriate indications for indwelling urethral catheter use

Patient has acute urinary retention or bladder outlet obstruction

Need for accurate measurements of urinary output in critically ill patients

Perioperative use for selected surgical procedures:

Patients undergoing urologic surgery or other surgery on contiguous structures of the genitourinary tract

Anticipated prolonged duration of surgery (catheters inserted for this reason should be removed in postanesthesia care unit)

Patients anticipated to receive large-volume infusions or diuretics during surgery

Need for intraoperative monitoring of urinary output

To assist in healing of open sacral or perineal wounds in incontinent patients

Patient requires prolonged immobilization (eg, potentially unstable thoracic or lumbar spine, multiple traumatic injuries such as pelvic fractures)

To improve comfort for end-of-life care if needed

Examples of inappropriate uses of indwelling catheters

As a substitute for nursing care of the patient or resident with incontinence

As a means of obtaining urine for culture or other diagnostic tests when the patient can voluntarily void

For prolonged postoperative duration without appropriate indications (eg, structural repair of urethra or contiguous structures, prolonged effect of epidural anesthesia)

Equipment

For intermittent catheterization, clean (nonsterile) technique may be considered with no difference in risk of CA-ASB or CA-UTI. However, indwelling urethral catheters should be inserted using aseptic (sterile) technique and with sterile equipment. Current data do not support the routine use of coated hydrophilic versus uncoated catheters, and further studies need to be conducted before any conclusion can be made.[96] A closed catheter drainage system with ports in the distal catheter for needle aspiration should be used and institution-specific strategies developed to ensure that disconnection of the catheter junction is minimized. The drainage bag is always kept below the level of the bladder. Preconnected Foley insertion systems may be considered but no data exist that this reduces CA-UTI. However, use of complex closed drainage system or application of tape at the catheter–drainage tube junction is not recommended.

Systems approach

Unit-wide and hospital-wide policies may be useful in infection prevention. More than 56% of hospitals do not have a system in place for monitoring patients with Foley catheters, and 74% do not monitor duration of catheterization. Shortened duration of catheterization via nursing directed interventions and bundling of catheter care have been shown to decrease rates of CA-UTI.[86,97,98]

Medical adjuncts and prophylaxis

Although there is some evidence that cranberry products and extracts decrease SUTIs in young women with recurrent UTIs, there is no clear evidence to recommend the generalized use of cranberry extracts and products for prevention of CA-UTIs.[99] Likewise, methenamine salts may be considered for the reduction of CA-ASB and CA-UTI in patients after gynecologic surgery who have an indwelling urinary catheter for 1 week or less; however, methenamine salts should not be used routinely for patients with long-term intermittent or indwelling Foley catheters. If methenamine salts are used, the urinary pH should be 6.0 or less, but there are insufficient data to recommend how best to achieve that pH goal. Systemic antimicrobials should not be used for routine prophylaxis because of the increased risk for selecting out antimicrobial-resistant organisms. Likewise, prophylactic antibiotics for either catheter placement or removal are not recommended for reduction of CA bacteriuria.

Catheter care

Reduction of urethral meatal colonization, a source for ascending bacterial infection, seems to be an excellent target for reduction of CA-UTIs. However, large randomized controlled trials do not support benefit to daily meatal cleaning with povidone-iodine solution, silver sulfadiazine, polyantibiotic ointment or cream, or soap and water. Irrigation of catheters with antimicrobial solutions may reduce CA-ASB in select patient populations, but its routine use is not recommended. There is insufficient evidence for routine catheter change in patients with functional long-term indwelling Foley catheters.

Summary: CA-UTIs

CA-UTIs are one of the most common health care–associated infections and can result in significant morbidity and prolongation of hospital stay. Critically ill patients tend to have a higher proportion of CA-ASB and CA-UTIs. It is important to recognize the indications for indwelling urinary catheters, and to remove them promptly once the indications are no longer valid. Proper catheter care and nursing bundles can reduce the incidence for CA-UTIs.

SSI

Epidemiology

SSI is a common infection in surgical patients, occurring in about 3% of all surgical procedures and in up to 20% of patients undergoing emergency intra-abdominal procedures. SICU patients can be particularly prone to this HAI. Severe skin and soft tissue infections, including those related to SSI, frequently require management in the ICU, in part related to associated septic shock or toxic shock syndrome or associated organ failure.[100] Beginning in 2012, hospitals participating in the CMS Inpatient Prospective Payment System will be required to report SSI data through NHSN, and these data will be included in the Inpatient Quality Reporting data, which are publicly reported by CMS at the Hospital Compare Web site.[101]

Risk Factors

SSI risk is strongly associated with wound classification, being low for the clean (class 1) and clean-contaminated (class 2, defined as gastrointestinal or genitourinary tract entered in a controlled manner) incisions and high for the contaminated (class 3, defined as open traumatic wounds, infected urine or bile, gross spillage from the gastrointestinal tract) and dirty-infected (class 4) incisions. Traditionally, SSI rates calculated by the CDC and NHSN have been risk-stratified using a risk index (NHSN Risk Index) of 3 equally weighted factors: the American Society of Anesthesiologists score, wound classification, and procedure duration.[102] However, for some procedures, these variables are not associated with SSI risk, are not equally important in the risk they confer, and are candidates for replacement by other, more important risk factor variables that should be taken into account. A set of new risk models was recently developed using existing data elements collected through NHSN, was associated with improved predictive performance, and will update the NHSN SSI risk index.[103] Laparoscopic surgery is associated with decreased SSI risk.

Diagnosis

SSI is categorized into superficial incisional, deep incisional, and organ/space SSI (intra-abdominal abscess or empyema, **Fig. 13**).[104] SSI rates should be followed for 30 days postoperatively, and for 1 year postoperatively in patients with implants.

Treatment

There are 4 fundamental management principles that are key to a successful outcome in caring for patients with severe skin infections, including SSI[105]:

1. Early diagnosis and differentiation of necrotizing versus nonnecrotizing skin infection, including SSI

2. Early initiation of appropriate empiric broad-spectrum antimicrobial therapy, including anti-MRSA antibiotics, and consideration of risk factors for specific pathogens

3. Source control (ie, early aggressive surgical intervention for drainage of abscesses and debridement of necrotizing soft tissue infections)

4. Pathogen identification and appropriate de-escalation of antimicrobial therapy

Antimicrobial therapy is an essential element for skin infections. The choice of antimicrobial agent for empiric treatment of SSI should be guided by the site and type of infection, but in critically ill patients should include empiric parenteral anti-MRSA antimicrobial therapy.[106] Guidelines for the antimicrobial treatment of complicated skin

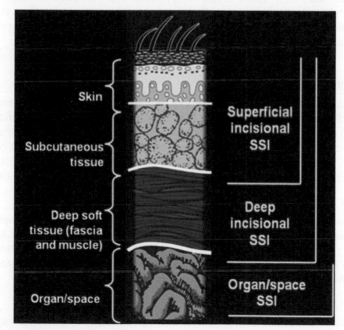

Fig. 13. SSI classification by the CDC.

infections provide comprehensive recommendations regarding antimicrobials.[107,108] The most common causative pathogens in SSI are gram-positive pathogens, with *S aureus* as the most common SSI pathogen, with increasing rates of MRSA. In abdominal procedures, SSIs are caused roughly equally by gram-positive and gram-negative organisms. In transplant recipients, *Enterococci* are the most commonly isolated pathogens, and fungal SSIs are more common.

Prevention

The Surgical Care Improvement Project (SCIP) was created in 2003 as a collaborative effort to reduce morbidity and mortality in surgical patients. The SCIP-INF quality measures are focused on SSI prevention and listed below.

INF-1	Prophylactic antibiotics received within 1 hour before surgical incision (2 hours if receiving vancomycin)
INF-2	Prophylactic antibiotic selection: patient received appropriate recommended antibiotic for their specific surgical procedure
INF-3	Prophylactic antibiotics are discontinued within 24 hours after surgery end time (48 hours for cardiac surgery patients)
INF-4	Cardiac surgery patients with controlled 6 AM postoperative blood glucose level (≤200 mg/dL)
INF-6	Surgery patients with appropriate surgical site hair removal (clippers or depilatory or those not requiring surgical site hair removal)

Antimicrobial prophylaxis for SSI prevention is the most important component of the SCIP-INF measures. For an antibiotic to be effective prophylaxis for SSI, it should (1) cover the most likely pathogens that cause SSI for the particular procedure; (2) be administered such that tissue levels of antibiotic are sufficient to have antibiotic activity at the time of incision; and (3) carry minimal risk to the patient in terms of cost and side effects. SCIP provides a list of approved antibiotics for surgical procedures annually.

VTE
Epidemiology

VTE remains one of the most common preventable causes of in-hospital mortality. In the United States, approximately 600,000 cases of symptomatic VTE and 300,000 VTE-related deaths occur annually.[109] Two-thirds of these cases occur in hospitalized patients, and critically ill patients are at the highest risk for developing DVT or PE. The incidence of DVT can range from 28% to 32% in mixed medical-surgical ICU patients to as high as 60% in trauma patients or 70% in acute ischemic stroke patients.[110]

Risk Factors

The Virchow triad describes the 3 fundamental risks factors for development of VTE: venous stasis, endothelial injury, and hypercoagulable state. Clinical risk factors for VTE in ICU patients are common (**Table 5**).[111] We use the Caprini Risk Assessment Model as a tool to quantify an individual's risk for VTE, and guide decision making regarding the appropriate VTE prophylaxis regimen (**Fig. 14**).[112]

Diagnosis

SICU patients with suspected DVT should undergo venous duplex compression ultrasonography (CUS) of the 4 extremities as the best diagnostic test. D-dimer assay has

Table 5 ICU acquired risk factors for development of VTE	
General Medical Risk Factors	**ICU Acquired Risk Factors**
Advanced age	Immobilization
Malignancy	Stroke
Recent surgery	Trauma
Previous VTE	Mechanical ventilation
Pregnancy	Invasive procedures/tests
Obesity	CVCs
Oral contraceptives	Sepsis
Nephrotic syndrome	Heart failure
Inherited or acquired hemophilia	Vasopressor use
Inflammatory bowel disease	Cardiopulmonary failure

Data from Chan CM, Shorr AF. Venous thromboembolic disease in the intensive care unit. Semin Respir Crit Care Med 2010;31(1):39–46. PMID: 20101544.

a high sensitivity (98%) and modest specificity (50%), so is useful for excluding DVT but not useful for confirming diagnosis. It should not be used in surgical patients, pregnant women, or patients who have cancer. If CUS is positive, anticoagulation treatment should be initiated without performing any additional studies. However, if the initial CUS is negative, a follow-up CUS should be repeated at 1 week; 2 negative CUS scans rule out DVT (**Fig. 15**). In patients for whom CUS is not feasible or nondiagnostic, computed tomography (CT) venography or magnetic resonance venography may be useful for diagnosis. In the case of isolated distal DVT, serial testing is recommended to rule out proximal extension. Patients who have suspected recurrence of DVT on the ipsilateral extremity should undergo CUS as an initial diagnostic modality; however, if the CUS is abnormal but nondiagnostic, further evaluation should be performed with venography. Pregnant patients with symptoms of DVT should be evaluated with CUS, followed by duplex ultrasonography of the iliac vein if CUS is negative.[113] Patients with suspicion for upper extremity DVT should be initially evaluated with Doppler CUS. If clinical suspicion is high, but initial ultrasonography is negative for DVT, further evaluation with moderate or highly sensitive D-dimer, serial ultrasonography, or venography is necessary. In ICU patients with possible PE, CT pulmonary angiography is indicated.

Treatment

Choice of therapy

Patients diagnosed with acute proximal DVT should be initiated on parenteral anticoagulation therapy; options are low-molecular-weight heparin (LMWH), fondaparinux, intravenous unfractionated heparin (IV-UFH). If the clinical suspicion is high, or if there is a delay of more than 4 hours to obtaining diagnostic test results, it is recommended that anticoagulation therapy be initiated empirically; however, if the clinical index of suspicion is low, then anticoagulation therapy should be withheld until diagnostic test results are available. Isolated DVT of the distal lower extremity veins generally does not require anticoagulation therapy unless there is development of extension on follow-up CUS (over 2 weeks) or if the patient has severe symptoms or risk factors for clot extension.[114]

Dosing

LMWH or fondaparinux is preferred over IV-UFH and subcutaneous (SC) UFH. In acute episodes of VTEs, treatment with once-daily dosing of LMWH is preferred

Deep Vein Thrombosis (DVT)
Prophylaxis Orders
(For use in Elective General Surgery Patients)

Thrombosis Risk Factor Assessment
(Choose all that apply)

BIRTHDATE
NAME
CPI No.
SEX M F VISIT No. ____________

Each Risk Factor Represents 1 Point

- ☐ Age 41-60 years
- ☐ Swollen legs (current)
- ☐ Varicose veins
- ☐ Obesity (BMI >25)
- ☐ Minor surgery planned
- ☐ Sepsis (<1 month)
- ☐ Acute myocardial infarction
- ☐ Congestive heart failure (<1 month)
- ☐ Medical patient currently at bed rest
- ☐ History of inflammatory bowel disease
- ☐ History of prior major surgery (<1 month)
- ☐ Abnormal pulmonary function (COPD)
- ☐ Serious Lung disease including pneumonia (<1 month)
- ☐ Oral contraceptives or hormone replacement therapy
- ☐ Pregnancy or postpartum (<1 month)
- ☐ History of unexplained stillborn infant, recurrent spontaneous abortion (≥ 3), premature birth with toxemia or growth-restricted infant
- ☐ Other risk factors____________

Subtotal:

Each Risk Factor Represents 2 Points

- ☐ Age 61-74 years
- ☐ Arthroscopic surgery
- ☐ Malignancy (present or previous)
- ☐ Laparoscopic surgery (>45 minutes)
- ☐ Patient confined to bed (>72 hours)
- ☐ Immobilizing plaster cast (<1 month)
- ☐ Central venous access
- ☐ Major surgery (>45 minutes)

Subtotal:

Each Risk Factor Represents 3 Points

- ☐ Age 75 years or older
- ☐ History of DVT/PE
- ☐ Positive Factor V Leiden
- ☐ Family History of thrombosis*
- ☐ Positive Prothrombin 20210A
- ☐ Positive Lupus anticoagulant
- ☐ Elevated serum homocysteine
- ☐ Heparin-induced thrombocytopenia (HIT) (Do not use heparin or any low molecular weight heparin)
- ☐ Elevated anticardiolipin antibodies
- ☐ Other congenital or acquired thrombophilia

If yes: Type____________
* most frequently missed risk factor

Subtotal:

Each Risk Factor Represents 5 Points

- ☐ Stroke (<1 month)
- ☐ Multiple trauma (<1 month)
- ☐ Elective major lower extremity arthroplasty
- ☐ Hip, pelvis or leg fracture (<1 month)
- ☐ Acute spinal cord injury (paralysis) (<1 month)

Subtotal:

TOTAL RISK FACTOR SCORE:

FACTORS ASSOCIATED WITH INCREASED BLEEDING
Patient may not be a candidate for anticoagulant therapy & SCDs should be considered.
Active Bleed, Ingestion of Oral Anticoagulants, Administration of glycoprotein IIb/IIIa inhibitors, History of heparin induced thrombocytopenia

CLINICAL CONSIDERATIONS FOR THE USE OF SEQUENTIAL COMPRESSION DEVICES (SCD)
Patient may not be a candidate for SCDs & alternative prophylactic measures should be considered.
Patients with Severe Peripheral Arterial Disease, CHF, Acute Superficial DVT

Total Risk Factor Score	Risk Level	Incidence of DVT	Prophylaxis Regimen
0-1	Low Risk	2%	☐ Early ambulation
2	Moderate Risk	10-20%	Choose the following medication OR compression devices: ☐ Sequential Compression Device (SCD) ☐ Heparin 5000 units SQ BID
3-4	Higher Risk	20-40%	Choose ONE of the following medications +/- compression devices: ☐ Sequential Compression Device (SCD) ☐ Heparin 5000 units SQ TID ☐ Enoxaparin/Lovenox: ☐ 40mg SQ daily (WT < 150kg, CrCl > 30mL/min) ☐ 30mg SQ daily (WT < 150kg, CrCl = 10-29mL/min) ☐ 30mg SQ BID (WT > 150kg, CrCl > 30mL/min) (Please refer to Dosing Guidelines on the back of this form)
5 or more	Highest Risk	40-80%	Choose ONE of the following medications PLUS compression devices: ☐ Sequential Compression Device (SCD) ☐ Heparin 5000 units SQ TID (Preferred with Epidurals) ☐ Enoxaparin/Lovenox (Preferred): ☐ 40mg SQ daily (WT < 150kg, CrCl > 30mL/min) ☐ 30mg SQ daily (WT < 150kg, CrCl = 10-29mL/min) ☐ 30mg SQ BID (WT > 150kg, CrCl > 30mL/min) (Please refer to Dosing Guidelines on the back of this form)

- ☐ Ambulatory Surgery - No orders for venous thromboembolic prophylaxis required
- ☐ VTE Prophylaxis Contraindicated, Reason: ____________

Joseph A. Caprini, MD, MS, FACS, RVT
VTE Risk Factor Assessment Tool

Physician Signature	Dr. #	Date	Time
Processed By:	Date/Time:		

White-Medical Record Yellow-MIS Pink-Pharmacy | University of Michigan Health System | DVT Prophylaxis Regimen

Fig. 14. Caprini VTE risk assessment tool to determine appropriate VTE prophylaxis. University of Michigan DVT prophylaxis orders using the Caprini Risk Assessment Model to guide (1) patient risk stratification for development of VTE, and (2) selection of appropriate DVT prophylaxis regimen.

over twice-daily dosing. Local considerations such as cost, availability, and familiarity of use dictate the choice between fondaparinux and LMWH. Patients placed on IV-UFH should have an initial bolus of 80 units/kg followed by initial drip rate at 18 units/kg/h (bolus 70 units/kg followed by 15 units/kg/h for cardiac or stroke patients); alternatively patients may be placed on fixed initial bolus dose of 5000 units followed by 1000 units/h. Patients with renal insufficiency (creatinine clearance <20 mL/min) should receive reduced doses of LMWH. Conversely, in morbidly obese patients with VTE and weight greater than 100 kg, fondaparinux dosing should be increased

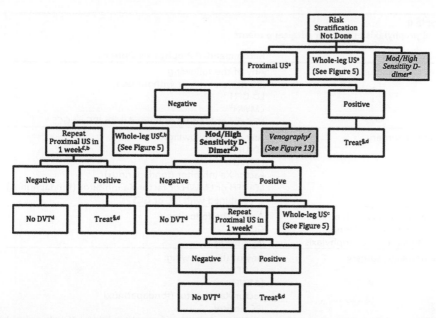

Fig. 15. Recommendations for evaluation of suspected first lower extremity DVT: risk stratification not performed. (*From* Bates SM, Jaeschke R, Stevens SM, et al. American College of Chest Physicians. Diagnosis of DVT: antithrombotic therapy and prevention of thrombosis, 9th ed: American College of Chest Physicians Evidence-Based Clinical Practice Guidelines. Chest 2012;141(Suppl 2):e395S; with permission.)

from the usual dose of 7.5 mg to 10 mg daily. In the absence of a need for rapid anticoagulation reversal, vitamin K antagonist (VKA) therapy, such as warfarin, should be started on day 1 or 2 of parenteral anticoagulation therapy. Parenteral anticoagulation should be continued for a minimum of 5 days and the international normalized ratio INR is 2.0 or more. The goal therapeutic range is an INR of 2.0 to 3.0 (target INR of 2.5). In patients who have an acute proximal DVT of the leg but have contraindications to anticoagulation, placement of an inferior venal cava filter is recommended, with subsequent initiation of anticoagulation once bleeding risk is resolved.[115]

Duration

Patients with a first episode of VTE (DVT or PE) should be treated for 3 months. If the VTE was unprovoked (ie, no risk factors), continuation of therapy may be reassessed after 3 months. Patients with recurrent VTE and who have a low bleeding risk should undergo extended anticoagulation therapy. VKAs are recommended in most patients with DVT; however, patients with VTE and cancer should be treated with LMWH. Compression stockings are recommended as adjunct treatment of patients with acute DVT.[116]

PE

In patients who have PEs without associated hypotension, the treatment algorithm is similar to DVT treatment. However, patients who have PE with associated hypotension should undergo (in order of preference) thrombolytic therapy, catheter-assisted thrombolectomy, or surgical pulmonary embolectomy.

Table 6
VTE prophylaxis option for surgical patients

Surgery Type	Recommended Prophylaxis Options[a]
Intracranial neurosurgery	Any of the following: IPC devices with or without GCS LD-UFH LMWH[b] LD-UFH or LMWH[b] combined with IPC or GCS
General surgery	Any of the following: LD-UFH LMWH Factor Xa inhibitor (fondaparinux) LD-UFH or LMWH or factor Xa inhibitor (fondaparinux) combined with IPC or GCS
General surgery with a reason for not administering pharmacologic prophylaxis	Any of the following: GCS IPC devices
Gynecologic surgery	Any of the following: LD-UFH LMWH Factor Xa inhibitor (fondaparinux) IPC devices LD-UFH or LMWH or factor Xa inhibitor (fondaparinux) combined with IPC or GCS
Urologic surgery	Any of the following: LD-UFH LMWH Factor Xa inhibitor (fondaparinux) IPC devices GCS LD-UFH or LMWH or factor Xa inhibitor (fondaparinux) combined with IPC or GCS
Elective total hip replacement	Any of the following started within 24 h of surgery: LMWH Factor Xa inhibitor (fondaparinux) Warfarin
Elective total knee replacement	Any of die following: LMWH Factor Xa inhibitor (fondaparinux) Warfarin IPC devices VFP
Hip fracture surgery	Any of the following: LD-UFH LMWH Factor Xa inhibitor (fondaparinux) Warfarin
Elective total hip replacement with a reason for not administering pharmacologic prophylaxis	Any of the following: IPC devices VFP

(continued on next page)

Table 6 (*continued*)	
Surgery Type	**Recommended Prophylaxis Options**[a]
Hip fracture surgery with a reason for not administering pharmacologic prophylaxis	Any of the following: GCS IPC devices VFP
Specifications Manual for National Hospital Impatient Quality Measures Discharges 04-01-11 (2Q11) through 12-31-11 (4Q11)	

Abbreviations: GCS, graduated compression stockings; VFP, venous foot pump.
[a] Patients who receive neuraxial anesthesia or have a documented reason for not administering pharmacologic prophylaxis may pass the performance measure if either appropriate pharmacologic or mechanical prophylaxis is ordered.
[b] Current guidelines recommend postoperative LMWH for intracranial neurosurgery.

Upper extremity DVT

In general, upper extremity DVTs are treated in the same manner as lower extremity DVTs. The development of a UE DVT associated with CVCs does not mandate catheter removal if it is still functional and there is an ongoing need for central venous access. If the catheter remains indwelling for longer than 3 months, then anticoagulation therapy should be extended.

Table 7 Recommendations for thromboprophylaxis in various risk groups		
	Risk and Consequences of Major Bleeding Complications	
Risk of Symptomatic VTE	**Average Risk (~1%)**	**High Risk (~2%) or Severe Consequences**
Very low (<0.5%)	No specific prophylaxis	
Low (~1.5%)	Mechanical prophylaxis, preferably with IPC	
Moderate (~3.0%)	LD-UFH, LMWH, or mechanical prophylaxis, with IPC	Mechanical prophylaxis, preferably with IPC
High (~6.0%)	LD-UFH or LMWH plus mechanical prophylaxis with ES or IPC	Mechanical prophylaxis, preferably with IPC, until risk of bleeding diminishes and pharmacologic prophylaxis can be added
High-risk cancer surgery	LD-UFH or LMWH plus mechanical prophylaxis with ES or IPC and extended-duration prophylaxis with LMWH after discharge	Mechanical prophylaxis, preferably with IPC, until risk of bleeding diminishes and pharmacologic prophylaxis can be added
High risk, LDUH and LMWH contraindicated or not available	Fondaparinux or low-dose aspirin (160 mg); mechanical prophylaxis, preferably with IPC; or both	Mechanical prophylaxis, preferably with IPC, until risk of bleeding diminishes and pharmacologic prophylaxis can be added

See **Table 5** for details about risk stratification for VTE.
Abbreviation: ES, elastic stockings.
Data from Gould MK, Garcia DA, Wren SM, et al; American College of Chest Physicians. Prevention of VTE in nonorthopedic surgical patients: antithrombotic therapy and prevention of thrombosis, 9th ed: American College of Chest Physicians Evidence-Based Clinical Practice Guidelines. Chest 2012;141(Suppl 2):e227S–77S. PMID: 22315263.

Special considerations

Patients with symptomatic thrombosis of hepatic or splanchnic veins (eg, portal, mesenteric, or splenic veins) should be treated with anticoagulation; however, asymptomatic patients should not be treated.

Reversal of Anticoagulation

In patients who require cessation of anticoagulation for anticipated major surgery or interventional procedure, VKAs should be stopped 5 days before surgery, and resumption of VKAs 12 to 24 hours after procedure and adequate hemostasis. Patients with mechanical heart valve, atrial fibrillation, or VTE at high risk for a thromboembolic event, bridging anticoagulation with a parenteral agent is advised; low-risk patients do not require bridging anticoagulation therapy. Patients who are on therapeutic SC-LMWH should have their anticoagulation stopped 24 hours before major surgery/intervention. Patients undergoing surgery with a high risk of bleeding should not resume anticoagulation therapy until 48 to 72 hours postoperatively.[117] In patients who are on VKAs and have an acute bleeding episode requiring reversal, 4-factor prothrombin complex concentrate (PCC) is the recommended treatment. In addition, patients should receive slow IV injection of vitamin K 5 to 10 mg.

Prevention

Patients who are critically ill are at high risk for development of VTE. ICU patients should receive pharmacologic thromboprophylaxis (either LMWH or low-dose UFH [LD-YFH]) in addition to mechanical prophylaxis with intermittent pneumatic compression (IPC) devices. Perioperative prophylaxis options for patients undergoing surgery are summarized in **Table 6**. In patients with high bleeding risk, mechanical prophylaxis with IPC is sufficient until bleeding risk decreases, at which point they should also receive chemoprophylaxis (**Table 7**).

Summary: VTE

VTE is a source of major morbidity and mortality in hospitalized patients. Critically ill patients represent a population who are at increased risk for VTE and should receive appropriate VTE prophylaxis. Routine screening for DVT is not recommended. However, in patients for whom there is a high index of suspicion, duplex CUS is a good screening modality. Treatment should be initiated for proximal VTE events, initially with parenteral anticoagulation; VKAs should be used once the patient no longer has bleeding risk. PCC is the recommended treatment of VKA-related bleeding.

SUMMARY

Critically ill patients in ICUs are subject to many complications associated with the advanced therapy required for treatment of their serious illnesses. Many of these complications are HAIs and are related to indwelling devices. These complications include VAP, CLABSI, and CA-UTI. SSI is also a common complication amongst SICU patients. VTE, including DVT and PE, is another common complication in critically ill patients. All efforts should be undertaken to prevent these complications in surgical critical care, and national efforts are under way for each of these complications.

REFERENCES

1. Klevens RM, Edwards JR, Richards CL Jr, et al. Estimating health care-associated infections and deaths in U.S. hospitals, 2002. Public Health Rep 2007;122(2):160–6.

2. Darouiche RO, Raad II, Heard SO, et al. A comparison of two antimicrobial-impregnated central venous catheters. Catheter Study Group. N Engl J Med 1999;340(1):1–8.
3. Safdar N, Maki DG. Risk of catheter-related bloodstream infection with peripherally inserted central venous catheters used in hospitalized patients. Chest 2005; 128(2):489–95.
4. Liem TK, Yanit KE, Moseley SE, et al. Peripherally inserted central catheter usage patterns and associated symptomatic upper extremity venous thrombosis. J Vasc Surg 2012;55(3):761–7.
5. Horan TC, Andrus M, Dudeck MA. CDC/NHSN surveillance definition of healthcare-associated infection and criteria for specific types of infections in the acute care setting. Am J Infect Control 2008;36:309–32.
6. Mermel LA, Allon M, Bouza E, et al. Clinical practice guidelines for the diagnosis and management of intravascular catheter-related infection: 2009 update by the Infectious Diseases Society of America. Clin Infect Dis 2009;49:1–45.
7. Rosenthal MB. Nonpayment for performance? Medicare's new reimbursement rule. N Engl J Med 2007;357(6):1573–5.
8. Pronovost P, Needham D, Berenholtz S, et al. An intervention to decrease catheter-related bloodstream infections in the ICU. N Engl J Med 2006;355: 2725–32.
9. Clancy CM. Progress on a national patient safety imperative to eliminate CLABSI. Am J Med Qual 2012;27(2):170–1.
10. Centers for Disease Control and Prevention. Vital signs: central line-associated blood stream infections–United States, 2001, 2008, 2009. MMWR Morb Mortal Wkly Rep 2011;60:243–8.
11. O'Grady NP, Alexander M, Burns LA, et al, Healthcare Infection Control Practices Advisory Committee. Guidelines for the prevention of intravascular catheter-related infections. Am J Infect Control 2011;39(4 Suppl 1):S1–34.
12. O'Grady NP, Alexander M, Burns LA, et al, Healthcare Infection Control Practices Advisory Committee (HICPAC). Guidelines for the prevention of intravascular catheter-related infections. Clin Infect Dis 2011;52(9):e162–93.
13. Casey AL, Mermel LA, Nightingale P, et al. Antimicrobial central venous catheters in adults: a systematic review and meta-analysis. Lancet Infect Dis 2008;8:763–76.
14. Timsit JF, Schwebel C, Bouadma L, et al, Dressing Study Group. Chlorhexidine-impregnated sponges and less frequent dressing changes for prevention of catheter-related infections in critically ill adults: a randomized controlled trial. JAMA 2009;301(12):1231–41.
15. Restrepo MI, Anzueto A, Arroliga AC, et al. Economic burden of ventilator-associated pneumonia based on total resource utilization. Infect Control Hosp Epidemiol 2010;31(5):509–15.
16. Magnotti LJ, Croce MA, Fabian TC. Is ventilator-associated pneumonia in trauma patients an epiphenomenon or a cause of death? Surg Infect (Larchmt) 2004;5(3):237–42.
17. O'Keefe GE, Caldwell E, Cuschieri J, et al. Ventilator-associated pneumonia: bacteremia and death after traumatic injury. J Trauma Acute Care Surg 2012; 72(3):713–9.
18. Napolitano LM. Perspectives in surgical infections: what does the future hold? [review]. Surg Infect (Larchmt) 2010;11(2):111–23.
19. Arozullah AM, Khuri SF, Henderson WG, et al. Development and validation of a multifactorial risk index for predicting postoperative pneumonia after major noncardiac surgery. Ann Intern Med 2001;135(10):847–57.

20. Napolitano LM. Use of severity scoring and stratification factors in clinical trials of hospital-acquired and ventilator-associated pneumonia. Clin Infect Dis 2010; 51(Suppl 1):S67–80.

21. Ozhathil DK, Li Y, Smith JK, et al. Colectomy performance improvement within NSQIP 2005-2008. J Surg Res 2011;171(1):e9–13.

22. Hubmayr RD, Burchardi H, Elliot M, et al. Statement of the 4th International Consensus Conference in Critical Care on ICU-Acquired Pneumonia–Chicago, Illinois, May 2002. Intensive Care Med 2002;28:1521.

23. Johanson WG, Pierce AK, Sanford JP. Changing pharyngeal bacterial flora of hospitalized patients: emergence of gram-negative bacilli. N Engl J Med 1969;281:1137.

24. de Jonge E, Schultz MJ, Spanjaard L, et al. Effects of selective decontamination of digestive tract on mortality and acquisition of resistant bacteria in intensive care: a randomized controlled trial. Ann Intern Med 2003;362:1011.

25. Adair CG, Gorman SP, Feron BM, et al. Implications of endotracheal tube biofilm for ventilator-associated pneumonia. Intensive Care Med 1999;25:1072.

26. American Thoracic Society, Infectious Diseases Society of America. Guidelines for the management of adults with hospital-acquired, ventilator-associated, and healthcare-associated pneumonia. Am J Respir Crit Care Med 2005;171(4): 388–416.

27. Available at: http://www.cdc.gov/nhsn/PDFs/vae/CDC_VAE_Communications Summary-for-compliance_20120313.pdf. Accessed April 20, 2012.

28. Meduri GU. Diagnosis and differential diagnosis of ventilator-associated pneumonia. Clin Chest Med 1995;16:61.

29. Fàbregas N, Ewig S, Torres A, et al. Clinical diagnosis of ventilator associated pneumonia revisited: comparative validation using immediate post-mortem lung biopsies. Thorax 1999;54:867.

30. Wunderink RG, Woldenberg LS, Zeiss J, et al. The radiologic diagnosis of autopsy-proven ventilator-associated pneumonia. Chest 1992;101:458.

31. Kollef MH, Bock KR, Richards RD, et al. The safety and diagnostic accuracy of minibronchoalveolar lavage in patients with suspected ventilator-associated pneumonia. Ann Intern Med 1995;122:743.

32. Shorr AF, Sherner JH, Jackson WL, et al. Invasive approaches to the diagnosis of ventilator-associated pneumonia: a meta-analysis. Crit Care Med 2005;33:46.

33. Klompas M. Does this patient have ventilator-associated pneumonia? JAMA 2007;297(14):1583–93.

34. Luyt CE, Combes A, Reynaud C, et al. Usefulness of procalcitonin for the diagnosis of ventilator-associated pneumonia. Intensive Care Med 2008;34(8): 1434–40.

35. Ramirez P, Garcia MA, Ferrer M, et al. Sequential measurements of procalcitonin levels in diagnosing ventilator-associated pneumonia. Eur Respir J 2008;31(2): 356–62.

36. Linssen CF, Bekers O, Drent M, et al. C-reactive protein and procalcitonin concentrations in BAL fluid as a predictor of ventilator-associated pneumonia. Ann Clin Biochem 2008;45:293–8.

37. Gibot S, Cravoisy A, Levy B, et al. Soluble triggering receptor expressed on myeloid cells and the diagnosis of pneumonia. N Engl J Med 2004;350(5): 451–8.

38. Determann RM, Millo JL, Gibot S, et al. Serial changes in soluble triggering receptor expressed on myeloid cells in the lung during development of ventilator-associated-pneumonia. Intensive Care Med 2005;31(11):1495–500.

39. Anand NJ, Zuick S, Klesney-Tait J, et al. Diagnostic implications of soluble triggering receptor expressed on myeloid cells-1 in BAL fluid of patients with pulmonary infiltrates in the ICU. Chest 2009;135(3):641–7.
40. Oudhuis GJ, Beuving J, Bergmans D, et al. Soluble triggering receptor expressed on myeloid cells-1 in bronchoalveolar lavage fluid is not predictive for ventilator-associated pneumonia. Intensive Care Med 2009;35(7):1265–70.
41. Meduri GU, Johanson WG Jr. International Consensus Conference: clinical investigation of ventilator-associated pneumonia. Chest 1992;102:551S.
42. CDC. National Nosocomial Infections Surveillance (NNIS) system report, data summary from January 1990–May 1999, issued June 1999. Am J Infect Control 1999;27:520–32.
43. Fridkin S, Weibel SF, Weinstein RA. Magnitude and prevention of nosocomial infections in the intensive care unit. Infect Dis Clin North Am 1997;11:479–96.
44. Hidron AI, Edwards JR, Patel J, et al, National Healthcare Safety Network Team, Participating National Healthcare Safety Network Facilities. NHSN annual update: antimicrobial-resistant pathogens associated with healthcare-associated infections: annual summary of data reported to the National Healthcare Safety Network at the Centers for Disease Control and Prevention 2006-2007. Infect Control Hosp Epidemiol 2008;29:996–1011.
45. Hanberger H, Walther S, Leone M, et al, EPIC II Group of Investigators. Increased mortality associated with methicillin-resistant Staphylococcus aureus (MRSA) infection in the intensive care unit: results from the EPIC II study. Int J Antimicrob Agents 2011;38(4):331–5.
46. Park DR. The microbiology of ventilator-associated pneumonia. Respir Care 2005;50(6):742–63 [discussion: 763–5].
47. Napolitano LM, Brunsvold ME, Reddy RC, et al. Community-acquired MRSA pneumonia and ARDS: 1-year followup. Chest 2009;136(5):1407–12.
48. Hidron AI, Low CE, Honig EG, et al. Emergence of community-acquired MRSA strain USA300 as a cause of necrotizing community-onset pneumonia. Lancet Infect Dis 2009;9:384–92.
49. Kallen AJ, Brunkard J, Moore Z, et al. Staphylococcus aureus community-acquired pneumonia during the 2006-2007 influenza season. Ann Emerg Med 2009;53(3):358–65.
50. Labandeira-Rey M, Couzon F, Boisset S, et al. Staphylococcus aureus Panton-Valentine leukocidin causes necrotizing pneumonia. Science 2007;315:1130–3.
51. Wenzel RP, Bearman G, Edmond MB. Community-acquired methicillin-resistant Staphylococcus aureus (MRSA): new issues for infection control. Int J Antimicrob Agents 2007;30:210–2.
52. Rello J, Ollendorf DA, Oster G, et al. Epidemiology and outcomes of ventilator-associated pneumonia in a large US database. Chest 2002;122:2115.
53. Iregui M, Ward S, Sherman G, et al. Clinical importance of delays in the initiation of appropriate antibiotic treatment for ventilator-associated pneumonia. Chest 2002;122:262.
54. Habarth S, Garbino J, Pugin, et al. Inappropriate initial antimicrobial therapy and its effect on survival in a clinical trial of immunomodulating therapy for severe sepsis. Am J Med 2003;115(7):529–35.
55. Luna CM, Vujacich P, Niederman MS, et al. Impact of BAL data on the therapy and outcome of ventilator-associated pneumonia. Chest 1997;111:676.
56. Kollef MH, Sherman G, Ward S, et al. Inadequate antimicrobial treatment of infections: a risk factor for hospital mortality among critically ill patients. Chest 1999;115(2):462–74.

57. Teixeira PJ, Seligman R, Hertz FT, et al. Inadequate treatment of ventilator-associated pneumonia: risk factors and impact on outcomes. J Hosp Infect 2007;65(4):361–7.

58. Chan JD, Dellit TH, Choudhuri JA, et al. Active surveillance cultures of methicillin-resistant *Staphylococcus aureus* as a tool to predict methicillin-resistant *S. aureus* ventilator-associated pneumonia. Crit Care Med 2012; 40(5):1437–42.

59. Chastre J, Wolff M, Fagon JY, et al. Comparison of 8 vs 15 days of antibiotic therapy for ventilator-associated pneumonia in adults: a randomized trial. JAMA 2003;290:2588.

60. Demoule A, Girou E, Richard JC, et al. Increased use of noninvasive ventilation in French intensive care units. Intensive Care Med 2006;32(11):1747–55.

61. Muscedere J, Dodek P, Keenan S, et al, VAP Guidelines Committee and the Canadian Critical Care Trials Group. Comprehensive evidence-based clinical practice guidelines for ventilator-associated pneumonia: prevention. J Crit Care 2008;23(1):126–37.

62. Wip C, Napolitano L. Bundles to prevent ventilator-associated pneumonia: how valuable are they? Curr Opin Infect Dis 2009;22(2):159–66.

63. Drakulovic MB, Torres A, Bauer TT, et al. Supine body position as a risk factor for nosocomial pneumonia in mechanically ventilated patients: a randomised trial. Ann Intern Med 1999;354:1851.

64. van Nieuwenhoven CA, Vandenbroucke-Grauls C, van Tiel FH, et al. Feasibility and effects of the semirecumbent position to prevent ventilator-associated pneumonia: a randomized study. Crit Care Med 2006;34(2):396–402.

65. Alexiou VG, Ierodiakonou V, Dimopoulos G, et al. Impact of patient position on the incidence of ventilator-associated pneumonia: a meta-analysis of randomized controlled trials. J Crit Care 2009;24(4):515–22.

66. Bouza E, Perez MJ, Munoz P, et al. Continuous aspiration of subglottic secretions in the prevention of ventilator-associated pneumonia in the postoperative period of major heart surgery. Chest 2008;134(5):938–46.

67. Dezfulian C, Shojania K, Collard HR, et al. Subglottic secretion drainage for preventing ventilator-associated pneumonia: a meta-analysis. Am J Med 2005; 118(1):11–8.

68. Diaz E, Rodríguez AH, Rello J, et al. Ventilator-associated pneumonia: issues related to the artificial airway. Respir Care 2005;50(7):900–6 [discussion: 906–9].

69. DeRiso AJ, Ladowski JS, Dillon TA, et al. Chlorhexidine gluconate 0.12% oral rinse reduces the incidence of total nosocomial respiratory infection and non-prophylactic systemic antibiotic use in patients undergoing heart surgery. Chest 1996;109:1556.

70. Koeman M, van der Ven AJ, Hak E, et al. Oral decontamination with chlorhexidine reduces the incidence of ventilator-associated pneumonia. Am J Respir Crit Care Med 2006;173(12):1348–55.

71. Chlebicki MP, Safdar N. Topical chlorhexidine for prevention of ventilator-associated pneumonia: a meta-analysis. Crit Care Med 2007;35(2):595–602.

72. Genuit T, Bochicchio G, Napolitano LM, et al. Prophylactic chlorhexidine oral rinse decreases ventilator-associated pneumonia in surgical ICU patients. Surg Infect (Larchmt) 2001;2(1):5–18.

73. Lorente L, Lecuona M, Jiménez A, et al. Ventilator-associated pneumonia with or without toothbrushing: a randomized controlled trial. Eur J Clin Microbiol Infect Dis 2012;31(10):2621–9.

74. Pobo A, Lisboa T, Rodriguez A, et al, RASPALL Study Investigators. A randomized trial of dental brushing for preventing ventilator-associated pneumonia. Chest 2009;136(2):433–9.
75. Kollef MH, Afessa B, Anzueto A, et al, NASCENT Investigation Group. Silver-coated endotracheal tubes and incidence of ventilator-associated pneumonia: the NASCENT randomized trial. JAMA 2008;300(7):805–13.
76. Garrard CS, A'Court CD. The diagnosis of pneumonia in the critically ill. Chest 1995;108(Suppl 2):17S–25S.
77. Girard TD, Kress JP, Fuchs BD, et al. Efficacy and safety of a paired sedation and ventilator weaning protocol for mechanically ventilated patients in intensive care (Awakening and Breathing Controlled trial): a randomised controlled trial. Lancet 2008;371(9607):126–34.
78. de Smet AM, Kluytmans JA, Cooper BS, et al. Decontamination of the digestive tract and oropharynx in ICU patients. N Engl J Med 2009;360:20.
79. D'Amico R, Pifferi S, Leonetti C, et al. Effectiveness of antibiotic prophylaxis in critically ill adult patients: systematic review of randomised controlled trials. BMJ 1998;316:1275.
80. Silvestri L, van Saene HK, Casarin A, et al. Impact of selective decontamination of the digestive tract on carriage and infection due to Gram-negative and Gram-positive bacteria: a systematic review of randomised controlled trials. Anaesth Intensive Care 2008;36:324.
81. Wunderink RG. Welkommen to our world. Emergence of antibiotic resistance with selective decontamination of the digestive tract. Am J Respir Crit Care Med 2010;181:426.
82. Rumbak MJ, Newton M, Truncale T, et al. A prospective, randomized, study comparing early percutaneous dilational tracheotomy to prolonged translaryngeal intubation (delayed tracheotomy) in critically ill medical patients. Crit Care Med 2004;32(8):1689–94.
83. Terragni PP, Antonelli M, Fumagalli R, et al. Early vs late tracheotomy for prevention of pneumonia in mechanically ventilated adult ICU patients: a randomized controlled trial. JAMA 2010;303(15):1483–9.
84. Cuthbertson BH. The TracMan trial presented at Critical Care Canada Forum on October 28, 2009, Toronto, Ontario, Canada. Available at: http://www.criticalcarecanada.com/pdf/CCCF%202009%20Final%20Programme%20Wednesday.pdf. Accessed April 20, 2012.
85. Barsanti MC, Woeltje KF. Infection prevention in the intensive care unit. Infect Dis Clin North Am 2009;23(3):703–25.
86. Oman KS, Makic MB, Fink R, et al. Nurse-directed interventions to reduce catheter-associated urinary tract infections. Am J Infect Control 2012;40(6):548–53.
87. Gould CV, Umscheid CA, Agarwal RK, et al, Healthcare Infection Control Practices Advisory Committee. Guideline for prevention of catheter-associated urinary tract infections 2009. Infect Control Hosp Epidemiol 2010;31(4):319–26.
88. Hooton TM, Bradley SF, Cardenas DD, et al, Infectious Diseases Society of America. Diagnosis, prevention, and treatment of catheter-associated urinary tract infection in adults: 2009 International Clinical Practice Guidelines from the Infectious Diseases Society of America. Clin Infect Dis 2010;50(5):625–63.
89. Griffiths R, Fernandez R. Strategies for the removal of short-term indwelling urethral catheters in adults. Cochrane Database Syst Rev 2007;(2):CD004011.
90. Available at: http://www.cdc.gov/HAI/pdfs/toolkits/CAUTItoolkit_3_10.pdf. Accessed April 20, 2012.

91. Laupland KB, Bagshaw SM, Gregson DB, et al. Intensive care unit-acquired urinary tract infections in a regional critical care system. Crit Care 2005;9(2):R60–5.

92. Available at: http://www.cdc.gov/nhsn/pdfs/pscManual/7pscCAUTIcurrent.pdf. Accessed April 20, 2012.

93. Joint Commission on Accreditation of Healthcare Organizations. Approved: new infection-related National Patient Safety Goal for 2012: catheter-associated urinary tract infections pose high risk. Jt Comm Perspect 2011;31(7):6–7.

94. Available at: http://www.jointcommission.org/assets/1/18/r3_report_issue_2_9_22_11_final.pdf. Accessed April 20, 2012.

95. Niel-Weise BS, van den Broek PJ. Urinary catheter policies for short-term bladder drainage in adults. Cochrane Database Syst Rev 2005;(3):CD004203.

96. Moore KN, Fader M, Getliffe K. Long-term bladder management by intermittent catheterisation in adults and children. Cochrane Database Syst Rev 2007;(4):CD006008.

97. Marra AR, Sampaio Camargo TZ, Gonçalves P, et al. Preventing catheter-associated urinary tract infection in the zero-tolerance era. Am J Infect Control 2011;39(10):817–22.

98. Andreessen L, Wilde MH, Herendeen P. Preventing catheter-associated urinary tract infections in acute care: the bundle approach. J Nurs Care Qual 2012; 27(3):209–17.

99. Jepson RG, Craig JC. Cranberries for preventing urinary tract infections. Cochrane Database Syst Rev 2008;(1):CD001321.

100. Sarkar B, Napolitano LM. Necrotizing soft tissue infections. Minerva Chir 2010; 65(3):347–62.

101. US Department of Health and Human Services (HHS). HHS action plan to prevent healthcare associated infections: appendices. Appendix G. Available at: http://www.hhs.gov/ophs/initiatives/hai/appendices.html. Accessed April 5, 2012.

102. Culver DH, Horan TC, Gaynes RP, et al. Surgical wound infection rates by wound class, operative procedure, and patient risk index. Am J Med 1991;91: S152–7.

103. Mu Y, Edwards JR, Horan TC, et al. Improving risk-adjusted measures of surgical site infection for the national healthcare safety network. Infect Control Hosp Epidemiol 2011;32(10):970–86.

104. Horan TC, Gaynes RP, Martone WJ, et al. CDC definitions of nosocomial surgical site infections, 1992: a modification of CDC definitions of surgical wound infections. Am J Infect Control 1992;20:271–4.

105. Napolitano LM. Severe soft tissue infections. Infect Dis Clin North Am 2009; 23(3):571–91.

106. Napolitano LM. Early appropriate parenteral antimicrobial treatment of complicated skin and soft tissue infections caused by methicillin-resistant *Staphylococcus aureus*. Surg Infect (Larchmt) 2008;9(Suppl 1):s17–27.

107. May AK, Stafford RE, Bulger EM, et al, Surgical Infection Society. Treatment of complicated skin and soft tissue infections. Surg Infect (Larchmt) 2009;10(5): 467–99.

108. Stevens DL, Bisno AL, Chambers HF, et al, Infectious Diseases Society of America. Practice guidelines for the diagnosis and management of skin and soft-tissue infections. Clin Infect Dis 2005;41(10):1373–406.

109. Mitchell JD, Collen JF, Petteys S, et al. A simple reminder system improves venous thromboembolism prophylaxis rates and reduces thrombotic events for hospitalized patients1. J Thromb Haemost 2012;10(2):236–43.

110. Chan CM, Shorr AF. Venous thromboembolic disease in the intensive care unit. Semin Respir Crit Care Med 2010;31(1):39–46.
111. Dalen JE. Pulmonary embolism: what have we learned since Virchow? Natural history, pathophysiology, and diagnosis. Chest 2002;122:1440–56.
112. Gould MK, Garcia DA, Wren SM, et al, American College of Chest Physicians. Prevention of VTE in nonorthopedic surgical patients: antithrombotic therapy and prevention of thrombosis, 9th ed: American College of Chest Physicians Evidence-Based Clinical Practice Guidelines. Chest 2012;141(Suppl 2): e227S–77S.
113. Bates SM, Jaeschke R, Stevens SM, et al, American College of Chest Physicians. Diagnosis of DVT: antithrombotic therapy and prevention of thrombosis, 9th ed: American College of Chest Physicians Evidence-Based Clinical Practice Guidelines. Chest 2012;141(Suppl 2):e351S–418S.
114. Guyatt GH, Akl EA, Crowther M, et al, American College of Chest Physicians Antithrombotic Therapy and Prevention of Thrombosis Panel. Executive summary: antithrombotic therapy and prevention of thrombosis, 9th ed: American College of Chest Physicians Evidence-Based Clinical Practice Guidelines. Chest 2012;141(Suppl 2):7S–47S.
115. Holbrook A, Schulman S, Witt DM, et al, American College of Chest Physicians. Evidence-based management of anticoagulant therapy: antithrombotic therapy and prevention of thrombosis, 9th ed: American College of Chest Physicians Evidence-Based Clinical Practice Guidelines [review]. Chest 2012; 141(Suppl 2):e152S–84S.
116. Kearon C, Akl EA, Comerota AJ, et al, American College of Chest Physicians. Antithrombotic therapy for VTE disease: antithrombotic therapy and prevention of thrombosis, 9th ed: American College of Chest Physicians Evidence-Based Clinical Practice Guidelines. Chest 2012;141(Suppl 2):e419S–94S.
117. Douketis JD, Spyropoulos AC, Spencer FA, et al, American College of Chest Physicians. Perioperative management of antithrombotic therapy: antithrombotic therapy and prevention of thrombosis, 9th ed: American College of Chest Physicians Evidence-Based Clinical Practice Guidelines. Chest 2012; 141(Suppl 2):e326S–50S.

Heparin-Induced Thrombocytopenia

Stephen Lanzarotti, MD[a],*, John A. Weigelt, MD, DVM[b]

KEYWORDS

- Heparin-induced thrombocytopenia • Thrombosis • Platelets • PF-4
- Direct thrombin inhibitor

KEY POINTS

- Heparin-induced thrombocytopenia is an immune process, triggered by the administration of a heparin molecule, which binds to a platelet-specific protein—platelet factor 4.
- The antigenic complex of heparin–PF4 induces an immunoglobulin response, which binds the antigen as well as platelets, contributing to both thrombocytopenia and thrombosis.
- Diagnosing the condition requires clinical suspicion, platelet count monitoring, and identification of the causative antibody.
- Treatment involves stopping all heparin administration and starting alternative anticoagulation therapy.

INTRODUCTION

Anticoagulation therapy in the hospital is widespread and many patients will be exposed to heparin at some time during their hospitalization. Proper medication use requires an understanding of the medication's indications and side effects. The purpose of this article is to review heparin-induced thrombocytopenia (HIT), which is a commonly misunderstood complication from heparin-therapy.

Thrombosis related to heparin administration has been described for almost as long as heparin has been used in the clinical setting. Heparin was discovered in the 1930s at Johns Hopkins Hospital and found widespread clinical use as an anticoagulant in the early 1950s. In 1959, Dr Rodger E. Weismann described a series of 10 patients who developed thromboses after heparin administration. An immunologic cause for the thrombosis was suggested as early as 1964 by Dr Brooke Roberts at the University

Stephen Lanzarotti, MD, has nothing to disclose. Stephen Lanzarotti, MD, has received no funding for the production of this article.
[a] Evansville Surgical Associates, St. Mary's Hospital, 520 Mary Street Suite 520, Evansville, IN 47710, USA; [b] Division of Trauma and Critical Care, Medical College of Wisconsin, 8701 Watertown Plank Road, Milwaukee, WI 53226, USA
* Corresponding author.
E-mail address: stephen.lanzarotti@stmarys.org

of Pennsylvania. Once platelet counts became available in the 1970s, the association between the thrombosis and thrombocytopenia became evident.[1] Dr Glen R. Rhodes described HIT as a distinct clinical entity and identified the associated antibody.[2] HIT is still prevalent today, but misdiagnosis of the syndrome, as well as misunderstanding of the disease process contributes to its continuing morbidity for the hospitalized patient.

The purpose of this article is to review HIT, especially its pathophysiology, diagnostic challenges, and therapeutic options. This article also discusses the current recommendations for surveillance of HIT, as well as special clinical circumstances relating to the disease. At the end of this article, three patient scenarios are presented to allow the reader to evaluate their understanding of the disease in regard to clinical situations.

PATHOPHYSIOLOGY

There are two described entities relating to HIT. HIT type I is a nonimmunogenic phenomenon, in which a self-limited thrombocytopenia occurs and spontaneously normalizes. There are no thrombotic complications and there is no need to stop heparin. It is also referred to as heparin-associated thrombocytopenia. There are no long-term effects from this form.[3,4]

HIT type II is an immune process, triggered by the administration of a heparin molecule that binds to a platelet-specific protein called platelet factor 4 (PF-4). The antigenic complex of heparin–PF-4 induces an IgG response that can bind both the antigen and platelets, contributing to thrombocytopenia and thrombosis. When there is an associated thrombosis, the disease may be called heparin-induced thrombocytopenia with thrombosis (HITT). Diagnosing the condition requires clinical suspicion, platelet count monitoring, and identification of the causative antibody. Treatment involves stopping all heparin-administration and starting alternative anticoagulation therapy as necessary.[3,4] HIT Type II is the entity discussed in this article.

The Antigen

One portion of the antigen is the heparin molecule itself. Unfractionated heparin (UFH) is a large, heavily sulfated glycosaminoglycan with a strong negative charge. It exists as a polymer with a molecular weight ranging from 3 kDa to 30 kDa, with a median range of 15 kDa. Heparin acts as a cofactor with antithrombin III to inhibit several coagulation factors, but has its strongest effect against thrombin (activated factor II) and somewhat less activity against activated factor X. There are several factors that effect heparin's metabolism, specifically its route of administration, dose concentration, and its ability to bind nonselectively to endothelium. Heparin is broken down in the circulation, as well as being excreted by the kidney. UFH is produced in two forms: one from bovine lung tissue and the other from porcine gut tissue. The bovine form has been shown to produce a higher incidence of HIT.[5] UFH is given subcutaneously or intravenously for either prophylaxis or therapeutic reasons.

Low-molecular-weight heparin (LMWH) is derived from UFH, and consists of shorter chains with a molecular weight between 2 and 9 kDa, with an average of 5 kDa. It has greater therapeutic activity against activated factor X than thrombin. It is only given by the subcutaneous route and can be used either prophylactically or therapeutically. Renal excretion is linear and not dose dependent.

UFH's size and sulfation to saccharide ratio makes it an ideal antigen. Heparin itself is not antigenic because it shares a similar biochemical makeup to that of heparan sulfate, a proteoglycan that is normally found throughout the body. Heparin is one determinant in the antigenic complex that initiates the disease process. In order for heparin to initiate the immunologic response, it must bind to PF-4, a protein that is stored and secreted by the α-granule of the platelet. Owing to heparin's highly negative charge, it binds well to most structures within the bloodstream, including the PF-4 molecule that normally exists in the bloodstream.

The PF-4 molecule is an α-granule particle that is stored and released by the platelet. It is a highly positively charged particle and a member of the C-X-C cytokine family. Other members of the C-X-C cytokine family, including but not limited to IL-8 and platelet basic protein, can also react with the heparin molecule and produce the HIT antibody.[6]

Once the heparin–PF-4 complex exists, it can generate an immune response. In a naïve individual, the response can happen no sooner than 4 to 14 days. Once the antigen is cleared, the antibody production stops, but antibody activity can be present for up to 100 days. If the antigen has not initiated an immune response by at least 2 weeks after initial exposure, the risk of an immunologic response is minimal.

The Antibody

Once the antigen is recognized, antibody formation begins through the humoral arm of the immune system. IgM, IgA, and IgG antibodies are all formed, but it is the IgG antibodies that have clinical significance. They take approximately 5 days from initial exposure to develop. Antibody formation is stimulated as long as the antigen exists, and production stops once the antigen is cleared from the system. LMWH has less ability to produce the antibody because of its smaller size and lower sulfation to saccharide ratio. However, if LMWH does generate an antibody response, it has the same effect as UFH, and the antibody produced by UFH will cross-react with the antigen produced by LMWH–PF-4 antigen. Once the antigen is cleared, the antibody is undetectable in serum after about 100 days. This antigenic response is not anamnestic. Thus, a subsequent heparin exposure once the antibody is cleared does not initiate a stronger response. It is unclear why this occurs. The implication of no anamnestic response is that a person's risk for a second occurrence of HIT does not seem to be higher once the antibody is cleared.

As many as 20% to 60% of people exposed to heparin will develop the heparin–PF-4 antibody, but only a small percentage of individuals will actually progress to the clinical syndrome.[7,8] This phenomenon has been described as the iceberg model of HIT antibody detection (see later discussion).

The Effects

The IgG antibody binding to the heparin–PF-4 epitope initiates the disease process. The very long heparin molecule can bind many PF-4 molecules, creating a long chain of epitopes, each which can react with a separate antibody. Once the immune complex forms, the Fc portion of the anti-heparin or PF-4 IgG antibody binds to the platelet membrane or the endothelial cell through an Fc receptor located on the surface membrane. The IgG-Fc portion binds to the Fc receptor on the target activating it. If the platelet becomes activated, it releases its granules, propagating platelet aggregation and further activation. If bound to the endothelium, procoagulant factors will be released, which initiates the coagulation cascade. The long complex of heparin–PF-4, with its multiple antibodies attached can activate multiple platelets and/or endothelial cells. Activated platelets induce other platelets to aggregate and initiate the coagulation cascade, including direct activation of thrombin. Thrombin is a procoagulant, which significantly increases the risk for spontaneous thrombosis.[9]

The immune complex-platelet groups not included in thrombosis are cleared from the circulation by the reticuloendothelial system. Thrombocytopenia occurs as platelets are consumed in thrombosis or as the immune complex-platelet groups are removed from the circulation.[10]

The Disease

Thrombocytopenia is seen in 80% to 90% of patients, and thrombosis occurs in up to 75% of the patients diagnosed with HIT.[11] Thrombosis most frequently occurs in the venous system, but can also present in the arterial system, with a ratio of 4 to 1. Pulmonary embolism is the most common presentation of HIT.[12] It seems that arterial thromboses occur at places with endothelial damage or atherosclerosis, and usually form a white clot which was originally thought to be a hallmark of this disease. Skin thromboses at sites of subcutaneous heparin injections are nearly pathognomonic of the disease.[13]

The diagnosis of a new or propagating thrombosis while on therapeutic or prophylactic anticoagulation should generate significant concern for this disease process. Nontraditional types of thrombosis should also raise suspicion of HIT. These include dural venous sinus thrombosis, adrenal vein thrombosis with or without subsequent adrenal hemorrhage and adrenal insufficiency, recurrent clotting of a continuous venovenous dialysis circuit, or acute myocardial infarction or stroke. The more severe a thrombosis, the more the clinician should entertain the thought that the patient could have HIT. Significant thrombosis can occur even when the platelet count is greater than 100,000/μL, and in 15% of patients, a thrombotic event can precede thrombocytopenia.[14]

The presence of the HIT antibody places the patient at the highest risk for spontaneous thrombosis compared with any other congenital or acquired thrombotic disease. For patients who are not anticoagulated and do not already have a thrombosis at the time of diagnosis, the cumulative 30-day risk of thrombosis is just over 52%.[12]

HIT thrombocytopenia is usually not as severe as other drug-induced thrombocytopenias. The platelet count begins to drop once the antibody is active (average is 5 days postexposure).[10] The nadir range is between 20,000 to 100,000/μL, with a median value around 60,000/μL. This is in contrast to other types of drug-induced thrombocytopenia in which the initial decrease is more immediately related to exposure, and the nadir is usually less than 20,000/μL.[15] The thrombocytopenia does not seem to predispose the patient to spontaneous bleeding, unless there is another, underlying bleeding diathesis. There is no indication to give platelets based on the thrombocytopenia alone, unless there is concomitant bleeding. Once the heparin is stopped, the platelet count returns to normal levels in about 4 days. Suspicion of the disease should be highest when platelet counts drop to less than 50% below baseline.[16] Using platelet counts below 150,000/μL as an indicator for HIT is no longer part of the clinical suspicion for the diagnosis.

HIT can occur with any type of heparin exposure, but UFH carries a higher risk than LMWH.[17] Higher dosages and long-term use carry higher risks, and intravenous administration seems to have a stronger causative effect. Heparin flushes and heparin-bonded devices also have been implicated in the disease.[18] Cardiac and orthopedic surgical procedures have been associated with the highest rates of the disease.

DIAGNOSIS

One common misconception is that HIT can be diagnosed with clinical evidence alone, or independently, with the documented presence of the PF-4 antibody. In truth, it takes both, along with good clinical judgment to appropriately diagnose this condition.

Clinical Evaluation

The evaluation of the patient suspected of HIT comprises understanding of the four Ts: the Timing of onset, the severity of Thrombocytopenia, the presence of Thrombosis, and oTher causes for thrombocytopenia. A pretest scoring system, which is detailed below, can assist the clinician in considering which patients should be further evaluated for HIT.

The timing of the platelet count decline relative to heparin exposure is important to understand. If a person is naïve to heparin exposure, it takes a minimum 4 to 5 days for the clinically significant IgG antibody to be produced. However, because the antibody can exist for up to 100 days, the onset of signs and symptoms will be immediate after another heparin exposure when the antibody is already present. Patients with circulating antibody can develop an acute inflammatory reaction to injected heparin, consisting of tachycardia, diaphoresis, dyspnea, chest pain, and fever, which can mimic an acute pulmonary embolus. If a patient has this type of reaction after heparin injection, the clinician must immediately consider the patient as having HIT, obtain a platelet count, and discontinue the heparin.[19] An acute drop with rapid recovery in the platelet count can occur and identification of thrombocytopenia in this clinical scenario is highly suggestive of HIT. This syndrome is called rapid-onset HIT.

Another atypical presentation is the delayed onset of HIT. These patients are in the hospital and exposed to heparin. They are then discharged within the next few days before any clinical indication they may be developing the disease and are discharged without additional heparin. They return to the hospital within the next few days with a new thrombosis. These patients have developed a very high titer of the antibody and have a delayed presentation, even though the heparin stimulus has been discontinued. Patients who present with a thrombotic episode within 2 weeks of being discharged from the hospital after receiving heparin should generate a significant concern for the diagnosis of HIT and should be screened before starting heparin.[20]

To evaluate a patient suspected of HIT, begin with the scoring system shown in **Table 1**. Evaluate each row and assign its numerical value (0–2 points) per patient criteria. If the total for all four columns is less than or equal to 3, the patient is very unlikely to have HIT and does not need to be tested for the antibody. If the score is between 4 and 5, there is a reasonable possibility that the patient has HIT, and the serologic evaluation should be sent. Depending on the clinical suspicion, the heparin should be stopped and alternative anticoagulation therapy should be started if necessary. If the score is greater than or equal to 6, there is a high probability for HIT and heparin should be stopped, alternative anticoagulation should be initiated, and the antibody test should be sent.[21]

This tool has been validated in clinical studies, specifically showing a high negative predictive value for those with low (≤3) scores. However, in patients with intermediate (score 4–5) or high (>6) scores, there seems to be a high positive predictive value, but not as significant as the negative predictive value for the low score.[8] There are also good correlations with serologic studies to prove or disprove the presence of the antibody.[22,23]

Laboratory Evaluation

Confirmation of the disease process entails proving the antibody is present. However, the presence of the antibody alone does not inherently diagnose HIT. The clinical and laboratory evaluation of HIT is described as an iceberg model. The number of patients developing the antibody far exceeds the number of patients with clinical manifestations of HIT. The patient with the clinical signs and symptoms along with a confirmatory

Table 1
The 4T pretest scoring system for HIT

	2 Points	1 Point	0 Points
Thrombocytopenia	Platelet count decrease >50% and platelet nadir ≥20	Platelet count decrease 30%–50% or platelet nadir 10–19	Platelet count decrease <30% or platelet nadir <10
Timing of platelet count decrease	Clear onset between days 5–10 or platelet decrease ≤1 d (prior heparin exposure within 100 d)	Consistent with days 5–10 decrease, but not clear (eg, missing platelet counts); onset after day 10; or decrease ≤1 d (prior heparin exposure 30–100 d ago)	Platelet count decrease <4 d without recent exposure
Thrombosis or other sequelae	New thrombosis (confirmed); skin necrosis; acute systemic reaction postintravenous UFH (UFH) bolus	Progressive or recurrent thrombosis; nonnecrotizing (erythematous) skin lesions; suspected thrombosis (not proven)	None
Other causes for thrombocytopenia	None apparent	Possible	Definite

Adapted from Lo CK, et al. Evaluation of pretest clinical score (4 T's) for the diagnosis of heparin induced thrombocytopenia in two clinical settings. J Thromb Haemost 2006;4:760; with permission.

functional antibody assay represents the tip of the iceberg of the percentage of patients with positive antibody and clinical disease.

The newest and most rapid screening test is the PIFA Heparin/PF-4 Rapid Assay (Akers Biosciences, Inc, Thorofare, New Jersey, USA), a microparticle, immunofiltration, single-use system. It can detect the presence of HIT antibodies in fresh serum within minutes by the presence or absence of color change on the test strip (http://www.akersbiosciences.com/products/us/heparin/index.php).

The standard assay is the ELISA test, the commonly known PF-4 antibody assay. This assay is rapid, readily available, and detects the presence of all antibodies that can react with the heparin–PF-4 epitope, including the IgM, the IgA, and IgG antibodies. It has a reasonably high sensitivity, but a low specificity for the disease because it cannot separate which antibodies are significant. It is performed and read out as an optic density (OD) and the lower limit is usually set at 0.4 OD. If the reading is greater than 0.4 OD, the test is read as positive. If the reading is greater than 1.0 OD, there is enough concentration of clinically significant antibody to consider the patient as positive for the disease and a confirmatory test is not necessary unless the clinical presentation is questionable. If the reading is greater than 2.0 OD, no further testing is indicated and HIT can be confirmed solely with this test.

Once antibody presence is proven, a confirmatory evaluation can be used in clinically unclear patients to identify if a clinically significant antibody exists. The next step in testing is to prove the antibody can activate platelets. Functional platelet assays are time-consuming, difficult to set up, and done in fewer centers than the ELISA assay. A common type of functional assay is the serotonin release assay, which uses serotonin radiolabeled platelets as the substrate. The patient's serum is mixed with the platelets, heparin is added, and, if there is a significant antibody present, the platelets will release the serotonin. The supernatant is evaluated for presence of the radiolabeled serotonin and reported as percent activity. The lower limit of normal is 20%, so any number higher is considered positive.

The sensitivity of the ELISA is greater than 90%, whereas the specificity is 50% to 70%. The specificity of many functional assays is greater than 95%, but the sensitivity is less than 90%. Together, the two assays are near 100% sensitive and specific.[16]

The usual scenario to generate a HIT diagnosis includes thrombocytopenia 4 to 14 days after initiation of heparin, with a nadir around 60,000/μL, and at least a 50% drop from baseline. All other causes of thrombocytopenia are excluded. Thrombosis might be present, but is not necessary for diagnosis. The patient has a positive serologic test, confirmed by a positive functional assay.

Once the diagnosis of HIT is confirmed, or even highly suspected, all heparin must be immediately stopped. Because the rate of spontaneous thrombosis remains high, simply stopping heparin is not enough, the patient needs to be treated because they are now in an extremely prothrombotic state with a thrombosis incidence of greater than 50% within 30 days of diagnosis.[12] Treatment consists of using an alternate anticoagulation strategy.

INCIDENCE AND SCREENING

The incidence of HIT varies in the hospitalized population, and depends on whether the patient has a medical or surgical illness, type of heparin, and duration of heparin exposure. The highest risk for HIT belongs to orthopedic patients undergoing hip fracture repair, hip, or knee replacement, receiving UFH. That risk has been reported as high as 4.5%. The same patient population receiving LMWH has a risk of around 0.5%. Cardiac surgery patients also are high risk with a reported incidence of up to

3%. Cardiac transplant patients have the highest risk at 11%. It is interesting that cardiac surgical patients form the antibody more frequently, but orthopedic patients represent the highest risk patient population for HIT.[24] General surgical patients receiving UFH have a risk of about 3%, whereas the same patient population receiving LMWH has a risk of about 0.3%.[25] Critical care patients have a risk of 0.5% and HIT is the least common cause of thrombocytopenia in this patient population.[20] The general medical population receiving UFH has a risk of 0.3% to 2.0%, but cardiac patients receiving UFH for coronary interventions have a frequency of 1.5% or higher.[25–27] Obstetric patients have the lowest risk for HIT at less than 0.1%. For all patients receiving either UFH or LMWH, the overall risk for HIT is around 1.2%. The chronic hemodialysis patient population has an ELISA antibody prevalence of 12%, but the rate of HIT in the dialysis population is very low.[25] HIT in the chronic hemodialysis patient is usually related to an additional exposure of heparin for some type of procedure and not to the usual heparin exposure of chronic hemodialysis. However, patients who are on chronic hemodialysis and possess the HIT antibody seem to have a higher mortality than hemodialysis patients without the antibody do.[28]

Because thrombocytopenia is the heralding event of this disease, screening the patient population at risk is considered prudent, but the level of evidence supporting the frequency of testing for screening is not strong. Both the American College of Chest Physicians (ACCP) and the College of American Pathologists have published recommendations regarding platelet count monitoring on patients receiving heparin.[19,29] Both recommendations are essentially the same. Here are the recommendations from the ACCP clinical practice guidelines from the 9th edition of *Antithrombotic therapy and prevention of thrombosis*:[29]

- For patients receiving heparin in whom clinicians consider the risk of heparin-induced thrombocytopenia (HIT) to be greater than 1% (based on 4T score), we suggest that platelet count monitoring be performed every 2 or 3 days from day 4 to 14 (or until heparin is stopped, whichever occurs first) (Grade 2C)
- For patients receiving heparin in whom clinicians consider the risk of HIT to be less than 1%, we suggest that platelet counts not be monitored. (Grade 2C)

TREATMENT AND THERAPEUTIC MODALITIES

Once the diagnosis of HIT is confirmed or strongly suggested, therapy to prevent or treat the thrombotic complications must be initiated. Simply stopping the heparin is not sufficient because the patient has a very high risk of spontaneous thrombosis if they do not already have a thrombotic complication.[12] Whether or not a thrombotic complication has already occurred, alternative anticoagulation treatments must be started to prevent either initiation, or propagation and worsening of the thrombosis.[3,30]

The approved initial therapy for HIT includes several classes of medications, including the direct thrombin inhibitors (DTI), Factor Xa inhibitors (heparinoids and pentasaccharides), and vitamin K antagonists (VKA).[30] The medications must be given in therapeutic dosages because a severely prothrombotic state is being treated, even if no thrombotic complications have yet occurred. The length of treatment depends on the presence of thrombosis.

LMWH is absolutely contraindicated as an alternative anticoagulation strategy for HIT, even if HIT was caused by UFH, because the antibody will cross-react with the LMWH and propagates the thrombosis.

Ancrod (Viprinex), a medication derived from pit viper venom, as well as the glycoprotein (Gp) IIb/IIIa inhibitors have been trialed for use in HIT, and have either shown no efficacy, or worsened the thrombotic complications or bleeding tendencies. They have no role in the treatment of HIT or HITT.

DTIs

The DTIs are recombinant or synthetic molecules derived from hirudin, the anticoagulant found in the salivary gland of the leech *Hirudo medicinalis*. They act directly on thrombin, and can bind to both free and bound thrombin. In contrast, anti-thrombin III/heparin can only act on unbound thrombin. The two medications currently approved for HIT therapy are lepirudin and argatroban. A third DTI, bivalirudin, is indicated for percutaneous coronary intervention (PCI) in patients with HIT.

DTIs include

- Lepirudin (Refludan) was the first recombinant therapy developed. It exists as a bivalent inhibitor which acts on thrombin's two exosites, which are both active in many of thrombin's biologic activities. Lepirudin is provided as a continuous intravenous infusion. It is mostly excreted by the kidneys, so it is not useful in patients with renal failure. However, there are renal adjustments available in dosing. Therapeutic levels are monitored by the activated partial thromboplastin time (APTT), and the therapeutic goal is a clotting time 1.5 to 2.0 times the normal APTT clotting time. The main side effect from lepirudin administration is an anaphylactic reaction when bolus injections are given.
- Argatroban is a synthetic molecule that is also provided as a continuous infusion. It is a monovalent molecule, acting only on thrombin's exosite responsible for propagation of coagulation. It is metabolized by the liver and is monitored with the APTT. Argatroban affects the prothrombin time-international normalized ratio (PT/INR), which can make the transition to VKA difficult. Goal APTT is 1.5 to 3.0 times normal clotting time for the APTT. Argatroban is indicated as therapy for HIT, and also for PCI in patients with documented HIT or HITT.
- Bivalirudin (Angiomax) is a synthetic, bivalent molecule that does not have Food and Drug Administration (FDA) approval for treatment of HIT or HITT, but there are some ongoing studies to detect its efficacy in the treatment of this disease. It has a unique method of metabolism, in which 80% of the molecule is cleaved to an inactive state by thrombin itself, and 20% is renally cleared, contributing to its extremely rapid plasma clearance. Its only indication at this time is for PCI in patients with HIT or HITT. Its efficacy is monitored with the APTT or activated clotting time.
- Oral DTIs, including dabigatran (Pradaxa) and ximelagatran (Exanta), are not currently approved for use in patients with HIT.
- Desirudin (Iprivask), a newer DTI given by the subcutaneous route, has not been approved for treatment in HIT.

FACTOR XA INHIBITORS

The only factor Xa inhibitor-approved therapy for HIT is danaparoid (Orgaran), but it is not available in the United States. The pentasaccharides are not approved for HIT therapy, but have shown efficacy in the management of both treatment as a bridge to VKA, as well as for deep venous thrombosis (DVT) prophylaxis in patients with a documented HIT antibody.

Factor Xa inhibitors include

- Danaparoid (Orgaran) is a heparinoid derived from porcine gut mucosa. Its active components are heparan, dermatan, and chondroitin sulfate. There is no heparin or heparin fragments. It is administered subcutaneously, and has no intravenous component. It can be administered both in prophylactic and therapeutic doses. Factor Xa levels are used to follow its effects.

- Pentasaccharides are small molecules that act on Factor Xa. They are dosed only subcutaneously, and can be given in prophylactic or therapeutic dosages. The FDA has not approved any pentasaccharide for use in treatment of HIT or HITT, but there are some small studies that have shown efficacy in patients with documented HIT.[31] Pentasaccharides might have efficacy for DVT prophylaxis in the patient with a moderate clinical suspicion of HIT who is awaiting confirmation of an antibody test but the clinician does not wish to convert to a DTI for treatment while awaiting results. There is some concern that the HIT antibody will cross-react with the pentasaccharides. However, the molecule seems to be too small to generate a significant thrombotic potential. There is one documented instance of fondaparinux (Arixtra) as the causative agent for HIT.[26]

VKAS

VKAs are the group of agents that act against vitamin K-dependent factors (factor II, VII, IX, X, and proteins C and S) by inhibiting the enzyme vitamin K epoxide reductase, which acts to reduce Vitamin K after it carboxylates the coagulation factors mentioned above. It is used only in the chronic management of HIT and is absolutely contraindicated during the acute phase of HIT or HITT. VKAs are monitored by the INR. The goal is to maintain the INR at two to three times normal.

During the acute phase of HIT, thrombin is activated, which shifts the coagulation cascade toward a procoagulant state. Protein C and its cofactor, protein S, act to inhibit thrombin. The half-life of protein C is significantly shorter than the other vitamin K-dependent factors. Using the VKA in the acute phase will deplete protein C faster than thrombin. Once protein C is inhibited, thrombin activity is enhanced. This can result in systemic thrombosis, which may lead to the condition called venous limb gangrene, coumarin-induced skin necrosis, or other significant life-threatening or limb-threatening thromboses. It is imperative that if HIT is diagnosed in the acute phase and a VKA has been initiated before resolution of the thrombocytopenia (return of platelet count to at least 150,000/μL), vitamin K should be given to reverse the effects of the VKA and limit the chance of venous limb gangrene.[30]

VKAs can be started once the platelet count returns to normal on the alternative anticoagulation therapy and there have been at least 5 days of concurrent treatment with non-heparin anticoagulation and VKA therapy. The non-heparin therapy can be discontinued after at least 5 days of overlap and a stable, therapeutic INR.[30]

LENGTH OF THERAPY

There is no consensus statement regarding length of therapy for HIT with or without thrombosis. What is clear is that once HIT is diagnosed, full anticoagulation therapy must be undertaken using a non-heparin anticoagulant at therapeutic doses and then transitioned to VKA. Many experts suggest that if there are no thrombotic events, treatment be continued for the duration the antibody exists or 100 days maximum. If a thrombotic event occurs, the judgment of duration must be made by the clinician, based on current evidence regarding length of therapy for treatment of thromboses.

SPECIAL CIRCUMSTANCES

There are several special circumstances involving patients with documented HIT requiring anticoagulation therapy, as well as special patient populations who may have difficult therapeutic management options.[32,33]

These patient populations include

- Patients with current or historical evidence of HIT who require cardiopulmonary bypass (CPB)

    The first step is to check for the presence of the antibody by ELISA. Three scenarios exist:

    1. The antibody is undetectable. If there is no antibody present, it is likely safe for the patient to undergo CPB with the normal heparin doses. Because there does not seem to be an anamnestic response to heparin in patients with a history of HIT, it would seem that the patient is at the same risk as the general population regarding production of HIT antibodies. This patient should be monitored for thrombocytopenia in the postoperative period.
    2. There is detectable antibody and normal platelet counts (subacute HIT). Re-exposure to heparin must be avoided and the patient should either be delayed until the antibody is, at best, weakly detectable by ELISA. Or, alternate anticoagulation may be used for the procedure and postoperative period.
    3. For acute HIT (antibody plus thrombocytopenia), no heparin should be used. The same principles apply as for the subacute patient and, unfortunately, there are few data to support the ideal agent or therapeutic levels of DTI for CPB. However, the current ACCP guidelines suggest a regimen for alternative anticoagulation in the patient population requiring CPB, but the levels of recommendation are not very strong. For patients requiring PCI, argatroban and bivalirudin have been approved for antithrombotic adjuncts in the patient with HIT.

- Patients requiring vascular procedures with current or historical evidence of HIT

    This patient population can be treated the same as the cardiac patient. If there is no or even weak antibody detected by ELISA, it should be safe to use heparin. There are no good data to suggest which DTI is preferred and what therapeutic level must be achieved in the patient with a HIT antibody requiring surgical intervention. There is no approved indication for the use of DTI in noncoronary vascular interventions, whether open or endovascular. The safest route is to wait until the antibody clears, if possible.

- Patients with remote history of HIT requiring DVT prophylaxis

    If no antibody exists, UFH or LMWH are safe, ensuring that routing monitoring for thrombocytopenia is undertaken. If the patient also has a history of thrombosis, he or she may be at increased risk of developing another thrombosis whether or not the original thrombosis was related to HIT. Pentasaccharides, danaparoid, and even warfarin (in the subacute phase) have all shown good efficacy for chemical prophylaxis in this patient population.

- Patients who are pregnant patient and have HIT

    Pentasaccharides do not cross the placenta and are likely safe. VKAs are con traindicated in pregnancy, and lepirudin and argatroban may cross the placenta.

- The patient is a child

    There are no current trials of DTI with children.

SUMMARY

HIT is an immune process, triggered by the administration of a heparin molecule, which binds to a platelet-specific protein—PF-4. The antigenic complex of heparin–PF-4 induces an IgG response that binds the antigen as well as platelets, contributing to thrombocytopenia and thrombosis. Diagnosing the condition requires clinical suspicion, platelet count monitoring, and identification of the causative antibody. Treatment involves stopping all heparin administration and starting alternative anticoagulation therapy.

Here are some patient situations that allow the reader to think about this disease from a clinical standpoint.

- Patient 1 is a 27-year-old man involved in a high-speed motor vehicle crash with polytrauma, including an open femur fracture, crushed spleen requiring damage control laparotomy, and a flail chest requiring a chest tube and prolonged invasive ventilation. UFH is started for DVT prophylaxis on hospital day 2. On hospital day 4, his platelet count is 40,000/μL. A PF-4 antibody is sent and returns weakly positive. Does this patient have HIT?
  - Discussion: This patient has multiple reasons for thrombocytopenia, and has a very low probability of HIT as a diagnosis. His weakly positive ELISA test is of no significance. No further workup or therapy is warranted.
- Patient 2 is a 74-year-old woman who undergoes elective sigmoid resection for diverticulitis. She has a history of coronary artery disease, peripheral vascular disease, and hypertension. Preoperative platelet count is normal at 160,000/μL. LMWH is started for DVT prophylaxis in the preoperative area, and continued for her hospital stay. On hospital day 6, she develops unilateral leg edema. Duplex ultrasound reveals a deep vein thrombosis. Therapeutic heparin intravenous infusion is initiated. On hospital day 7, her platelet count is noted to be 60,000/μL. She subsequently develops shortness of breath and a chest CT scan reveals a pulmonary embolus. The PF-4 antibody is drawn and sent, but will take two days to return a result. What is the appropriate next step?
  - Discussion: This patient is an older woman with a DVT and PE on heparin therapy after elective sigmoid resection. She has a high enough concern for HITT that all heparin should be stopped and alternative anticoagulation started. She should be transitioned to VKA after her platelet count returns to normal and she has been covered with both DTI and VKA for at least 5 days, provided her antibody assay returns positive. The length of therapy should be based on current guidelines for thrombotic therapy.
- Patient 3 is a 62-year-old dialysis-dependent man, who is admitted to the hospital with a lower extremity arterial thrombus. A therapeutic heparin drip is started. On hospital day 4, his platelet count is noted to be 85,000/μL, and his baseline is 110,000/μL. PF-4 antibody is sent and the result returns as positive. Does this patient have HIT?
  - Discussion: This patient is a chronic hemodialysis patient with a new arterial thrombus, mild thrombocytopenia, and positive ELISA assay. This patient has a low probability for HIT in that he receives chronic heparin, and has not been exposed to a separate source of heparin before his thrombosis. Arterial thrombosis is fairly common in this patient population and the thrombocytopenia is likely reflective of the consumption from the clot. However, this assay should be confirmed by a functional platelet assay and, if positive, he has confirmed HIT and will need alternative anticoagulation. The presence of the HIT antibody may put him at higher risk of mortality compared with other hemodialysis patients without the antibody.

REFERENCES

1. Warkentin TE. History of heparin induced thrombocytopenia. In: Warkentin TE, Greinacher A, editors. Heparin induced thrombocytopenia. 3rd edition. New York: Marcel Dekker publisher; 2004. p. 2–5.
2. Rhodes GR, Dixon RH, Silver D. Heparin induced thrombocytopenia: eight cases with thrombotic-hemorrhagic complications. Ann Surg 1977;186:752–8.
3. Hassan Y, Awaisu A, Aziz NA, et al. Heparin-induced thrombocytopenia and advances in its therapy. J Clin Pharm Ther 2007;32:535–44.
4. Pravinkumar E, Webster NR. HIT/HITT and alternative anticoagulation: current concepts. Br J Anaesth 2003;90:676–85.
5. Francis JL, Palmer GJ III, Moroose R, et al. Comparison of bovine and porcine heparin in heparin antibody formation after cardiac surgery. Ann Thorac Surg 2003;75:17–22.
6. Safraz A, Iqbal O, Tobu M, et al. Immunobiology and pathophysiology of heparin induced thrombocytopenia/thrombosis syndrome—an update. Turk J Haematol 2002;19(2):127–31.
7. Lo GK, Sigouin CS, Warkentin TE. What is the potential for overdiagnosis of heparin induced thrombocytopenia? Am J Hematol 2007;82:1037–43.
8. Lo GK, Juhl D, Warkentin TE. Evaluation of pretest clinical score (4 Ts) for the diagnosis of heparin induced thrombocytopenia in two clinical settings. J Thromb Haemost 2006;4:759–65.
9. Greinacher A, Warkentin TE. Treatment of heparin induced thrombocytopenia: an overview. In: Warkentin TE, Greinacher A, editors. Heparin induced thrombocytopenia. 3rd edition. New York: Marcel Dekker publisher; 2004. p. 339.
10. Warkentin TE. Clinical picture of heparin induced thrombocytopenia in: heparin induced thrombocytopenia. 3rd edition. New York: Marcel Dekker publisher; 2004. p. 55–9.
11. Greinacher A, Farner B, Kroll H, et al. Clinical features of heparin induced thrombocytopenia including risk factors for thrombosis: a retrospective analysis of 408 patients. Thromb Haemost 2005;94:132–5.
12. Warkentin TE, Kelton JG. A 14 year study of heparin induced thrombocytopenia. Am J Med 1996;101:502–7.
13. Warkentin TE, Roberts RS, Hirsch J, et al. Heparin induced skin lesions and other unusual sequelae of the heparin induced thrombocytopenia syndrome. Chest 2005;127:1857–61.
14. Warkentin TE. Clinical presentations of heparin induced thrombocytopenia. Semin Hematol 1998;35:9–16.
15. Aster RH, Bougie DW. Drug induced immune thrombocytopenia. N Engl J Med 2007;357:580–7.
16. Hirsch J, Raschke R. Heparin and low molecular weight heparin: the Seventh ACCP Conference on Antithrombotic and Thrombolytic Therapy. Chest 2004; 126(Suppl):188S–203S.
17. Warkentin TE, Levine MN, Hirsch J, et al. Heparin induced thrombocytopenia in patients treated with low molecular weight heparin or unfractionated heparin. N Engl J Med 1995;332:1330–5.
18. Mureebe L, Graham JA, Bush RL, et al. Risk of heparin induced thrombocytopenia from heparin bonded vascular prostheses. Ann Vasc Surg 2007;21:719–22.
19. Warkentin TE. Platelet count monitoring and laboratory testing for heparin induced thrombocytopenia: recommendations of the College of American Pathologists. Arch Pathol Lab Med 2002;126:1415–23.

20. Selleng K, Warkentin TE, Greinacher A. Heparin induced thrombocytopenia in intensive care patients. Crit Care Med 2007;35:1165–76.
21. Warkentin TE, Heddle NM. Laboratory diagnosis of immune heparin induced thrombocytopenia. Curr Hematol Rep 2003;2:148–57.
22. Pouplard C, Gueret P, Fouassier M, et al. Prospective evaluation of the '4Ts' score and particle gel immunoassay specific to heparin/pf4 for the diagnosis of heparin induced thrombocytopenia. J Thromb Haemost 2007;5:1373–9.
23. Gruel Y, Regina S, Pouplard C. Usefulness of pretest clinical score (4Ts) combined with immunoassay for the diagnosis of heparin induced thrombocytopenia. Curr Opin Pulm Med 2008;14(5):397–402.
24. Warkentin TE, Sheppard JI, Horsewood P, et al. Impact of the patient population on the risk for heparin induced thrombocytopenia. Blood 2000;96(5):1703–8.
25. Jang IK, Hursting MJ. When heparins promote thrombosis. Circulation 2005;111: 2671–83.
26. Warkentin TE, Maurer BT, Aster RH. Heparin induced thrombocytopenia associated with fondaparinux. N Engl J Med 2007;365:2653–4.
27. Smythe MA, Koerber JM, Mattson JC. The incidence of recognized heparin induced thrombocytopenia in a large, tertiary care teaching hospital. Chest 2007;131:1644–9.
28. Carrier M, Rodger MA, Fergusson D, et al. Increased mortality in hemodialysis patients having specific antibodies to the platelet factor 4 complex. Kidney Int 2008;73(2):213–9.
29. Guyatt GH, Akl EA, Crowther M, et al. Antithrombotic therapy and prevention of thrombosis, 9th edition: American College of Chest Physicians Evidence-Based Clinical Practice Guidelines. Chest 2012;141(Supp 2):26s–8s.
30. Warkentin TE, Greinacher A, Koster A, et al. Treatment and prevention of heparin-induced thrombocytopenia; American College of Chest Physicians Evidence-Based Clinical Practice Guidelines (8th edition). Chest 2008;133(Suppl 6): 340S–80S.
31. Lobo B, Finch C, Howard A, et al. Fondaparinux for the treatment of patients with acute heparin induced thrombocytopenia. Thromb Haemost 2008;99:2–3.
32. Hassell K. The management of patients with heparin induced thrombocytopenia who require anticoagulant therapy. Chest 2005;127(Suppl 2):1S–8S.
33. Di Nisio M, Middeldorp S, Buller H. Direct thrombin inhibitors. N Engl J Med 2005; 353:1028–40.

Optimizing Drug Therapy in the Surgical Intensive Care Unit

William J. Peppard, PharmD, BCPS[a], Sarah R. Peppard, PharmD, BCPS[b], Lewis Somberg, MD[c],*

KEYWORDS

- Pharmacology • Sedation • Delirium • Antibiotic • Paralytic • Anticoagulation

KEY POINTS

- Given the multiple variables in ICUs that affect pharmacokinetics and pharmacodynamics, an understanding of drug properties and pharmacotherapy is essential to optimize care.
- Appropriate pharmacotherapy, as a supplement to surgical intervention, can improve patient outcomes in surgical ICUs (SICUs).

INTRODUCTION

Drug therapy has evolved dramatically in recent decades to keep pace with the needs of evolving critical care patients. Drug therapies have become increasingly complex requiring specialized training to optimize care. Pharmacokinetic and pharmacodynamic principles are of high importance in ICUs given the heterogeneity of the patient population. Multiple variables affect the dose, route, and frequency of drug administration needed to achieve a given physiologic response (**Table 1**).[1,2]

Falling outside the therapeutic window may lead to treatment failures and/or toxicity, both of which may contribute to increased morbidity and mortality. Several organizations, including the Society of Critical Care Medicine, have endorsed an interdisciplinary model to optimize patient care in ICUs.[3]

This article provides a review of commonly prescribed medications in SICUs, focusing on sedatives, antipsychotics, neuromuscular blocking agents (NMBAs),

This work received no financial support.
The authors have nothing to disclose.
[a] Department of Pharmacy, Froedtert Hospital, 9200 West Wisconsin Avenue, Milwaukee, WI 53226, USA; [b] Department of Pharmacy Practice, Concordia University Wisconsin School of Pharmacy, 12800 North Lake Shore Drive, Mequon, WI 53097–2418, USA; [c] Division of Trauma/Critical Care, Department of Surgery, Medical College of Wisconsin, 8701 Watertown Plank Road, Milwaukee, WI 53226, USA
* Corresponding author.
E-mail address: lsomberg@mcw.edu

Table 1
Physiologic variables known to effect pharmacokinetics and pharmacodynamics

Physiologic Variable	Effect on Drug	Dosing Modification Required
Hepatic dysfunction	Decreased metabolism, increased risk of coagulopathy	Decrease dose/frequency, conservative anticoagulation
Renal dysfunction	Decreased clearance, decreased protein binding	Decrease dose/frequency, avoid nephrotoxins
Advanced age	Decreased metabolism and clearance, increased sensitivity to drug	Decrease dose/frequency, avoid medications on Beers list
Malnutrition (hypoalbuminemia)	Decreased protein binding	Decrease dose/frequency
Hypothermia	Decreased metabolism, intracellular electrolyte shift	Decrease dose/frequency, conservative electrolyte supplementation
Burns	Hypermetabolic state, alteration in protein binding, increased Vd	Increase dose/frequency
Head injury	Increased clearance	Increase dose/frequency
Obesity	Increased Vd for lipophilic drugs	Increase dose
Pregnancy	Increased Vd	Increase dose, avoid teratogens
Volume overload	Increased Vd, decreased SC and IM absorption	Increase dose, avoid SC and IM routes of administration

Abbreviations: SC, subcutaneous; Vd, volume distribution; IM, intramuscular.
Data from Jacobi J, Fraser GL, Coursin DB, et al. Clinical practice guidelines for the sustained use of sedatives and analgesics in the critically ill adult. Crit Care Med 2002;30(1):119–41.

cardiovascular agents, anticoagulants, and antibiotics. A brief overview of pharmacology is followed by practical considerations to aid prescribers in selecting the best therapy within a given category of drugs to optimize patient outcomes.

SEDATIVES

The indication for pharmacologic sedation in ICUs varies but is often associated with the need to control anxiety and agitation, especially for those patients requiring mechanical ventilation (MV) or for procedural sedation.[4] Pharmacologic sedation should only be used after reversible causes of agitation, such as hypoxemia, hypotension, hypoglycemia, uncontrolled pain, and withdrawal from drugs or alcohol, are corrected. It is imperative to ensure that the environment and analgesia are optimized, including nonpharmacologic measures, such as frequent and continued reorientation.[5]

An objective scale should be used to titrate sedation to a predefined goal, especially in patients requiring sedation during MV. The most common validated scales used in ICUs are the Richmond Agitation–Sedation Scale (RASS) and the Ramsay scale.[6–8] Historically, sedatives have been used to achieve deep sedation (RASS −2 to −3 or Ramsay 4–5), but contemporary practice strives to achieve a much lighter level of sedation (RASS 0 to −1 or Ramsay 2–3), which minimizes negative consequences of deep and prolonged sedation. Negative consequences of oversedation include increased incidence and duration of delirium, long-term cognitive dysfunction, increased duration of MV, and prolonged ICU and hospital length of stay (LOS). Daily sedation vacations allow sedative drugs to clear from the patient's system and enable more reliable neurologic assessment. When accompanied by protocol-driven breathing trials, sedation vacations demonstrate improved outcomes as measured by decreased duration of MV, decreased ICU LOS, and decreased mortality.[9] Given that the RASS and the Ramsay scale are of no value in chemically paralyzed patients, bispectral index (BIS) monitoring, which is a numeric algorithmic analysis of an electroencephalogram, may be considered. The use of BIS is not well studied outside the operating room.

Many clinical factors affect drug selection, such as the indication for sedation, physiologic parameters that affect drug distribution, metabolism and elimination, adverse effects of the drug, institution formulary and guidelines, anticipated duration of sedation, and prescriber preference. Sedatives commonly used in ICUs are reviewed, with a focus on efficacy, safety, and variables to consider when determining the drug of choice for a given clinical circumstance (**Table 2**).

Propofol

Propofol (Diprivan) possesses hypnotic, anxiolytic, and amnestic properties but lacks analgesic effects.[10,11] Additionally, it acts as an anticonvulsant, decreases cerebral oxygen consumption, and reduces intracranial pressure (ICP). As a result, propofol is particularly useful in postsurgical patients, patients in status epilepticus, and those with traumatic brain injury resulting in elevated ICP. Propofol has several proposed mechanisms of action; it acts on multiple receptors to interrupt neural transmission in the central nervous system (CNS), including γ-aminobutyric acid (GABA), N-methyl-D-aspartate (NMDA), glycine, nicotinic, and muscarinic receptors.

Table 2
Sedative overview

Drug	Onset of Action (IV)	Use	Dose	Safety Considerations
Propofol	~1 min	RSI, PS, short-term sedation	RSI, PSI: 0.5–1 mg/kg Infusion: 5–65 µg/kg/min	PRIS with prolonged and high dose
Midazolam	2–5 min	RSI, PS, short-term sedation	PRN: 0.02–0.08 mg/kg q1–2 h Infusion: 0.04–0.2 mg/kg/h	Accumulation with prolonged and high dose, DDIs
Lorazepam	5–20 min	Short-term, and long-term sedation	PRN: 0.02–0.06 mg/kg q2–4 h Infusion: 0.01–0.1 mg/kg/h	PG toxicity, titrate slowly to avoid oversedation
Flumazenil	1–2 min	BZD reversal	0.2 mg q1–2 min	Over reversal may precipitate seizure
Dexmed-etomidine	5–10 min	Short-term sedation	Infusion: 0.2–1.5 µg/kg/min	Lacks amnestic properties, hypotension
Ketamine	<1 min	RSI, PS	PRN: 0.5–2 mg/kg	Emergence reaction
Etomidate	<1 min	RSI, PS	PRN: 0.3 mg/kg	Adrenal suppression

Abbreviations: DDIs, drug-drug interactions; PRN, as-needed intermittent dosing; PRIS, propofol infusion syndrome; PS, procedural sedation; RSI, rapid sequence intubation.

Data from Jacobi J, Fraser GL, Coursin DB, et al. Clinical practice guidelines for the sustained use of sedatives and analgesics in the critically ill adult. Crit Care Med 2002;30(1):119–41.

The high lipid solubility of propofol allows for rapid distribution into the CNS, resulting in an onset of action of approximately 1 minute. Its rapid hepatic metabolism yields a short half-life, allowing for rapid emergence from sedation within a few minutes after a single dose. Emergence is seen within 10 to 30 minutes after a short-term (<72 hours) continuous infusion, making frequent neurologic assessment feasible when targeting light sedation. Accumulation may occur secondarily to the drug's lipophilicity; the emergence time becomes prolonged (3–4 hours) with extended duration of infusion (>72 hours). Targeting deeper levels of sedation also yields a significantly longer emergence time and is generally discouraged. Clinical trials find propofol similar to midazolam for sedation in ICUs as measured by safety and efficacy, although time to wakefulness was consistently shorter in the propofol group.[12–16] Acquisition cost for propofol is higher than with either midazolam (Versed) or lorazepam (Ativan) but less than dexmedetomidine (DEX) (Precedex). Propofol use has not yet been associated with the development of delirium.

Respiratory depression, hypotension (attributed to systemic vasodilation, especially in hypovolemic patients), arrhythmias, and hypertriglyceridemia are common dose-dependent adverse effects of propofol. Although less severe at doses used for procedural sedation (1 mg/kg) compared with those used for induction and maintenance of anesthesia or continuous sedation (2–2.5 mg/kg), they remain clinically significant. Low-dose propofol used concurrently with ketamine (Ketalar) can lessen the impact of these adverse effects (discussed later).[17] Propofol is suspended in a 10% lipid emulsion containing egg lecithin and soybean oil and should be avoided in patients with known allergies to these compounds. The lipid content also results in unintentional caloric intake and should be factored into nutritional assessments accordingly.

Propofol can be administered by intravenous (IV) push for procedural sedation or as a continuous IV infusion for ongoing sedation in ICUs. Propofol infusion syndrome (PRIS) may occur with prolonged and/or high-dose infusions.[18] PRIS, defined as metabolic acidosis and cardiac dysfunction, along with one of the following: rhabdomyolysis, hypertriglyceridemia, or renal failure, was reported in 1.1% of patients in one prospective trial.[19] Although rare, the clinical significance is high and can be life threatening, with mortality rates ranging from 18% to 83%.[19,20] Rate and duration of infusion are strong risk factors for the development of PRIS, and it is recommended that infusions greater than 65 µg/kg/min for longer than 48 hours be avoided.[19] Other contributing factors include underlying mitochondrial disease or fatty acid oxidation defects, young age, critical illness of the CNS or respiratory origin, exogenous catecholamine or glucocorticoid administration, or inadequate carbohydrate intake.[19] When using high-dose or prolonged infusion of propofol, it is recommended that triglycerides, pH, lactate, and creatine kinase be followed at least daily, because abnormal values are associated with the development of PRIS. Propofol should immediately be discontinued if PRIS is suspected, although complications and even death may ensue after propofol discontinuation because there is no antidote for PRIS.

Benzodiazepines

Benzodiazepines (BZDs) have been used for decades in ICUs. They possess anxiolytic, amnestic, sedative, and anticonvulsant properties.[4,10] These actions are modulated by BZDs binding to GABA receptors, resulting in neuronal inhibition. BZDs are efficacious for rapid sequence intubation (RSI), procedural sedation, sedation during MV, and substance withdrawal. They vary by potency, duration of action, and lipid solubility, making certain BZDs more suitable for specific indications. High lipid solubility, as seen with midazolam and diazepam (Valium), yields rapid onset of action due to the increased blood-brain barrier permeability whereas the more water-soluble lorazepam has a slower onset of effect on the CNS. Midazolam and lorazepam are commonly used for sedation in ICUs, lorazepam and diazepam for seizures or alcohol withdrawal, and diazepam for muscle spasms. Alcohol withdrawal protocols, such as the Clinical Institute Withdrawal Assessment for Alcohol, are not well validated in ICUs. They may be used in appropriate and communicative patients but should generally be avoided in most patients.

BZDs are metabolized in the liver by oxidative cytochrome P450 enzyme systems and/or by glucuronide conjugation. This is of particular importance in SICUs given that acute inflammation after elective surgery is associated with a significant decline in cytochrome P450 activity, thereby directly affecting the metabolism of BZDs.[21] Doses should be adjusted downward accordingly.

Hypotension is a common adverse effect seen with BZDs, especially in patients who are critically ill, elderly, or have hepatic dysfunction. To minimize the impact of hemodynamic changes, initial dosing should be conservative and titrated slowly to effect. Although BZDs are effective sedatives, they are associated with increased risk for developing delirium.[22-24] Delirium is associated with increased mortality.[25,26] It is unclear how these data will affect future use of BZDs in ICUs.

Midazolam

Midazolam is a short-acting BZD commonly used in ICUs.[4] It can be used intermittently, usually dosed 2 mg to 4 mg IV every 1 to 2 hours (0.02–0.08 mg/kg) and titrated to effect or titrated as a continuous infusion (0.04–0.2 mg/kg/h) to maintain more consistent sedation if intermittent dosing fails. Due to its high lipophilicity, it quickly and readily crosses the blood-brain barrier and rapidly induces its sedative effects but is not a desirable option as a single dose for the treatment of an acute seizure due to its rapid redistribution out of the CNS. It is useful as a continuous infusion for patients with status epileptics. Midazolam distributes extensively to adipose, leading to drug accumulation over time and an increasing duration of action with prolonged use. To prevent excessive accumulation, midazolam should only be used for short-term sedation (<72 hours) and used with caution in those with renal failure. In these patients, it is not uncommon for time to wakefulness after cessation of drug to be measured in days, not hours, if not dosed appropriately.

Midazolam is hepatically metabolized to active metabolites, which accumulate extensively in patients with renal failure. It is subjected to significant drug-drug interactions as both a substrate and inhibitor of several cytochrome P450 pathways, including 3A4. The azole antifungals, macrolides, and nondihydropyridine calcium channel blockers (CCBs) may result in increased midazolam levels, whereas carbamazepine (Tegretol) and rifampin (Rifadin) may result in reduced midazolam levels. Drug dosages need to be adjusted accordingly and more careful monitoring may be required.

Lorazepam

Lorazepam is a long-acting BZD with approximately 2 to 3 times the potency of midazolam. It is effective when dosed intermittently, usually at a starting dose of 1 mg to 2 mg every 2 to 4 hours as needed.[4] If the intermittent dosing strategy fails, lorazepam may also be used as a continuous infusion after an appropriate loading dose for long-term sedation (>72 hours) but should be dosed with caution. A standard starting infusion rate is 4 mg/h. Owing to its long half-life, it is not easily titrated. Conventional frequent titration is every 5 to 15 minutes and results in an initially slow clinical response but ultimately leads to deep oversedation because the second, third, fourth, and fifth dose adjustments are made before the physiologic effects of the first dose adjustment are fully observed. Intermittent boluses may be administered during an infusion, but the infusions should be titrated no more frequently than every 8 hours. Lorazepam remains in the CNS longer than midazolam or diazepam, making it a good agent for the acute treatment of seizures.

The IV formulation of lorazepam contains propylene glycol (PG) as a diluent that accumulates in the setting of renal failure. PG toxicity primarily manifests as an anion gap metabolic acidosis and CNS depression.[27,28] Because these signs may be easily overlooked in a critically ill patient, proactive monitoring is necessary. In place of serum PG concentrations, a calculated osmol gap of greater than 10 mOsm/L to 12 mOsm/L may be used to identify patients with PG accumulation.[27,28] Risk factors include infusions greater than 0.1 mg/kg/h, a history of alcohol abuse, hepatic or renal dysfunction, and concomitant metronidazole usage.[28]

Flumazenil

Flumazenil (Romazicon) is an effective BZD antidote. It attenuates BZD sedative and respiratory depressive effects. It acts in the CNS by competitively inhibiting the BZD binding site of the GABA receptor. Flumazenil use should be avoided if at all possible and reserved for patients whose BZD toxicity is life threatening. The starting dose is 0.2 mg IV given over 30 seconds with an onset of action of 1 to 2 minutes and peak effects in about 6 minutes. Additional doses may be given every 1 minute until the desired level of consciousness is achieved, up to a maximum of 3 mg. Partial responders at 3 mg may be advanced to a maximum dosage of 5 mg. If a response is not seen at that dose, then BZD toxicity is unlikely. Some BZDs have a longer duration of action than flumazenil, necessitating redosing, which may be done safely at 20-minute intervals. Rapid BZD reversal may result in acute withdrawal for patients with BZD dependence, which may present as seizure or severe agitation.

Dexmedetomidine

DEX selectively stimulates centrally acting, α_2-adrenergic receptors with sympatholytic, sedative, and analgesic properties but lacks GABA effects.[29] Mechanistically, it is similar to clonidine but has a significantly higher affinity for the α_{2a} receptor. Adverse hemodynamic effects, however, such as bradycardia, sinus arrest, and hypotension, may occur. These effects are more pronounced in patients with labile hemodynamics at baseline or those requiring concurrent vasopressor therapy and are more likely to occur when administering a loading dose. For this reason, a loading dose is no longer routinely recommended. These effects may still be seen, however, with the maintenance infusion regardless of loading dose. A starting dose of 0.4 µg/kg/h is reasonable for most patients and should be titrated in increments of 0.1 µg/kg/h no more frequently than every 10 to 15 minutes to a maximum of 1.5 µg/kg/h.

The quality of sedation induced by DEX differs significantly from that of other sedative drugs. Patients are generally calm and sedated but arousable and even interactive, whereas BZDs and propofol often render patients sedated with limited, if any, interactive ability. DEX exhibits some analgesic properties, although concurrent use of analgesics is still indicated. More importantly, DEX lacks amnestic properties. As a result, DEX should not be used as a sole sedative in the setting of neuromuscular blockade where deeper sedation and amnesia are desired. Unlike BZDs and propofol, DEX has minimal effect on respiratory drive and does not suppress electroencephalogram. Therefore, BIS monitoring is not an appropriate means of measuring sedation for these patients.

In the critical care setting, DEX has been compared with lorazepam and midazolam in registration trials, resulting in Food and Drug Administration (FDA) approval for short-term sedation in intubated patients.[30,31] These studies suggest DEX is a safe and effective alternative and may yield shorter duration of MV and ICU LOS. In a subsequent economic analysis, the reduced duration of MV and ICU LOS were believed responsible for significantly lower total ICU costs compared with midazolam infusion.[32] Controversy exists surrounding the suggestion that DEX is associated with less delirium and coma in mechanically ventilated patients. Due to poor study design and composite endpoints used, further investigation is warranted to definitively answer this question. Subsequent studies demonstrate DEX to be similar to midazolam and propofol in maintaining light to moderate sedation in patients receiving prolonged MV. Duration of MV was reduced in patients receiving DEX compared with midazolam but not compared with propofol.[33] The safety and efficacy of DEX have not been established in trauma patients.[34]

Current research is focused on finding the optimal population for the use of DEX, for example, defining its role for optimizing sedation while minimizing delirium and in patients at high-risk for alcohol withdrawal. Most data are limited to animal studies and human case reports, but additional human data are forthcoming.[35] Additional data support the use of DEX in cardiothoracic surgery patients. The routine use of DEX as a first-line therapy for sedation in all patients, however, has been slow to evolve.

Ketamine

Ketamine is a nonbarbiturate anesthetic that also possesses analgesic properties.[36] The precise mechanism of action is not fully elucidated, but it is believed to bind to NMDA receptors in the CNS and to interact with opiate, norepinephrine, serotonin, and muscarinic cholinergic receptors as well.[36] The most common adverse effects are emergence phenomena (described as nightmares, hallucinations, delirium, and visual disturbances), transient elevations in blood pressure (BP), including ICP, and heart rate, respiratory drive stimulation, and emesis. It should be avoided in patients with elevated ICP, active myocardial ischemia, or a history of coronary artery disease when alternatives, such as etomidate or BZDs, are available. Its role in procedural sedation at a dose of 1 mg/kg IV is largely limited in the adult population due to the high incidence (10%–20%) of emergence phenomena, although these phenomena are less common (<2%) in pediatrics.[36,37] Ketamine may be used synergistically with propofol for procedural sedation, allowing for lower doses of each to be used (0.5 mg/kg each).[17] In addition to using lower doses, it is believed that the addition of ketamine mitigates some of the hypotensive and respiratory depressive effects of propofol. Ketamine was prospectively compared with etomidate for RSI and found to have similar efficacy and safety, except for a higher percentage of etomidate patients developing adrenal insufficiency.[38] The investigators concluded ketamine is a safe and valuable alternative to etomidate for endotracheal intubation in critically ill patients and should be considered in those with sepsis.

When used at lower doses as a continuous infusion (10–40 mg/h), it may be used as an adjunct to opioids for analgesia and is opioid sparing.[36] This practice is of particular benefit in the perioperative setting. Although an oral formulation is not commercially available and is poorly bioavailable, it may be compounded from the IV formulation and used as a bridge to wean off a continuous infusion. Emergence phenomena are much less common at these lower doses.

Etomidate

Etomidate (Amidate) is a short-acting hypnotic with GABA effects. Its minimal cardiovascular and respiratory effects make it an ideal agent for RSI and induction for anesthesia. Historically it was used as a continuous infusion for the maintenance of sedation, but it was later associated with increased mortality when used in this manner.[39] It was subsequently identified that etomidate suppresses the hypothalamus-pituitary-adrenal axis, thus resulting in adrenal suppression. Its use as a continuous infusion is obsolete; however, its role for RSI is still prominent but not without controversy. Although safe and effective for most patients, some data suggest that even a single dose (0.3 mg/kg) for RSI may contribute to worse outcomes in critically ill septic patients.[40,41] Conservative management dictates avoiding the drug in these patients as long as therapeutic alternatives, such as BZDs or ketamine, are available.

PSYCHOTROPHICS

Delirium is manifested by an acute onset of fluctuating disturbances in consciousness, accompanied by inattention, disorganized thinking, and perceptual disturbances. It may be hyperactive, hypoactive, or manifest features of both.[42] The development of delirium is of particular concern in ICUs because it is associated with increased morbidity, prolonged neurologic deficits, mortality, and health care cost.[26,43–47] Risk factors are multifactorial and can be divided into host factors, factors of acute illness, and iatrogenic and environmental factors. Nonpharmacologic interventions focus on minimizing the impact of these factors by correcting reversible causes, optimizing the environment, and initiating early ambulation.[48,49] Pharmacologic interventions are focused in 2 areas: the prevention and treatment of delirium.

A standardized tool for the detection of delirium is recommended for use in ICUs.[4] The Confusion Assessment Method for the Intensive Care Unit (CAM-ICU) and Intensive Care Delirium Screening Checklist (ICDSC) have been validated in ICUs and are commonly used. The CAM-ICU is a dichotomous scale simply identifying if delirium is present or not, whereas the ICDSC is a scale of 1 to 8; a score of greater than or equal to 4 has a 99% sensitivity correlation for a psychiatric diagnosis of delirium.[50–53] The 2 scales were prospectively compared with each other and yielded comparable results.[54] Given the numeric scale, the ICDSC may be better at determining patients trending toward and away from delirium and, therefore, may be more useful. Use of an objective tool allows for quick and reliable detection of delirium by both nurses and physicians.[55] A more comprehensive look at the disease state and treatment options may be found in one of several review articles.

Delirium Prevention

Two approaches for the pharmacologic prevention of delirium are described. First is the avoidance of certain precipitating drugs, such as sedatives (especially BZDs) and anticholinergics.[22–24] This also includes avoiding medications on the Beers list for elderly patients.[56,57] Although these medications are not clearly associated with increased mortality, it is generally accepted that minimizing these medications reduces adverse drug effects.[58] The second approach is to proactively administer drugs with the intent of delirium prophylaxis. A few drugs have been studied for the prevention of delirium in the perioperative setting, including the antipsychotics haloperidol (Haldol), risperidone (Risperdal), and olanzapine (Zyprexa).[59–61] Although outcomes demonstrated mixed results, a Cochrane review concluded that none of these agents is generally effective for the prevention of delirium.[49] Since the Cochrane review was published, a large (n = 457) prospective, double-blind, randomized, placebo-controlled trial compared haloperidol infusion to placebo for the prevention of delirium in noncardiac postoperative ICU elderly patients.[62] The incidence of delirium was 15.3% in the haloperidol group versus 23.2% in the placebo group. The impact of this study on practice is yet to be seen.

Cholinesterase inhibitors, donepezil (Aricept) and rivastigmine (Exelon) have also been studied in the prevention of delirium in ICU patients but have yielded negative results.[63,64] A recent meta-analysis of 24 trials using DEX failed to show a reduction in delirium.[65] Other pharmacologic approaches to delirium prevention have focused on minimizing sleep deprivation and optimizing the use of narcotics in the postoperative setting, but outcome data are limited.[66–69]

Delirium Treatment

The treatment of delirium should be initiated only after underlying causes are evaluated and corrected and after analgesia and sedation are optimized. Only a few small, prospective trials have evaluated the use of typical and atypical antipsychotics for the treatment of delirium. Although it is unclear which class yields better outcomes, it is generally accepted that the atypicals, which predominately work on serotonin receptors, are at least as well tolerated as typicals, which act on dopamine receptors (Table 3). All of these agents lack FDA approval for the treatment of ICU delirium; therefore, recommended doses are based on clinical experience and clinical trials in critically ill patients rather than package inserts (Table 4). Antipsychotic agents are associated with increased mortality when used in elderly patients with pre-existing dementia, and, therefore, all now carry a black box warning to this effect.

Typical Antipsychotics: Haloperidol and Chlorpromazine

Haloperidol is the most commonly prescribed typical antipsychotic, largely due to the high incidence of adverse effects associated with other typical agents. Haloperidol and chlorpromazine (Thorazine) can successfully treat agitation and delirium in hospitalized patients.[70] Haloperidol remains the drug of choice according to the Society of Critical Care Medicine, although these guidelines are more than a decade old; an update is expected later this year.[4] Haloperidol is dosed intermittently on an as-needed basis, loaded in a stacked fashion, scheduled, and as a continuous infusion, although the optimal dosing strategy has not yet been clearly defined.[70–72] QT prolongation remains a concern with haloperidol and, therefore, routine ECG monitoring is recommended. Proactive monitoring for neuroleptic malignant syndrome and extrapyramidal symptoms (EPSs) is also recommended. The drug should be immediately discontinued if these occur.

Atypical Antipsychotics: Quetiapine, Olanzapine, Risperidone, and Ziprasidone

With quetiapine (Seroquel), the predominantly antihistaminic mechanism of action, short half-life (which facilitates dose titration), low propensity to alter the QT interval,

Table 3						
Adverse drug effects of selected antipsychotics						
Drug	Anticholinergic	Sedation	EPS	Orthostatic Hypotension	Metabolic	QT Prolongation
Haloperidol	+	+++	+++	+	+	+++
Quetiapine	+	+++	+	+++	++	+
Risperidone	+	++	+++	+++	++	+
Olanzapine	+++	+++	+	+	+++	+
Ziprasidone	+	+	+	+	+	+++

Abbreviations: +, none to minimal activity; ++, moderate activity; +++, marked activity.

Table 4
Dosing of selected antipsychotics[a]

Drug	Common ICU Dose	Routes Available	Considerations
Haloperidol	2 mg IV, increasing dose q15–20 min prn until response achieved, then scheduled q4–6 h until delirium resolved and taper off; alternatively may continue IV or po q2–4 h prn in lieu of scheduled dosing	IM (often used IV but not FDA approved), po, liquid	QTc prolongation and torsades de pointes with higher doses, neuroleptic malignant syndromes, EPS
Quetiapine	25–50 mg po q6–12 h prn, increased by 25–50 mg daily to max of 400 mg/d	po	Sedation, hypotension
Risperidone	0.25–1 mg po q6–12 h prn, increased by 0.5–1 mg every 2–3 d to max dose 6 mg/d	po, liquid, ODT	EPS
Olanzapine	2.5–5 mg po q6–12 h prn, increased by 2.5–5 mg daily to max dose 20 mg/d	IM, po, ODT	Sedation
Ziprasidone	20–40 mg po q6–12 h prn, increased by 20 mg daily to max dose of 160 mg/d	IM, po	QTc prolongation

Abbreviations: IM, intramuscular; EPS, extrapyramidal; max, maximum; ODT, orally disintegrating tablet.

[a] Based on clinical experience and clinical trials in critically ill (nonelderly, nonpsychiatric, nondemented) patients, doses should be reduced by at least 50% when used in elderly patients. Regularly reassess for de-escalation to an as needed basis and discontinue once no longer clinically indicated.

and rare reports of EPSs make it a viable option for treatment of delirium. A small placebo-controlled prospective pilot study of the treatment of ICU delirium suggests that quetiapine when added to as-needed haloperidol results in faster delirium resolution, less agitation, and a greater rate of transfer to home or rehabilitation.[73] The drug is generally well tolerated, but robust efficacy and safety data are lacking. Larger studies are warranted to validate these findings.

Olanzapine is an effective alternative to haloperidol for the treatment of ICU delirium, although its undesirable sedative properties are of concern, especially in those with hypoactive delirium.[74,75] Although subsequent prospective studies found no difference between olanzapine, risperidone, and haloperidol for the treatment of delirium, none of the patients were in an ICU.[76,77] These results may not be applied to ICU patients; therefore, initial olanzapine findings have not been further validated.

A prospective pilot study randomized ICU patients to receive ziprasidone (Geodon), haloperidol, or placebo for the treatment of delirium.[78] Treatment with either antipsychotic did not improve the number of days alive without delirium or coma nor did it increase adverse outcomes compared with placebo.

Limited outcome data are available to aid practitioners in selecting antipsychotic therapy for the treatment of ICU delirium. Haloperidol remains the standard of care for the treatment of ICU delirium, although quetiapine offers a therapeutic alternative with potentially fewer adverse drug effects. Olanzapine may be considered an alternative to haloperidol and quetiapine, although concerns regarding sedation are legitimate and must be considered. Risperidone's role may be similar to olanzapine's, although concerns for EPSs and hypotension may limit its use. The role of ziprasidone in ICUs has not yet been defined, and concerns for ECG changes are legitimate. Once delirium has resolved, drug treatment is no longer indicated and should be discontinued. Minimizing patients' exposure to antipsychotic therapy is preferred, regardless of which agent is used.

NEUROMUSCULAR BLOCKING AGENTS

NMBAs have been used for many years in ICUs. As the name implies, these agents disrupt the transmission of impulses to the motor endplate, resulting in muscle paralysis. Single doses may be used for procedures, including RSI, line placement, and dressing changes. Short-term use during transport between and within health care facilities is described, which provides an element of safety when providers have limited access to patients, such as in an elevator, ambulance, or helicopter.[79] This practice is the standard of care for critically wounded military personnel during aeromedical evacuation. Commonly cited indications for long-term use are facilitating MV, ablation of muscle spasms (tetanus), control of ICP, and decreasing oxygen demand.[79] Placebo-controlled randomized trials are generally lacking for these agents. Most studies make the assumption that NMBAs are indicated and, therefore, compare one agent to another, or are dose-finding studies comparing different dosing strategies of the same agent. Given that the use of sustained NMBAs poses significant risks, it should only be considered after efforts to provide adequate sedation have failed to achieve the desired therapeutic goals. During NMBA use, clinicians should regularly assess for the opportunity to discontinue therapy. The adverse effects associated with the use of NMBAs are discussed.

Depolarizing Agent: Succinylcholine

NMBAs are divided into 2 main groups: depolarizing agents and nondepolarizing agents.[79] Depolarizing agents mimic acetylcholine (ACh) at the neuromuscular junction (NMJ), yielding sustained depolarization and prevention of muscle contractions. The depolarization of the postsynaptic membrane causes repetitive excitation of the motor end plate, resulting in fasciculation. Succinylcholine (Anectine) is the only available depolarizing agent in the United States. Its primary use is for RSI and it is used for this indication more than any other NMBA due to its rapid onset and short duration of action (**Table 5**).[80] Because succinylcholine is metabolized more slowly than ACh, its prolonged effect on muscle cells results in an extracellular shift of potassium, which may lead to dysrhythmias or even cardiac arrest.[81] On average, the rise in serum potassium is modest, at 0.5 meq/L, although it can be higher in patients predisposed to hyperkalemia (renal failure, burns, crush injury, and severe infection).[82–84] Succinylcholine should be avoided in these patients. It should also be avoided in patients with a family history of malignant hyperthermia. Other adverse effects include bradycardia, hypotension, and elevated intraocular pressure, but the drug is generally well tolerated.

Nondepolarizing Agents: Atracurium, Cisatracurium, Rocuronium, Vecuronium, and Pancuronium

Nondepolarizing agents, which resemble ACh, competitively inhibit ACh receptors in the NMJ; the prevention of ACh binding results in blockade of muscle contraction.

Table 5
Neuromuscular blockers used for rapid sequence intubation

Drug	Dose (mg/kg)	Onset (s)	Duration (min)	Comments
Succinylcholine	1.5	<60	10	Preferred agent; contraindicated in malignant hyperthermia; avoid in patients predisposed to hyperkalemia; higher doses needed in patients with myasthenia gravis
Rocuronium	0.6–1.2	60–90	25–50	Preferred agent when unable to use succinylcholine; may require a subsequent dose of sedative to outlast paralytic effects
Vecuronium	Avoid due to slow onset of action			
Cisatracurium	Avoid due to slow onset of action			
Atracuronium	Avoid due to histamine release (hypotension) and slow onset of action			
Pancuronium	Avoid due to vagolytic action (hypertension and tachycardia) and long duration of action			

Data from Murray MJ, Cowen J, DeBlock H, et al. Clinical practice guidelines for sustained neuromuscular blockade in the adult critically ill patient. Crit Care Med 2002;30(1):142–56.

Although these agents vary in onset and duration of action, they are generally too slow acting for routine RSI (**Table 6**).[79] The only exception to this is rocuronium (Zemuron), which exhibits an onset of action nearly as rapid as succinylcholine. Route of elimination and adverse effects are of highest importance when selecting an agent to be used as a continuous infusion, the primary role of nondepolarizing agents. The nondepolarizing agents are further divided in 2 subgroups, the benzylisoquiniliniums and the aminosteroidals.

The benzylisoquiniliniums, atracurium (Tracrium) and cisatracurium (Nimbex), are eliminated via Hofmann elimination, a spontaneous degradation in plasma and tissue at normal body pH and temperature, and by ester hydrolysis.[79] Elimination is not dependent on renal or hepatic function. Atracurium yields the active metabolite laudanosine, which may accumulate and induce seizures. It also causes mast cell degranulation, which releases histamine resulting in vasodilation and hypotension. This hypotensive effect has largely limited its use, especially in the critically ill patient population. These effects are also seen with cisatracurium but they are significantly less pronounced, thereby making it the preferred agent, especially in hemodynamically unstable patients. Tachyphylaxis is associated with prolonged use of both agents, whereby progressive upward dose titration is required to maintain neuromuscular blockade. Upward dose titration, especially in prolonged use, can have a significant impact on ICU drug costs.

The remaining NMBAs comprise the aminosteroidal group. With the exception of tubocurarine (Curare), Pancuronium (Pavulon) is the oldest NMBA and was the mainstay of therapy from the 1970s through the early 1980s because therapeutic alternatives were lacking. Although effective, pancuronium is poorly tolerated because of its vagolytic activity, which results in tachycardia, hypertension, and increased myocardial oxygen demand. Its long duration of action (60–100 minutes) makes it a difficult agent to effectively titrate. Vecuronium (Norcuon) became the mainstay of therapy with its introduction in 1984 and remains widely used today. It lacks vagolytic activity and, therefore, exerts minimal hemodynamic effects. In addition, its shorter duration of

Table 6
Neuromuscular blockers used for continuous infusion

Drug	Loading Dose (mg/kg)	Continuous Dose (µg/kg/min)	Onset of Action (min)	Duration of Action (min)	Elimination	Comments
Atracurium	0.4–0.5	2–15	2–3	20–35	Hofmann elimination (dependent on pH and temperature)	Tachyphylaxis associated with prolonged use; seizure risk due to accumulation of active metabolite laudanosine; histamine release results in hypotension
Cisatracurium	0.1	0.5–10	1.5–2	20–35	Hofmann elimination (dependent on pH and temperature)	Tachyphylaxis associated with prolonged use
Pancuronium	0.04–0.1	1–2	2–3	60–100	Renal 57%–89%; hepatic 15%; biliary (11%)	Vagolytic activity causes tachycardia, hypertension, and increased CO; significant accumulation in renal failure
Vecuronium	0.1	1–2	2.4–3.8	25–60	Biliary 30%–50%; hepatic 30%; renal 15%–30%	Accumulation seen in renal and hepatic failure
Rocuronium	0.4–0.5	4–16	1–1.5	25–50	Biliary extensive; renal up to 30%	Accumulation seen in renal failure

Data from Murray MJ, Cowen J, DeBlock H, et al. Clinical practice guidelines for sustained neuromuscular blockade in the adult critically ill patient. Crit Care Med 2002;30(1):142–56.

action (35–45 minutes) allows for easier dose titration. It is primarily eliminated via the bile, although hepatic and renal elimination play a significant role. Accumulation with continued administration may result in a prolonged effect in the setting of renal or hepatic failure. Rocuronium is similar to vecuronium with regard to tolerability and accumulation seen in the setting of renal failure. Its onset of action, however, is more rapid than any other nondepolarizing agent, making it a feasible option for RSI.

Adverse Drug Effects

The use of NMBAs is not without adverse effects. The most common complication is prolonged recovery, defined as a 50% to 100% longer time to recovery than predicted by pharmacologic parameters. This phenomenon is more commonly reported with pancuronium and vecuronium due to accumulation of NMBAs and/or active metabolites; however, this observation may be due in part to these agents having longer use in clinical practice compared with the newer benzylisoquiniliniums.[85] Another, more sinister, complication is acute quadriplegic myopathy syndrome. It is characterized by the triad of acute paresis, myonecrosis, and increased creatine kinase.[86,87] Caution should be used in the setting of concomitant corticosteroid administration due to its association with increased risk of developing acute quadriplegic myopathy syndrome.[79] ACh receptor upregulation, as seen in spinal cord injury, results in resistance to nondepolarizing agents but increased sensitivity to depolarizing agents. Conversely, down-regulation, as seen in myasthenia gravis, leads to increased sensitivity to nondepolarizing agents. Several medications may affect the action of NMBAs (**Box 1**). Most medications that interact have a potentiating effect on the action of NBMA, whereas fewer inhibit NMBA activity.[79,88]

Monitoring

Patients should be closely monitored during NMBA administration to assess the degree of neuromuscular blockade.[79,89] Peripheral nerve stimulation, as used in the operating room, is the most common method. Train-of-four of 1 to 2 out of 4, along with clinical assessment, is recommended for monitoring patients receiving NMBA.[79] Dosing of NMBA guided by train-of-four monitoring may yield faster recovery after paralysis, result in fewer adverse effects, and provide some pharmacoeconomic

---

Box 1
Medications affecting neuromuscular blocker activity

Potentiate	Antagonize
Antiarrhythmics: procainamide, quinidine, verapamil	Antiepileptics: carbamazepine, phenytoin
Antibiotics: aminoglycosides, tetracyclines, clindamycin	Other: ranitidine, theophylline
Cardiovascular medications: β-blockers, CCBs	
Cations: calcium, magnesium	
Immunosuppressants: cyclophosphamide, cyclosporine	
Inhaled anesthetics: desflurane, sevoflurane, isoflurane, halothane	
Local anesthetics	
Other: dantrolene, diuretics, lithium	

Data from Naguib M, Lien CA. Pharmacology of muscle relaxants and their antagonists. In: Miller RD, ed. Miller's anesthesia. 7th edition. Philadelphia: Churchill Livingstone; 2009. p. 859–912; and Murray MJ, Cowen J, DeBlock H, et al. Clinical practice guidelines for sustained neuromuscular blockade in the adult critically ill patient. Crit Care Med 2002;30(1):142–56.

benefits; however, data are conflicting. It is suggested that good clinical assessment alone may yield similar outcomes to those associated with train-of-four use.[90] Given the increased sophistication of mechanical ventilator processors, spontaneous respiration could be used as an indication of incomplete blockade and titrate NMBA accordingly irrespective of train-of-four results.

Sedation

NMBAs lack analgesic, sedative, and amnestic properties and, therefore, require concurrent use of a sedative agent possessing amnestic properties, such as propofol or BZDs. DEX lacks amnestic properties and should be avoided in these patients. The RASS and the Ramsay scale are not validated in paralyzed patients and should be avoided. The popularity of BIS has increased in recent years in patients receiving NMBA, although strong data are lacking. Its role remains controversial in ICUs. Some practitioners have suggested BIS only be used to increase sedation during paralysis but not to reduce sedation. Clinical assessment and thorough physical examination remain the standard for monitoring sedation in paralyzed patients.

Reversal Agents

The need for reversal of nondepolarizing NMBA is common, especially in the perioperative setting. The primary goal is to maximize nicotinic transmission while minimizing muscarinic side effects.[88] Therapy consists of an acetylcholinesterase inhibitor and an anticholinergic agent. Acetylcholinesterase inhibitors, such as neostigmine (Prostigmin), pyridostigmine (Mestinon), physostigmine, (Antilirium), and edrophonium (Reversol), act at the NMJ, allowing for more ACh to compete for binding with the NMBA. Neostigmine is most commonly used because of its less severe adverse effect profile compared with other agents. Unfortunately, the cholinesterase inhibitors are not specific for the NMJ and act at cholinergic receptors in other organ systems. The most prominent effects are on the cardiovascular system, which result in decreased heart rate and dysrhythmias, but the pulmonary, cerebral, gastrointestinal, genitourinary, and ophthalmologic systems may also be affected. These muscarinic actions may be attenuated or prevented by the coadministration of an anticholinergic agent, such as glycopyrrolate (Robinul) or atropine (Atreza). These agents are administered at a fixed dose relative to the ACh inhibitor. A common combination is neostigmine (2.5 mg) administered with glycopyrrolate (0.5 mg; 0.2 mg glycopyrrolate per 1 mg neostigmine). The anticholinergic (glycopyrrolate) should be given before the acetylcholinesterase inhibitor (neostigmine) to minimize the adverse effects manifested on the muscarinic receptors.

CARDIOVASCULAR AGENTS

Catecholamines, or sympathomimetics, exert their cardiovascular effects through their actions on α_1, α_2, β_1, β_2 and dopaminergic receptors. The type of physiologic effect that is elucidated from these agents is determined by the location of the receptor (**Table 7**) and the affinity of the agent for the specific adrenoceptor subtypes (**Table 8**).[91] The use of these catecholamines in the critical care setting is dictated by the underlying disease state and desired clinical effect; therefore, it is important to determine the cause of the shock state to appropriately choose a vasopressor or inotrope. Vasopressors should not be used in a hypovolemic patient until proper fluid resuscitation has been achieved to minimize potential toxicity from these agents (**Table 9**) and, in some situations, vasopressors should not be used at all. The use of vasopressors in hemorrhagic shock may lead to increased mortality and the

Table 7
Distribution of adrenoceptor subtypes and physiologic response

Adrenoceptor Type	Primary Location	Physiologic Response to Agonist Activity
α_1	Arteries, arterioles, veins	Arterial and venous constriction
α_2	Arteries, arterioles, veins CNS	Arterial and venous constriction Decreased BP
β_1	Heart	Increased contractility and heart rate (positive inotropic and chronotropic effects)
β_2	Vascular smooth muscle (blood vessels) Bronchial smooth muscle	Vasodilation Bronchodilation
D_1	Renal, coronary, and cerebral smooth muscle	Vasodilation
D_2	Nerve endings	Modulates neurotransmitter release
V_{1a}	Vascular smooth muscle	Vasoconstriction
V_2	Renal collecting duct	Water reabsorption

Data from Biaggioni I RD. Adrenoceptor agonists & sympathmimetic drugs. In: Katzung BM, S Trevor A, ed. Basic & clinical pharmacology. 11th edition. Ipswich (MA): McCraw-Hill Professional; 2009.p. 127–48; and Goodman LS. GA, Brunton LL. Adrenergic agniosts and antagonists. Goodman & Gillman's manual of pharmacology and therpeutics. Ipswich (MA): McGraw-Hill Professional; 2008.p. 148–87.

mainstay of therapy for these patients remains blood and fluid resuscitation.[92] Common vasopressors and inotropes and their appropriate use are discussed.

Vasopressors

Phenylephrine

Phenylephrine (Neo-Synephrine) is a direct-acting, predominately α_1-adrenergic receptor agonist with minimal affinity for β-adrenergic receptors (see **Table 8**). The vasoconstriction caused by α_1-adrenergic stimulation results in an increase in

Table 8
Adrenoceptor affinity and clinical effects of vasopressors and inotropes

Medication	Receptors							Clinical Effects			
	α_1	α_2	β	β_2	D_1	D_2	V_{1a}	CO	SVR	HR	BP
Phenylephrine	+++	+	0	0	0	0	0	↔/↑	↑↑	↔/↓	↑
Epinephrine[a]	+++	++	+++	++	0	0	0	↑↑	↔/↑	↑	↑
Norepinephrine[a]	+++	++	++	0	0	0	0	↔/↑	↑↑	↔/↑	↑
Dopamine[a]	++	++	++	+	+++	+++	0	↑	↑	↑	↔/↑
Dobutamine	0/+	0	+++	+	0	0	0	↑	↓	↑	↑/↓
Vasopressin	0	0	0	0	0	0	++	↔/↓	↑	↔/↓	↑

Abbreviations: 0, no effect; +, mild agonist effect; ++, moderate agonist effect; +++, marked agonist effect; ↔, no change; ↑, increased; ↓, decrease; HR, heart rate.
[a] The α_1 effects of epinephrine, norepinephrine, and dopamine are more prominent at high doses.
Data from Refs.[91,93,94,100]

Table 9
Inotropic and vasopressor clinical indication, dose range and major side effects

Drug	Clinical Indication	Dose Range	Major Side Effects
Phenylephrine	Hypotension; neurogenic shock with normocardia	Infusion: 0.4–3 µg/kg/min	Reflex bradycardia, peripheral vasoconstriction
Epinephrine	Septic/vasodilatory shock; cardiac arrest; symptomatic bradycardia	Infusion: 0.01–0.1 µg/kg/min Bolus: 1 mg IV Q 3–5 min (for pulseless patients only)	Ventricular arrhythmias, cardiac ischemia
Norepinephrine	Septic/vasodilatory/ cardiogenic shock	Infusion: 0.01–5 µg/kg/min	Arrhythmias, peripheral ischemia
Dopamine	Septic/vasodilatory/ cardiogenic shock	Infusion: 2–20 µg/kg/min	Ventricular arrhythmias, cardiac ischemia
Vasopressin	Septic/vasodilatory shock; cardiac arrest	Infusion: 0.01–0.1 Unit/min (maintenance 0.03–0.04 Unit/min) Bolus: 40 units IV (for cardiac arrest only)	Cardiac, peripheral, and splanchnic vasoconstriction
Dobutamine	Low CO, symptomatic bradycardia	Infusion: 2–20 µg/kg/min	Tachycardia
Milrinone	Low CO	Bolus: 50 µg/kg over 10–30 min Infusion: 0.125–0.75 µg/kg/min (dose adjustment required for renal impairment)	Ventricular arrhythmias, hypotension

Data from Refs.[91,93,94,100]

systemic vascular resistance (SVR) and ultimately a dose-dependent increase in BP. In the presence of normal cardiovascular reflexes, this rise in BP elicits a baroreceptor-mediated increase in vagal tone leading to a slowing of the heart rate HR. The resulting decrease in HR does not necessarily result in a lowering of cardiac output (CO).[91,93,94] The increased venous return related to phenylephrine use can lead to an increase in stroke volume; however, the effects on CO remain controversial in the literature.[95,96] These physiologic effects, along with its rapid onset and short duration of action, make phenylephrine a useful medication in the setting of hypotension, although it is not a first-line treatment for most types of shock due to limited outcome data.[91,97,98] Phenylephrine is specifically not recommended as a first-line agent for septic shock, and its use is not addressed in the cardiogenic shock guidelines.[97,98] Due to its alpha selectivity, however, the drug can be useful in certain patient populations. Phenylephrine is a good agent for neurogenic shock in the setting of normocardia and in patients with hypotension and concomitant aortic stenosis and is also an option in shock states when tachyarrhythmias limit the use of other vasopressors.[99]

Epinephrine
Epinephrine (ADRENALIN) is an endogenous catecholamine with high affinity for α-adrenergic and β-adrenergic receptors in cardiac and vascular smooth muscle. The β-adrenergic effects are more pronounced at lower doses (1–10 µg/min) whereas the

α_1-adrenergic effects are seen more with higher dosages (>10 µg/min).[91,93,94] The increase in systolic BP seen with epinephrine is a result of its positive inotropic and chronotropic actions on the heart (β_1 effects) and the vasoconstriction (α_1 effects) actions on blood vessels. Epinephrine also acts on β_2-adrenergic receptors in the vasculature leading to vasodilation, balancing the drugs overall effect on SVR. These physiologic effects make epinephrine an effective drug for shock states; however, the undesirable side effects of tachyarrhythmias, ischemia related to increased oxygen consumption, lactic acidosis, and hypoglycemia can limit its use.[100] Similar to phenylephrine, epinephrine is recommended as a second-line agent in patient's failing to respond to first-line therapies for septic shock.[98] Its use is not recommended in cardiogenic shock management outside of advanced cardiac life support (ACLS) where bolus dosing increases blood flow to the heart and brain during cardiopulmonary resuscitation and makes VF more susceptible to defibrillation.[97,101] In patients with neurogenic shock, epinephrine is an option for the treatment of symptomatic bradycardia.[99]

Norepinephrine

Norepinephrine (Levophed) is an agonist with similar potency to epinephrine at α_1-adrenergic and α_2-adrenergic receptors with less pronounced β-adrenergic receptor effects. Consequently, norepinephrine can cause potent vasoconstriction leading to increased BP and also produces a small (10%–15%) increase in CO and stroke volume.[100] Similar to other catecholamines, its vasoconstrictive effects have the potential to cause a decrease in renal, splanchnic, or peripheral blood flow, particularly in patients not adequately fluid resuscitated.[102] Norepinephrine is well studied in septic shock where it increases BP without causing deterioration of cardiac index and organ function.[103,104] The largest randomized trial to date showed no significant difference in 28-day mortality between norepinephrine and dopamine for the treatment of shock, rendering either agent a first-line vasopressor for septic shock.[98,105] Norepinephrine is also an option for the management of hypotension accompanying spinal cord injury as well as cardiogenic shock.[97,99]

Dopamine

Dopamine (Intropin), the natural precursor of norepinephrine, acts on dopaminergic and adrenergic receptors to varying degrees in a dose-dependent fashion (see **Table 8**). At lower doses (0.5–5 µg/kg/min) it stimulates mostly dopaminergic receptors leading to vasodilation of mesenteric and renal tissues and increased blood flow to these areas. The increase in blood flow caused by low-dose dopamine does not translate into a clinical benefit and its use is not recommended for protection from renal failure.[106] Moderate doses (5–10 µg/kg/min) stimulate β_1-adrenergic receptors resulting in an increase in HR and contractility. The α_1-adrenergic effects of dopamine predominate at high doses (≥10 µg/kg/min), leading to vasoconstriction and an increase in BP.[100] Dopamine increases in BP and CO primarily due to its increase in stroke volume and HR; therefore, it is often an option in the setting of hypotension and cardiac compromise. These effects also lead to tachycardia and arrhythmias, a major limitation of dopamine therapy. Dopamine continues to be recommended along with norepinephrine as a first-line therapy for the treatment of septic shock.[98] It is also recommended as a potential agent for the management of hypotension along with bradycardia in spinal cord injury and for increasing CO in the setting of hypotension for patients in cardiogenic shock.[97,99]

Vasopressin

Vasopressin (Pitressin) is a peptide hormone that is synthesized in the hypothalamus, stored in the pituitary gland, and released in response to hypotension or increased plasma osmolality.[100] It stimulates vasopressin (V_{1a}) receptors, causing smooth muscle contraction and vasoconstriction, and vasopressin (V_2) receptors, enhancing renal collecting duct permeability and water reabsorption, leading to an increase in SVR and a reflexive increase in vagal tone. Vasopressin also increases responsiveness of the vasculature to catecholamines. The addition of low doses of vasopressin (0.01–0.04 units/min) to catecholamine therapy in patients with vasopressor-refractory septic shock decreases catecholamine requirements.[107,108] Vasopressin remains effective in the setting of acidosis, whereas catecholamines do not. A fixed dose of vasopressin (0.03–0.04 units/min) is a safe and effective adjunctive therapy to norepinephrine in fluid-resuscitated patients with septic shock and this therapy is recommended in the surviving sepsis guidelines.[98,109] Vasopressin is typically not titrated and is given as a fixed dose because higher doses of vasopressin are associated with splanchnic, digital, and cardiac ischemia. Its use should be reserved for situations where alternative vasopressors have failed.[110] Vasopressin is not recommended in the treatment of cardiogenic shock outside the setting of ACLS.[97,101]

Inotropes

Dobutamine

Dobutamine (Dobutrex) is a synthetic catecholamine with a strong affinity for both β_1-adrenergic receptors and β_2-adrenergic receptors. It binds in a 3:1 ratio to the β_1-adrenergic receptors and β_2-adrenergic receptors leading to its inotropic effects. It has a variable effect on BP secondary to its modest effects on the α_2-adrenergic and β_2-adrenergic receptors, usually leading to a net vasodilation.[100] Vasoconstriction increasingly dominates at higher infusion rates.[100] Monitoring CO and other clinical measures of tissue perfusion are typically used to guide dosing. Dobutamine is the drug of choice in patients with a low-output syndrome with reasonable BP.[97] However, It can significantly increase myocardial oxygen consumption and therefore, can potentially induce ischemia.[100] Dobutamine also has a role the in treatment of septic shock as the first-line therapy for patients with a low-output state but adequate filling pressures.[98] Reference is not made to dobutamine in the spinal cord injury guidelines.[99]

Milrinone

Milrinone (Primacor) is a phosphodiesterase inhibitor whose inotropic activity is caused by a prevention of the breakdown of intercellular cyclic adenosine monophosphate.[100] Due to its mechanism of action, milrinone tends to have fewer chronotropic and arrhythmogenic effects compared with the catecholamines; however, its effects on vascular smooth muscle cells can cause vasodilation leading to an exacerbation of hypotension.[100] The side effect of hypotension and its long half-life (2–4 hours) limits its use in ICUs to patients whose adrenergic receptors are downregulated or desensitized due to chronic heart failure (HF) or chronic β-agonist administration.[98] The use of milrinone is not commented on in any of the current consensus guidelines for the treatment of septic, cardiogenic, or neurogenic shock.[97–99]

Acute Hypertension

Acute hypertension in ICUs is common, often iatrogenic in nature, and is associated with a high risk of acute end-organ damage and bleeding, especially in the perioperative setting.[111] Hypertensive emergencies are defined by severe elevations in BP, typically systolic BP greater than 180mmHg or diastolic BP greater than 120 mm Hg, in the presence of end-organ damage, such as neurologic changes, hypertensive encephalopathy, myocardial ischemia or infarction, renal insufficiency, and so forth.[112] The therapeutic goal for these patients is to lower the mean arterial pressure by 20% to 25% within 60 minutes, avoiding a precipitous or excessive decrease in BP. If a patient remains stable, the BP can further be reduced to systolic BP 160 mm Hg and diastolic BP of 100 mm Hg to 110 mm Hg over the next 2 to 6 hours. The ultimate goal is to be at a patient's baseline BP in 24 to 48 hours.[112] To reduce BP in a controlled and predictable manner, it is important to understand the IV drug options available. The agent of choice depends on the clinical presentation (**Box 2**, **Table 10**).[113] Hypertensive urgencies also require therapeutic intervention; however, they can often be managed with oral therapy and do not necessarily require admission to an ICU. The pharmacology of common IV antihypertensives and their appropriate use are discussed.

Nicardipine

Nicardipine (Cardene), a second-generation dihydropyridine CCB, is highly selective for vascular smooth muscle and causes vasodilation, leading to a reduction in BP and a decrease in afterload. It has strong selectivity for cerebral and coronary vessels and, therefore, is useful in the setting of cerebral and cardiac ischemia.[114–119] Nicardipine has demonstrated ability to increase stroke volume and coronary blood flow with a favorable effect on myocardial oxygen balance; however, it is contraindicated in patients with advanced aortic stenosis.[120–122] It has similar efficacy to sodium nitroprusside (Nipride) for perioperative BP control and the treatment of hypertensive emergencies and it is safe for patients with renal and hepatic disease (see **Box 2**).[123–125] The most common adverse effects associated with nicardipine are headache, nausea, vomiting, hypotension, and reflex tachycardia.[122]

Box 2
Preferred agents for hypertensive emergencies based on comorbidity

Comorbidity	Preferred Agent(s)
Acute aortic dissection	Esmolol (may add nicardipine or nitroprusside to IV β-blocker)
Acute HF	Nitroprusside, nitroglycerin
Acute intracerebral hemorrhage/acute ischemic stroke	Labetalol, nicardipine
Acute myocardial infarction	β-Blocker in combination with nitroglycerine (if HR <70 beats/min, nicardipine or clevidipine)
Acute pulmonary edema	Nitroprusside, nitroglycerin
Acute renal failure	Fenoldopam, nicardipine, clevidipine
Eclampsia or preeclampsia	Hydralazine, labetalol, nicardipine
Perioperative hypertension	Clevidipine, esmolol, nicardipine, nitroglycerin, nitroprusside
Sympathetic crisis or catecholamine toxicity	Nicardipine, fendoldopam, clevidipine (avoid unopposed β-blockade)

Data from Chobanian AV, Bakris GL, Black HR, et al. Seventh report of the joint national committee on prevention, detection, evaluation, and treatment of high blood pressure. Hypertension 2003;42(6):1206–52; and Marik PE, Varon J. Hypertensive crises: challenges and management. Chest 2007;131(6):1949–62.

Table 10
Commonly prescribed intravenous antihypertensives

Drug	Dose	Onset, Duration	Adverse Effects
Nicardipine	5–15 mg/h (max 15 mg/h) Titration: 2.5 mg/h every 5 min	5–10 min, 4–6 h (longer with prolonged infusion)	Headache, hypotension, nausea, vomiting, reflex tachycardia Contraindications: aortic stenosis Caution: angina/MI, acute HF
Clevidipine	1–2 mg/h (max 21 mg/h, short-term experience with 32 mg/h) Titration: double dose every 90 s	2–4 min, 5–15 min	Headache, AF, nausea, vomiting, acute renal failure Contraindications: soy/egg allergies, severe aortic stenosis, defective lipid metabolism Caution: HF, reflex tachycardia, rebound HTN
Nitroprusside	0.3–0.5 µg/kg/min (max 3 µg/kg/min) Titration: 0.5 µg/kg/min	Immediate, 2–3 min	Cyanide toxicity, methemoglobinemia Contraindications: renal, hepatic failure Caution: increased ICP
Nitroglycerin	5–10 µg/min (max 200 µg/min) Titration: 5 µg/min every 3–5 min	2–5 min, 5–10 min	Headache, tachyphylaxis, methemoglobinemeia Contraindications: concomitant use of phosphodiesterase inhibitors
Hydralazine	5–10 mg IV every 4–6 h (max 20 mg/dose)	5–30 min, 1–4 h	Reflex tachycardia, headache, flushing Caution: angina/MI, increased ICP, aortic dissection
Esmolol	0.5–1 mg/kg loading dose, 25–50 µg/kg/min (max 300 µg/kg/min)	1–2 min, 10–30 min	Bradycardia/heart block, bronchospasm Caution: concurrent β-blocker therapy, HF
Labetalol	20–80 mg IV every 15 min OR 0.5–2 mg/min (max 300 mg/24 h)	5–10 min, 3–6 h	Bradycardia/heart block, bronchospasm Caution: concurrent β-blocker therapy, HF
Fenoldopam	0.1 µg/kg/min (max 1.6 µg/kg/min)	<5 min, 30 min	Headache, flushing, tachycardia, dizziness, increased intraocular pressure Caution: glaucoma, sulfite allergy
Enalaprilat	0.625–1.25 mg IV every 4–6 h (max 5 mg every 6 h)	Within 30 min, 12–24 h	Renal insufficiency/ failure, hyperkalemia Contraindications: pregnancy, renal artery stenosis

Abbreviations: HF, heart failure; HTN, hypertension; MI, myocardial infarction.
Data from Refs.[112–116]

Clevidipine

Clevidipine (Cleviprex), a third-generation dihydropyridine CCB, acts specifically to vasodilate the arterioles and can reduce afterload without affecting cardiac-filling pressures or causing reflex tachycardia.[126] Due to its rapid onset and offset of action, clevidipine is useful when tight BP control is critical and has been studied most in the perioperative setting.[127–130] Clevidipine is rapidly metabolized by esterases in the blood, and, therefore, its metabolism is not affected by renal or hepatic function. It is commercially available in a lipid emulsion, which carries limitations with regard to allergies, total dosage, triglyceride monitoring, and risk of microbial growth.[113]

Sodium nitroprusside

Sodium nitroprusside is an arterial and venous vasodilator that decreases preload and afterload. Unlike CCBs, sodium nitroprusside dilates large-capacitance vessels.[116] It decreases cerebral blood flow while increasing ICPs and is not recommended in patients with hypertensive encephalopathy or after a cerebrovascular accident.[131,132] In patients with coronary artery disease, there is the potential that sodium nitroprusside can cause a reduced coronary perfusion pressure due to the theorized coronary steal mechanism and is not recommended in the setting of acute myocardial infarction.[133] It has a short onset and offset of action and is useful when rapid BP reduction is needed, such as the perioperative setting. Intra-arterial BP monitoring is strongly recommended with the use of sodium nitroprusside due to the drug's potency, rapid onset of action, and the development of tachyphylaxis.[116] There is a risk of cyanide toxicity when the drug is used in patients with renal or hepatic disease, at higher doses and for long periods of time; however, the coadministration of thiosulfate can help avoid toxicity.[116]

Nitroglycerin

Nitroglycerin (Nitro-Bid) is a potent venodilator and can cause arterial smooth muscle dilation at high doses.[113] It reduces BP by decreasing preload and in volume-depleted patients, and reduced preload can decrease CO.[134] This is an undesirable effect in patients with compromised myocardial, cerebral, or renal perfusion. Severe hypotension and reflex tachycardia are reported with nitroglycerin use in volume-depleted patients.[135] Administration of low doses of nitroglycerin (approximately 60 μg/min) can be beneficial as adjunct therapy for patients with hypertensive emergencies associated with acute coronary syndromes or acute pulmonary edema.[136]

Hydralazine

Hydralazine (Apresoline) causes relaxation of arteriolar smooth muscle leading to peripheral vasodilation and reduced cardiac afterload.[113] There is some evidence that hydralazine can cause reflex sympathetic stimulation leading to increases in HR and ICP; however, this effect can be blunted by coadministration of a β-receptor antagonist.[137–139] Hydralazine is administered as intermittent IV or intramuscular (IM) bolus doses. A single dose has an onset of action of up to 30 minutes and a prolonged pharmacologic effect on BP, up to 12 hours in some reports.[113,116,140] The unpredictability of the dose response as well as the prolonged duration of action limits the drug's utility as a first-line option for the treatment of hypertensive emergencies.

Esmolol

Esmolol (Brevibloc) is a short-acting, selective β₁-adrenergic receptor antagonist.[113,116] Due to its pharmacokinetic properties, esmolol is a good medication for heart rate control in the critically ill and is useful in decreasing the sympathetic discharge seen with severe postoperative hypertension accompanied by increased

HR, CO, and BP.[141–143] Esmolol is indicated for perioperative BP management and can be safely used in the setting of myocardial ischemia or infarction, although caution should be used in the setting of HF.[112,144]

Labetalol

Labetalol (Trandate) is a combined selective α_1-adrenergic and nonselective β-adrenergic antagonist. It blocks α-receptor to β-receptor activity in a ratio of 1:7 when given IV and because of the α-adrenergic activity, the decrease in CO related to the β-receptor blockade is minimized.[145,146] Cerebral, renal, and coronary blood flow are maintained with labetalol use and it is a drug of choice in the setting of pregnancy-induced hypertensive emergency due to limited placental drug transfer.[146] Caution should be used in the setting of reactive airway disease, decompensated HF, and second-degree or third-degree atrioventricular (AV) block.[112]

Fenoldopam

Fenoldopam (Corlopam) is a selective peripheral D_1-agonist causing vasodilation of peripheral arteries and the renal and mesenteric vasculature. It lowers BP and SVR while maintaining renal blood flow.[147] It is associated with a lower risk of the need for renal replacement therapy in patients at risk for acute renal impairment; however, the data for prophylaxis of contrast-induced nephropathy are not robust.[148,149] There is a dose-related increase in intraocular pressure with the drug and it should be avoided in patients with glaucoma.[147]

Enalaprilat

Enalaprilat (Vasotec) is an IV angiotensin-converting enzyme inhibitor that causes vasodilation due to decreased production of angiotensin II, a potent vasoconstrictor.[113] Enalaprilat is not commonly used in critically ill patients with hypertensive emergencies due to its variable onset and long duration of action. It should also be avoided in patients with acute MI, bilateral renal artery stenosis, and pregnancy.

Antiarrhythmic Agents

Atrial arrhythmias occur frequently in ICUs, whereas ventricular arrhythmias are less common but often much more serious and life threatening.[150] Arrhythmias in ICUs are often related to catecholamine excess (endogenous or exogenous), hypoxia, infections, cardiac ischemia, or electrolyte disturbances. Management of arrhythmia should focus on correction of underlying causes as well as drug therapy directed at the arrhythmia itself. In the setting of hemodynamic compromise due to arrhythmia, however, cardioversion should be performed.[101] This discussion focuses on the drug therapy options for the most commonly encountered arrhythmias in ICUs.

Atrial fibrillation

Atrial fibrillation (AF) is the most common narrow complex tachyarrhythmia encountered in ICUs and is particularly prevalent in surgical patients.[150,151] AF occurs in 20% to 50% of postcardiac surgery patients with a peak incidence on postoperative day 2.[152] Appropriate preoperative prophylaxis with β-blockers or amiodarone is recommended for the prevention of postoperative AF. There are 2 treatment strategies for rapid onset of new AF in hemodynamically stable patients: rate control, and cardioversion. Rate control can be achieved with β-blockers, CCBs, or digoxin, and the most common agent for chemical cardioversion is amiodarone.[150,152] Other antiarrhythmic agents, such as procainamide (Pronestyl), sotalol (Betapace), and ibutilide (Corvert), convert AF to sinus rhythm, but their safety profiles limit their use outside of expert consultation.[152] When using either strategy, it is important to consider the patient's anticoagulation needs in the setting of AF. Anticoagulation is usually initiated if AF persists greater than 48 hours.[152]

β-Blockers β-Blockers work to slow ventricular rate in AF and are particularly useful in the setting of increased adrenergic tone.[152] There is some evidence that these agents are superior to CCB for establishing rate control.[141,153] Metoprolol (Lopressor) and esmolol are most commonly used in ICUs due to their IV formulations. Metoprolol is typically dosed 2.5 mg to 5 mg IV every 5 to 10 minutes for a total of 15 mg as BP tolerates. Esmolol can be a good option in more unstable patients due to its rapid onset and offset of action.[150]

Calcium channel blockers The nondihydropyridine CCBs, diltiazem (Cardizem) and verapamil (Calan), are also effective AV nodal blockers used for rate control in AF.[154–156] Both of these agents have a negative inotropic effect and should be used cautiously in HF.[157] Diltiazem is available in an IV formulation and is commonly used as a continuous infusion of 5 mg/h to 15 mg/h. IV diltiazem may cause hypotension, so caution should be used in hemodynamically unstable patients.

Digoxin Digoxin (Lanxin) controls ventricular response through a centrally mediated vagal mechanism as well as via direct action on the AV node, leading to HR control at rest. It has limited use in ICUs given the higher level of circulating catecholamines and the longer onset of action (at least 60 minutes).[152] For the treatment of AF, a loading dose of digoxin (0.25 mg every 2 hours up to a maximum of 1.5 mg) is recommended. Digoxin use is also limited by drug interactions and potential for arrhythmias, especially in elderly patients with compromised renal function.[158]

Amiodarone Amiodarone is considered a class III antiarrhythmic drug due to its potassium channel blockade; however, the drug also acts on sodium channels and calcium channels and has a negative chronotropic effect on cardiac nodal tissue.[159] The drug is used for both atrial and ventricular arrhythmias and is effective for conversion of AF as well as ventricular rate control in AF when other agents are ineffective, although the latter indications carry less evidence.[152,160] Amiodarone is not superior to other antiarrhythmic drugs for successful conversion of recent-onset AF, although it is relatively safe in patients with structural heart disease and left ventricular dysfunction.[152] Acute adverse effects of amiodarone include bradycardia, hypotension, and phlebitis. Concerns with thyroid, liver, lung, and ocular toxicity occur with long-term use.

Ventricular arrhythmias

Ventricular arrhythmias include ventricular tachycardia (VT), ventricular fibrillation (VF), and torsades de pointes. These arrhythmias are often life threatening and appropriate ACLS guidelines should be followed when they are encountered. As with atrial arrhythmias, unstable patients presenting with a ventricular arrhythmia should be candidates for immediate cardioversion.[101] In the setting of VF or pulseless VT, epinephrine (1 mg IV/intraosseous) may be given after the first defibrillation effort and high-quality cardiopulmonary resuscitation. Amiodarone (300 mg IV push) is also part of the ACLS VF/pulseless VT algorithm if defibrillation, cardiopulmonary resuscitation, and a vasopressor fail to produce a perfusing rhythm.[101] Amiodarone improves the rate of return of spontaneous circulation and hospital admission in refractory VF/pulseless VT. If torsades de pointes are encountered at any time, magnesium sulfate (2 g IV bolus) should be considered. In the setting of a stable, monomorphic VT, there are additional drug therapy options.

Adenosine Adenosine (Adenocard) directly inhibits that AV nodal refractory period and is indicated for regular narrow complex supraventricular tachycardias as well as regular wide complex tachycardias, if the cause of the latter cannot be determined.[101,159] Adenosine 6 mg to 12 mg IV push is relatively safe for both treatment and diagnosis of regular wide-complex tachycardias. In the setting of supraventricular tachycardias with aberrancy, adenosine converts the tachycardia into a sinus rhythm.[161,162] If the underlying rhythm is VT, there is no effect on the rhythm with adenosine administration and patients are then candidates for IV antiarrhythmic drugs or elective cardioversion.[101]

Procainamide Procainamide, a class Ia antiarrhythmic, is the first-line therapy for patients with stable, monomorphic VT due to its conversion rates compared with lidocaine (Xylocaine).[163] The side effects of QT prolongation and hypotension limit its use. Also, procainamide is contraindicated in patients with HF.[101] For this reason as well as its side effects, amiodarone is often used in its place.

Sotalol Sotalol has both β-adrenergic receptor activity and the ability to prolong the action potential.[159] Sotalol (100 mg IV over 5 minutes) is more effective at the conversion of a stable, monomorphic VT compared with lidocaine and is recommended with the same level of evidence as amiodarone for this indication.[101,164] Sotalol should be avoided in patients with prolonged QT interval and should be used cautiously in patients with HF due to its β-blocking activity.

ANTICOAGULANTS
Intravenous and Subcutaneous Anticoagulants

Unfractionated heparin
Unfractionated heparin (UFH) is an indirect parenteral anticoagulant often indicated for venous thromboembolism (VTE) prophylaxis as well as therapeutic anticoagulation.[165] The half-life of UFH is approximately 1.5 hours, allowing for frequent monitoring and rapid titration. This, along with rapid elimination from the body, makes UFH an attractive agent for use in critically ill patients. When dosed therapeutically, the anticoagulant effect of UFH is monitored using the activated partial prothrombin time to a goal of 1.5 to 2.5 times control.[165] Although this therapeutic goal is based on retrospective data from the 1970s, it is widely accepted today.[166] Activated clotting time is used to monitor the higher UFH doses given to patients undergoing cardiopulmonary bypass surgery, percutaneous coronary interventions, and extracorporeal membrane oxygenation. The dose of UFH can vary based on indication and the presence of thrombosis. Evidence suggests that patients with an active venous thrombosis require higher doses of UFH compared with patients requiring UFH infusions for prophylaxis of clot formation or for the treatments of acute coronary syndrome.[167,168] The use of an institution specific protocol for dosing and monitoring UFH is recommended to assure appropriate safety and efficacy. Patients requiring unusually high doses of UFH may be heparin resistant due to antithrombin III (AT III) deficiency or increased UFH clearance; the use of alternative anticoagulants may be indicated in these situations.

The use of UFH can be limited by hemorrhagic complications and its ability to induce heparin-induced thrombocytopenia (HIT). Fortunately, protamine sulfate can rapidly reverse the anticoagulant effects of heparin in the setting of hemorrhagic complications (**Table 11**). There is a slight risk of hypotension and bradycardia with protamine sulfate administration that can be minimized by slow administration over 10 minutes. HIT is an immune-mediated drug reaction related to heparin exposure that is associated with a high risk of thrombosis.[169] HIT is characterized by

Table 11
Common anticoagulants and reversal agents

Drug	Reversal Agents	Dose	Onset of Action	Precautions
UFH	Protamine sulfate	1 mg Protamine IV/100 units of UFH (max of 50 mg over 10 min)	5 min	Hypotension and bronchoconstriction
LMWH	Protamine sulfate	If LMWH given within 8 h: 1 mg of protamine IV/100 anti-Xa units of LMWH	5 min	
Fundaparinux	No antidote: hemodialysis slightly reduces plasma levels by ~ 20%; rFVIIa is option			
DTI	No antidote: rFVIIa and PCC likely ineffective; hemodialysis may remove ~60% of dabigatran			
Warfarin	Vitamin K (Phytonadione)	po: 1–10 mg IV: 1–10 mg over 10–20 min	po: ~24 h IV: 12–16 h	Anaphylaxis with IV formulation
	FFP	Variable (10–15 mL/kg IV)	Temporary effect (4–6 h)	Volume sensitive patients; risk of TRALI
	PCC	25–50 units/kg[a] IV (not exceeding rate of 10 mL/min)	Immediate	Thrombosis
	rFVIIa	30–90 µg/kg IV bolus over 2–5 min	10–20 min	Thrombosis
Rivaroxaban	No antidote: PCC (studied in health volunteers only)			

Abbreviations: FFP, fresh frozen plasma; TRALI, transfusion-related acute lung injury.
[a] Various other dosing strategies available (INR based and factor level based).
Data from Refs. [180,186,191,192,229–234]

a thrombocytopenia (platelet count <150 × 10^9/L) typically presenting 5 to 10 days after the initiation of UFH, with or without thrombosis. The 4Ts scoring tool is used to help practitioners predict the presence of HIT by looking for the timing of thrombocytopenia, the timing of the drop in platelet count, presence of thrombosis, and other potential causes of thrombocytopenia.[170,171] The diagnosis of HIT is confirmed by the presence of platelet-activating antiplatelet factor 4 antibodies and, occasionally, the serotonin release assay is used if additional confirmation is warranted.[169] Alternative anticoagulants, typically direct thrombin inhibitors (DTIs), are indicated in the setting of HIT.

Low-molecular-weight heparins

Low-molecular-weight heparins (LMWHs) are derived from UFH and have a more predictable dose response curve compared with UFH. Similar to UFH, they are used for thromboprophylaxis as well as therapeutic anticoagulation. LMWHs are dosed as a subcutaneous injection daily or twice daily depending on the indication and patient specific factors, such as weight and renal function. Monitoring with anti-Xa levels is not routinely recommended outside of LMWH use in obese patients, pregnancy, and in the setting of renal insufficiency.[172–174] The half-life of LMWHs of 3 to 6 hours is dose dependent and prolonged in patients with renal failure, which may limit the utility of these drugs in certain critical care populations.[165] Optimal dosing of LMWHs in patients with renal insufficiency is uncertain and use in this patient population is linked with increased bleeding risk.[25] For these reasons, UFH is the preferred agent when therapeutic anticoagulation is indicated in the setting of renal insufficiency.[165] There are some data, specifically for enoxaparin (Lovenox) and dalteparin (Fragmin), suggesting no increased bleeding risk with prophylactic LMWH dosing in patients with a creatinine clearance (CrCl) of less than 30 mL/min.[175–177] The dosing of LMWHs in obese patients is also controversial. Data that are available suggest dosing based on total body weight up to a weight of 144 kg with enoxaparin and 190 kg with dalteparin is appropriate.[178,179]

LMWHs carry a similar risk of bleeding complications compared with UFH; however, their use is associated with lower rates of nonhemorrhagic complications, such as HIT and osteoporosis.[165,180] There is not a proved method for neutralizing the anticoagulant effects of LMWH. Protamine sulfate administration is recommended for its partial neutralization activity of LMWH if given within an 8-hour window of the last LMWH dose.[165]

Fondaparinux

Fondaparinux (Arixtra) is a synthetic analog of the AT III–binding portion of UFH and LMWH that has an increased affinity for AT III. Similar to LMWH, fondaparinux has a predictable dose-response curve and is administered once daily in fixed doses. It has a half-life of approximately 17 hours and this can be extended up to 21 hours in elderly patients, which can limit its use in critically ill patients.[181] Fondaparinux is indicated for thromboprophylaxis as well as for the treatment of acute coronary syndromes, deep vein thrombosis, and pulmonary embolism.[165] The dosing is based on indication, patient weight, and renal function. Elimination of fondaparinux is almost completely dependent on renal clearance and, therefore, it is contraindicated in patients with a CrCl of less than 30 mL/min. Routine coagulation monitoring is not recommended; however, when determining the anticoagulant activity of fondaparinux, a fondaparinux-specific anti-Xa assay is used.

Fondaparinux carries a similar bleeding risk to UFH and LMWH. Protamine sulfate is ineffective in neutralizing its anticoagulant activity.[180] If uncontrolled bleeding does occur with fondaparinux therapy, administration of recombinant factor VIIa (rFVIIa) may be effective.[182] Fondaparinux is unlikely to cause HIT and there are case reports suggesting it can be used for HIT treatment, but additional safety and efficacy studies are needed.[169,183]

Direct thrombin inhibitors

Lepirudin (Refludan), bivalirudin (Angiomax), and argatroban are parenteral DTIs used for the treatment of HIT. Lepirudin has a half-life of approximately 60 minutes and it is renally eliminated. Dose reductions are required if CrCl less than 60 mL/min. It is contraindicated in renal failure. It is a good therapeutic option in patients with hepatic dysfunction.[184] Lepirudin can cause antibodies to develop in up to 40% of patients exposed to the drug. Anaphylaxis can occur if patients are re-exposed to the drug; therefore, alternatives should be considered in patients who have previously received lepirudin.[165]

In addition to HIT, bivalirudin is indicated for anticoagulation in patients undergoing percutaneous interventions for acute coronary syndrome. Bivalirudin has a short half-life of 25 minutes and is partially eliminated by the kidneys; dose reduction is recommended in patients to moderate to severe renal dysfunction.[165]

Argatroban is indicated for the treatment of HIT and can be used during percutaneous interventions when UFH is contraindicated due to recent history of HIT. It is primarily metabolized by the liver and must be used cautiously in patients with hepatic dysfunction. Conversely, it is a good option for patients with severe renal impairment.[165] Lower empiric dosing is recommended for critically ill patients to prevent prolonged or exaggerated anticoagulant effects. The half-life is 45 minutes and, as with all parenteral DTIs, activated partial prothrombin time is recommended for monitoring of the anticoagulant effect. All DTIs can interact with the laboratory assay for the international normalized ratio (INR), causing a falsely elevated INR.[165] This is seen especially with argatroban, and specific recommendations are available on how to appropriately transition to a vitamin K antagonist, such as warfarin (Coumadin).

There are no specific antidotes for DTIs should hemorrhagic complications arise. rFVIIa has been studied as a reversal agent in healthy volunteers; its use in bleeding patients is not established.[185] Hemodialysis can be an effective way to remove DTIs.

Oral Anticoagulants

Warfarin

Warfarin, a vitamin K antagonist, has been the only oral anticoagulant for the treatment and prevention of thromboembolic events until the recent addition of an oral DTI and a direct factor Xa inhibitor to the market. Of the oral anticoagulant options, warfarin has the most efficacy and safety data available, but the monitoring requirements and drug, food, and genetic interactions often complicate therapy. Owing to its half-life of 36 to 42 hours, warfarin can take up to a week for onset and offset of action, deeming the drug difficult to use in the critical care setting.[186] Fortunately, warfarin has several reversal options (see **Table 11**). The reversal strategy for warfarin depends on the indication for reversal and the urgency of the situation. Therapeutic reversal options include administration of vitamin K and blood derivatives, such as fresh frozen plasma, prothrombin complex concentrates (PCCs), and rFVIIa.[187–189]

Dabigatran

Dabigatran (Pradaxa) is approved for the prevention of stroke or systemic embolism in nonvalvular AF.[186] It is also used for prevention of VTE in the setting of total knee or hip arthroplasty although this indication is lacking in the United States. Compared with warfarin, dabigatran has a short half-life, 12 to 17 hours, and, therefore, bridging is not recommended with the initiation of therapy. No therapeutic monitoring is recommended with dabigatran therapy and determining the degree of anticoagulation with the drug can be challenging.[186] Measuring the ecarin clotting time is likely the most promising measure of dabigatran effect; however, this test is not readily available.[190] As with other DTIs, there is no antidote for dabigatran. The limited data available with using rFVIIa and PCCs suggest that these agents are ineffective in reversing bleeding related to dabigatran use. Hemodialysis may be effective in removing up to 60% of the drug.[191,192]

Rivaroxaban

Rivaroxaban (Xarelto) is a direct factor Xa inhibitor approved for VTE prophylaxis in patients undergoing total hip or knee replacement surgery and for stroke and VTE prevention in patients with nonvalvular AF. Compared with warfarin and dabigatran, rivaroxaban has a short half-life of 6 to 7 hours; however, factor Xa activity may not return to normal until up to 24 hours after the dose is given.[193] No antidote for rivaroxaban exists and due to its high protein binding, it is unlikely that the drug is dialyzable.[186] There are limited data evaluating the role of PCCs and rFVIIa in the setting of rivaroxaban use. One study showed restoration of prolonged PT and normalization of thrombin generation after PCC administration in healthy volunteers who had received rivaroxaban; however, the clinical implications of these findings are unknown.[192]

ANTIBIOTICS

Antibiotic therapies are of tremendous importance to ICU care. Inappropriate empiric therapy and delayed initiation of therapy contribute to increased mortality, development of resistance, increased health care costs, and lack of compliance with national standards.[98,194–201] Lack of compliance with national standards results in financial penalties on reimbursement. Antimicrobial drug development has been declining for years and the future does not look promising. Therefore, appropriate use of currently available antibiotics, referred to as antimicrobial stewardship, is imperative.[202,203] Although beyond the scope of this article, stewardship can be summarized as appropriate drug selection based on patient-specific risk factors, such as appropriate dose, route, and frequency; de-escalation based on culture and sensitivity reports; and duration of therapy compliant with evidence-based treatment guidelines. Following these stewardship principles, along with source control, yields optimal outcomes while minimizing unnecessary resistance and health care cost.[202] To aid prescribers, the Infectious Diseases Society of America has published treatment guidelines for major disease states available free of charge at www.idsociety.org. For appropriate dosing information, drug package inserts should be consulted.

β-Lactams

β-Lactam (BL) antibiotic is a general term used to describe antibiotics that contain a BL ring in their molecular structure.[204,205] BL antibiotics include penicillins, cephalosporins, β-lactam/β-lactamases (BLase) inhibitors. Each of these antibiotic classes manifests their activity on the bacterial cell wall, resulting in time-depending killing. Extended infusions may increase efficacy and reduce treatment costs. Patients with allergies to a specific BL should be considered at risk for allergic reactions to other BL antibiotics. In general, BL antibiotics are well tolerated. Potential adverse effects include hypersensitivity reactions, interstitial nephritis, drug fever, thrombocytopenia, possibly hemorrhagic complications as a result of disturbing synthesis of vitamin

K–dependent clotting factors, and biliary sludging for those that concentrate in the bile. The BL subgroups are discussed in more detail later.

Cephalosporins

The cephalosporin drug class has a reported allergic cross-reactivity of 5% to 10% to penicillin.[206,207] They should be avoided in those with serious or immediate reactions (anaphylaxis or bronchospasm) but may be tried in patients with mild or delayed reactions, although drug desensitization would be a safer approach.[208] Moving from first-generation to third-generation cephalosporins, the gram-negative activity is enhanced at the expense of some gram-positive activity, although all generations (including fourth) lack activity against enterococci (**Table 12**).[209] Cephalosporins have good tissue penetration and distribute well to organs. First-generation cephalosporins, such as cefazolin (Ancef), are commonly used for perioperative prophylaxis owing to their activity against skin flora, such as methicillin-sensitive *Staphylococcus aureus* (MSSA) and *S epidermitis*. Cefazolin may also be used therapeutically for routine gram-positive pathogens and has some activity against anaerobes associated with mouth flora. The term, cephamycin, is sometimes used to describe a subset of cephalosporins that have enhanced activity against anaerobes, including mouth and colon flora, such as second-generation cefoxoitin (Mefoxin) and cefotetan (Cefotan). Although second-generation cephalosporins have less gram-positive activity than first generations, they are good options for a mixed infection or perioperative prophylaxis for bowel surgery. Third-generations, such as ceftriaxone (Rocephin), can be used in combination with the antianaerobic metronidazole (Flagyl) to broaden the spectrum of activity. This combination is efficacious for uncomplicated and complicated intra-abdominal infections when multidrug-resistant pathogens are not suspected.[210] Fourth-generation cefepime (Maxipime) has the broadest spectrum of gram-negative activity and maintains activity against *Pseudomonas aeruginosa*, as does the third generation, ceftazidime (Fortaz), making them viable options for nosocomial infections, including pneumonia. The recently developed fifth-generation ceftobiprole (Zeftera) and ceftaroline (Teflaro) retained activity against methicillin-resistant *S aureus* (MRSA), including exotoxin-producing strains. Of the 2, only ceftobiprole maintains activity against *P aeruginosa*. Both agents have marginal activity against enterococci.

β-Lactam/β-Lactamase Inhibitors

Piperacillin/tazobactam (Zosyn) and ticarcillin/clavulanate (Timentin) offer an enhanced spectrum of activity compared with cefepime, particularly against anaerobes and gram-negative pathogens, like *P aeruginosa*.[205] Ampicillin/sulbactam (Unasyn) has a narrower spectrum as a result of the less potent BLase inhibitor sulbactam, which results in less gram-negative activity. All agents maintain activity against resistant organisms that are cephalosporinase producing and BLase producing, which would otherwise render cephalosporins ineffective. Only patients previously exposed to antibiotics and those at risk for resistant pathogens should receive these drugs empirically. These agents must be avoided in patients with BL allergies. Amoxcillin/clavulanate (Augmentin) is an oral option that allows for step-down therapy.

Carbapenems

Carbapenems maintain activity against a wide spectrum of bacteria, including those harboring resistance to other drug classes, such as cephalosporinases and extended-spectrum BLase.[205] As a result, this drug class should not be routinely used first line but reserved for complicated and resistant infections, similar to BL/BLase inhibitors. Cross-reactivity with penicillin allergy is less defined as compared

Table 12
Antimicrobial activity against select pathogens

Drug	Route	G(+)	G(−)	Anaerobes	Enterococcus	MRSA	Pseudomonas
Ceftazidime, cefepime	IV	+	+	−	−	−	+
Ceftaroline, ceftobiprole	IV	+	+	−	−	+	Ceftobiprole only
Moxifloxacin	po, IV	+	+	+	±	±	−
Ciprofloxacin, levofloxacin	po, IV	+	+	±	±	±	+
Ertapenem	IV	+	+	+	−	−	−
Meropenerr, imipenem-cilastatin, doripenem	IV	+	+	+	+	−	+
Ampicillin-sulbactam	IV	+	+	+	+	−	−
Amoxicillin-clavulunate	po	+	+	+	+	−	−
Piperacillin-–azobactam, ticarcillin-clavulanate	IV	+	+	+	+	−	+
Gentamicin, tobramycin, amikacin	IV	+	+	−	−	−	+
Vancomycin	IV	+	−	±	+	+	−
Linezolid	po, IV	+	−	±	+	+	−
Tigecycline	IV	+	+	+	+	+	−
Daptomycin	IV	+	−	±	+	+	−

Abbreviations +, reliable activity; −, lack of activity; G(+), gram-positive pathogens; G(−), gram-negative pathogens; po, oral.

with cephalosporins but is estimated as 10% or more.[211] Meropenem (Merrem), imipenem-cilastatin (Primaxin), and doripenem (Doribax) have similar spectrums of activity and are generally interchangeable. They maintain activity against most clinically significant gram-positive and gram-negative pathogens (including MSSA, enterococci, and *P aeruginosa*), and anaerobes. Ertapenem (Invanz) has a narrower spectrum, which lacks activity against enterococci and *P aeruginosa*. Its use may select out for these pathogens in clinical practice.

Carbapenems may reduce seizure threshold and should be avoided in high-risk patients. It has been suggested that meropenem may have the lowest risk of seizure in the drug class and is often used for infections related to the CNS.

Fluoroquinolones

Fluoroquinolones (FQs) most often used in practice are moxifloxacin (Avelox), levofloxacin (Levaquin), and ciprofloxacin (Cipro).[212] They have good tissue penetration and serve as empiric therapy for most infections when multidrug resistance is not suspected. Moxifloxacin has strong gram-positive activity, good gram-negative activity, and strong anaerobic activity but lacks urine penetration and should not be used for urinary tract infections. It lacks activity against *Clostridium difficile* and is associated with *C difficile* infection (CDI) outbreaks as a result of killing competitive flora in the bowel. Levofloxacin maintains good activity against most bacteria, whereas ciprofloxacin has strong gram-negative activity at the expense of only moderate gram-positive and anaerobic activity. These traits make ciprofloxacin a nice formulary complement to moxifloxacin. FQs often maintain in vitro activity against MSSA and MRSA but yield a high incidence of treatment failure and resistance; FQ use should be avoided for the treatment of these bacteria. Ciprofloxacin can treat *Enterococcus* in the urine where it achieves concentrations but should be avoided in other sites of infection. FQ should be avoided in patients at risk for seizures because they may reduce the seizure threshold. FQs have multiple drug interactions, in particular, in SICUs, warfarin (Coumadin), theophylline (Uniphyl), and specifically ciprofloxacin with tizanidine (Zanaflex); concurrent use should be avoided. They also prolong QTc interval and should be used cautiously with drugs with similar effects, such as fluconazole (Diflucan) and amiodarone (Cordarone).

Aminoglycosides

Aminoglycosides are among the most potent gram-negative antimicrobials available and have been used effectively for decades.[213] Resistance rates decrease from gentamicin (Garamycin) to tobramycin (Nebcin) to amikacin (Amikin) having the most robust activity profile. They remain the gold standard for gram-negative bacteremia owing to potency and concentration in the serum, although their empiric use has diminished as a result of less toxic therapeutic alternatives.[214] Aminoglycosides remain a reliable drug class for many multi-drug resistant pathogens. They may be used synergistically with BL antibiotics for resistant strains of *S aureus* and Enterococcus; the BL antibiotic disrupts the bacterial cell wall, allowing the aminoglycoside to penetrate the bacteria and manifest its activity. Dosing has evolved to extended interval, usually 5 mg/kg/d to 7 mg/kg/d (15–21 mg/kg/d for amikacin), to optimize the concentration-dependent killing.[215–217] A peak to minimal inhibitory concentration ratio of 10:1 has yielded increased survival.[214] Nephrotoxicity is common with a reported incidence as high as 20%; renal function should be closely monitored. Ototoxicity may also occur. Nephrotoxicity and ototoxicity may not be reversible. Pharmacist consultation has demonstrated increased efficacy with decreased toxicity and should routinely be considered.

MRSA Treatment Options

Infections caused by MRSA are associated with increased morbidity, mortality, and health care costs.[218] Fortunately, several treatment options are available. Vancomycin, a glycopeptide with a broad gram-positive spectrum, has been the cornerstone of MRSA treatment for decades.[219,220] Over time, the minimal inhibitory concentration has risen, but true resistance is rare. It also has activity against enterococci, but its use has induced the development of vancomycin-resistant enterococci (VRE), which is on the rise. For both staphylococci and enterococci, BL antibiotics should always be used if possible based on susceptibility results because their efficacy is greater than that of vancomycin for these bacteria. Nephrotoxicity associated with vancomycin is concerning; dosing should be patient-specific to minimize potential risk.[220] Most institutions have pharmacokinetic consult services that can optimize dosing to achieve evidence-based troughs (ranging from 10 to 20 µg/mL depending on indication) while minimizing adverse effects.[220]

Linezolid is well established for the treatment of nosocomial pneumonia and complicated skin and skin structure infections (SSTI).[221] It also maintains activity against VRE, although similar to vancomycin, resistance is on the rise. Limited data suggest superiority of linezolid over vancomycin for the treatment of pneumonia, but this remains controversial.[222] The oral formulation is well absorbed and offers a useful option for patients able to tolerate oral medications. The drug's weak monoamine oxidase inhibition increases the risk of serotonin syndrome, a rare but fatal complication, when used concurrently with other serotonergic agents. This combination should be avoided if possible. Adverse effects include optic neuropathy, peripheral neuropathy, and pancytopenia, commonly manifested as thrombocytopenia. Limiting the duration of treatment to less than 14 days reduces the likelihood of these complications.

Tigecycline (Tygacil) is a broad-spectrum glycylcycline approved for complicated intra-abdominal infections and SSTI infections.[218,223] It maintains activity against MRSA, VRE, and extended-spectrum BLase-producing pathogens. It lacks activity against *P aeruginosa*, however, which greatly limits its role as monotherapy. Owing to its similarities to tetracycline, it has been slow to gain acceptance for the treatment of serious life-threatening infections. An unexplained increase in all-cause mortality is observed in patients receiving tigecycline in both phase 3 and 4 studies. Also, tigecycline monotherapy should be avoided in patients with perforated bowel due to poorer outcomes reported in phase 3 trials. Its use is often limited to treating patients with BL allergies, intolerant to conventional therapy, or with polymicrobial infections. Side effects are minimal compared with other agents, most commonly manifested as nausea and vomiting.

Daptomycin (Cubicin) has good activity against MRSA but has little role in SICUs except for treatment of endocarditis or for complicated SSTI where other therapies have failed or are contraindicated.[224] Daptomycin is inactivated by pulmonary surfactant and should not be used to treat bacterial pneumonia. The most common serious adverse effects are myopathy and rhabdomyolysis for which baseline and weekly creatine kinase measurement is recommended. It is associated with the development of eosinophilic pneumonia. If any of these is observed, daptomycin should be immediately discontinued.

In addition to the previously discussed agents there are several other oral options with activity against community-associated MRSA, including Sulfamethoxazole-trimethoprim (Bactrim and Septra), doxycycline (Vibramycin), and clindamycin (Cleocin) (**Box 3**).[225] These agents are not usually used for severe nosocomial MRSA infection but are often used for community-acquired MRSA infections, usually SSTI.

> **Box 3**
> **Oral treatment options for MRSA**
>
> Sulfamethoxazole-trimethoprim
>
> Doxycycline
>
> Minocycline
>
> Clindamycin
>
> Levofloxacin[a]
>
> Ciprofloxacin[a]
>
> Linezolid
>
> [a] Good in vitro activity but limited outcome data and should not be considered a first-line therapy.
>
> *Data from* Peppard WJ, Daniels A, Fehrenbacher L, et al. Evidence based approach to the treatment of community-associated methicillin-resistant Staphylococcus aureus. Infect Drug Resist 2009;2:27–40.

Clostridium difficile Treatment Options

CDI is an increasingly common complication in health care, including ICUs. Treatment is determined by both episode (initial vs recurrent) and severity of infection (**Table 13**).[226] Metronidazole is the drug of choice for the initial episode of mild-to-moderate CDI and has the lowest acquisition cost of all treatment. Both IV and oral metronidazole are effective treatment options. Oral vancomycin is generally reserved for more severe infections due to demonstrated superiority compared with metronidazole. IV vancomycin is not effective for CDI; rectal therapy may be considered when oral therapy is not an option. Combination therapy may be considered in severe or complicated CDI.

Fungal Treatment Options

Fluconazole (Diflucan), an azole antifungal, remains the standard of care for most uncomplicated *Candida* infections in ICUs, but local susceptibility patterns must also be considered.[227] It maintains good activity against *Candida albicans*, the most prevalent species in ICUs, although its activity has decreased against *C glabrata* over the years, the second most prevalent species. Voriconazole (Vfend), another azole, has slightly enhanced activity against *Candida* species but not enough to warrant routine use beyond treatment of *Aspergillus* species.[227,228] Both agents are associated with elevations in liver enzymes and QTc prolongation but are generally well tolerated. For moderately severe to severe illness or in patients with recent azole exposure, empiric therapy should consist of an echinocandin rather than an azole.[227] Echinocandins have more potent activity against *Candida* than azoles and maintain activity against some *Aspergillus* species. Caspofungin (Cancidas), micafungin (Mycamine), and anidulafungin (Eraxis) are generally considered interchangeable in terms of activity spectrum and side-effect profile. They are generally well tolerated although they can be associated with elevation in liver enzymes.

DRUG SHORTAGES

In recent years, drug shortages have had an increasing impact on patient care; ICUs are not immune to these effects. Several organizations, such as the American Society of Health-System Pharmacists and the American Medical Association, have worked

Table 13
Treatment based on severity of *Clostridium difficile* infection

Severity	Treatment	Duration (days)	Level of Evidence	Comments
Initial episode of mild to moderate	Metronidazole (500 mg po 3 times daily)	10–14	A-I	Metronidazole is the drug of choice for the initial episode of mild-to-moderate CDI (A-I)
Initial episode of severe	Vancomycin (125 mg po 4 times daily)	10–14	B-I	IV vancomycin is ineffective for the treatment of CDI
Severe, complicated	Vancomycin (500 mg po 4 times daily) ± metronidazole (500 mg IV 3 times daily)	10–14	C-III	Rectal vancomycin (500 mg in 100 mL normal saline) may be added if ileus is present (C-III); consider colectomy for severely ill patients (B-II)
First recurrence	Same regimen as initial episode; treatment may differ based on stratification of disease severity	10–14	A-II; C-III	
Second or later recurrence	Vancomycin therapy using a tapered and/ or pulse regimen	Variable	B-III	Avoid metronidazole beyond first recurrence of CDI or for long-term chronic therapy due to risk of neurotoxicity (B-II)

Data from Cohen SH, Gerding DN, Johnson S, et al. Clinical practice guidelines for Clostridium difficile infection in adults: 2010 update by the society for healthcare epidemiology of America (SHEA) and the infectious diseases society of America (IDSA). Infect Control Hosp Epidemiol 2010;31(5):431–55.

closely with legislators and the FDA to promote sustained production of drugs and minimize or prevent future shortages. This process is slow and does not address immediate needs. It is recommended that prescribers work closely with clinical pharmacists to prospectively address and manage potential shortages. Clinical pharmacists should be used to help estimate drug supply, recommend alternative therapies, and provide education to prescribers when formulary changes are made to accommodate shortages.

SUMMARY

In summary, appropriate pharmacotherapy, as a supplement to surgical intervention, can improve patient outcomes in SICUs. Given the multiple variables in ICUs that affect pharmacokinetics and pharmacodynamics, however, an understanding of drug properties and pharmacotherapy is essential to optimize care. Collaboration between a clinical pharmacist and intensivist can help improve patient outcomes and provide delivery of safe and cost-effective drug therapy.

ACKNOWLEDGMENTS

We would like to recognize, Dave Herrmann, Ann Patten, Melissa Handcock, and Kate Oltrogge for their contributions.

REFERENCES

1. Moellering RC Jr. Principles of anti-infective therapy. In: Mandell GL, Bennett JE, Dolin R, editors. Principles and practice of infectious diseases, vol. 1, 5th edition. Philadelphia: Churchill Livingstone; 2000. p. 223–35.
2. Amsden GW, Ballow CH, Bertino JS. Pharmacokinetics and pharmacodynamics of anti-infective agents. In: Mandell GL, Bennett JE, Dolin R, editors. Principles and practice of infectious diseases, vol. 1, 5th edition. Philadelphia: Churchill Livingstone; 2000. p. 253–61.
3. Erstad BL, Haas CE, O'Keeffe T, et al. Interdisciplinary patient care in the intensive care unit: focus on the pharmacist. Pharmacotherapy 2011;31(2):128–37.
4. Jacobi J, Fraser GL, Coursin DB, et al. Clinical practice guidelines for the sustained use of sedatives and analgesics in the critically ill adult. Crit Care Med 2002;30(1):119–41.
5. Sessler CN, Varney K. Patient-focused sedation and analgesia in the ICU. Chest 2008;133(2):552–65.
6. Sessler CN, Gosnell MS, Grap MJ, et al. The Richmond agitation-sedation scale: validity and reliability in adult intensive care unit patients. Am J Respir Crit Care Med 2002;166(10):1338–44.
7. Ely EW, Truman B, Shintani A, et al. Monitoring sedation status over time in ICU patients: reliability and validity of the richmond agitation-sedation scale (RASS). JAMA 2003;289(22):2983–91.
8. Ramsay MA, Savege TM, Simpson BR, et al. Controlled sedation with alphaxalone-alphadolone. Br Med J 1974;2(5920):656–9.
9. Girard TD, Kress JP, Fuchs BD, et al. Efficacy and safety of a paired sedation and ventilator weaning protocol for mechanically ventilated patients in intensive care (Awakening and Breathing Controlled trial): a randomised controlled trial. Lancet 2008;371(9607):126–34.
10. Gommers D, Bakker J. Medications for analgesia and sedation in the intensive care unit: an overview. Crit Care 2008;12(Suppl 3):S4.
11. Ostermann ME, Keenan SP, Seiferling RA, et al. Sedation in the intensive care unit: a systematic review. JAMA 2000;283(11):1451–9.
12. Carrasco G, Cabre L, Sobrepere G, et al. Synergistic sedation with propofol and midazolam in intensive care patients after coronary artery bypass grafting. Crit Care Med 1998;26(5):844–51.
13. Carrasco G, Molina R, Costa J, et al. Propofol vs midazolam in short-, medium-, and long-term sedation of critically ill patients. A cost-benefit analysis. Chest 1993;103(2):557–64.
14. Hall RI, Sandham D, Cardinal P, et al. Propofol vs midazolam for ICU sedation: a Canadian multicenter randomized trial. Chest 2001;119(4):1151–9.
15. Ronan KP, Gallagher TJ, George B, et al. Comparison of propofol and midazolam for sedation in intensive care unit patients. Crit Care Med 1995;23(2):286–93.
16. Roekaerts PM, Huygen FJ, de Lange S. Infusion of propofol versus midazolam for sedation in the intensive care unit following coronary artery surgery. J Cardiothorac Vasc Anesth 1993;7(2):142–7.

17. Thomas MC, Jennett-Reznek AM, Patanwala AE. Combination of ketamine and propofol versus either agent alone for procedural sedation in the emergency department. Am J Health Syst Pharm 2011;68(23):2248–56.

18. Wong JM. Propofol infusion syndrome. Am J Ther 2010;17(5):487–91.

19. Roberts RJ, Barletta JF, Fong JJ, et al. Incidence of propofol-related infusion syndrome in critically ill adults: a prospective, multicenter study. Crit Care 2009;13(5):R169.

20. Bray RJ. Propofol infusion syndrome in children. Paediatr Anaesth 1998;8(6): 491–9.

21. Haas CE, Kaufman DC, Jones CE, et al. Cytochrome P450 3A4 activity after surgical stress. Crit Care Med 2003;31(5):1338–46.

22. Pandharipande P, Cotton BA, Shintani A, et al. Prevalence and risk factors for development of delirium in surgical and trauma intensive care unit patients. J Trauma 2008;65(1):34–41.

23. Pandharipande P, Shintani A, Peterson J, et al. Lorazepam is an independent risk factor for transitioning to delirium in intensive care unit patients. Anesthesiology 2006;104(1):21–6.

24. Pandharipande P, Ely EW. Sedative and analgesic medications: risk factors for delirium and sleep disturbances in the critically ill. Crit Care Clin 2006;22(2): 313–27, vii.

25. Lim W, Dentali F, Eikelboom JW, et al. Meta-analysis: low-molecular-weight heparin and bleeding in patients with severe renal insufficiency. Ann Intern Med 2006;144(9):673–84.

26. Ely EW, Shintani A, Truman B, et al. Delirium as a predictor of mortality in mechanically ventilated patients in the intensive care unit. JAMA 2004; 291(14):1753–62.

27. Barnes BJ, Gerst C, Smith JR, et al. Osmol gap as a surrogate marker for serum propylene glycol concentrations in patients receiving lorazepam for sedation. Pharmacotherapy 2006;26(1):23–33.

28. Yahwak JA, Riker RR, Fraser GL, et al. Determination of a lorazepam dose threshold for using the osmol gap to monitor for propylene glycol toxicity. Pharmacotherapy 2008;28(8):984–91.

29. Gerlach AT, Murphy CV, Dasta JF. An updated focused review of dexmedetomidine in adults. Ann Pharmacother 2009;43(12):2064–74.

30. Riker RR, Shehabi Y, Bokesch PM, et al. Dexmedetomidine vs midazolam for sedation of critically ill patients: a randomized trial. JAMA 2009;301(5): 489–99.

31. Pandharipande PP, Pun BT, Herr DL, et al. Effect of sedation with dexmedetomidine vs lorazepam on acute brain dysfunction in mechanically ventilated patients: the MENDS randomized controlled trial. JAMA 2007;298(22):2644–53.

32. Dasta JF, Kane-Gill SL, Pencina M, et al. A cost-minimization analysis of dexmedetomidine compared with midazolam for long-term sedation in the intensive care unit. Crit Care Med 2010;38(2):497–503.

33. Jakob SM, Ruokonen E, Grounds RM, et al. Dexmedetomidine vs midazolam or propofol for sedation during prolonged mechanical ventilation: two randomized controlled trials. JAMA 2012;307(11):1151–60.

34. Devabhakthuni S, Pajoumand M, Williams C, et al. Evaluation of dexmedetomidine: safety and clinical outcomes in critically ill trauma patients. J Trauma 2011; 71(5):1164–71.

35. Muzyk AJ, Fowler JA, Norwood DK, et al. Role of alpha2-agonists in the treatment of acute alcohol withdrawal. Ann Pharmacother 2011;45(5):649–57.

36. Aroni F, Iacovidou N, Dontas I, et al. Pharmacological aspects and potential new clinical applications of ketamine: reevaluation of an old drug. J Clin Pharmacol 2009;49(8):957–64.

37. Green SM, Roback MG, Kennedy RM, et al. Clinical practice guideline for emergency department ketamine dissociative sedation: 2011 update. Ann Emerg Med 2011;57(5):449–61.

38. Jabre P, Combes X, Lapostolle F, et al. Etomidate versus ketamine for rapid sequence intubation in acutely ill patients: a multicentre randomised controlled trial. Lancet 2009;374(9686):293–300.

39. Watt I, Ledingham IM. Mortality amongst multiple trauma patients admitted to an intensive therapy unit. Anaesthesia 1984;39(10):973–81.

40. Lipiner-Friedman D, Sprung CL, Laterre PF, et al. Adrenal function in sepsis: the retrospective Corticus cohort study. Crit Care Med 2007;35(4):1012–8.

41. Cuthbertson BH, Sprung CL, Annane D, et al. The effects of etomidate on adrenal responsiveness and mortality in patients with septic shock. Intensive Care Med 2009;35(11):1868–76.

42. Delirium diagnostic and statistical manual of mental disorders. 4th edition. Arlington (VA): American Psychiatric Association; 2000.

43. Ely EW, Gautam S, Margolin R, et al. The impact of delirium in the intensive care unit on hospital length of stay. Intensive Care Med 2001;27(12): 1892–900.

44. Lin SM, Liu CY, Wang CH, et al. The impact of delirium on the survival of mechanically ventilated patients. Crit Care Med 2004;32(11):2254–9.

45. Milbrandt EB, Deppen S, Harrison PL, et al. Costs associated with delirium in mechanically ventilated patients. Crit Care Med 2004;32(4):955–62.

46. Ouimet S, Kavanagh BP, Gottfried SB, et al. Incidence, risk factors and consequences of ICU delirium. Intensive Care Med 2007;33(1):66–73.

47. Thomason JW, Shintani A, Peterson JF, et al. Intensive care unit delirium is an independent predictor of longer hospital stay: a prospective analysis of 261 non-ventilated patients. Crit Care 2005;9(4):R375–81.

48. Banerjee A, Girard TD, Pandharipande P. The complex interplay between delirium, sedation, and early mobility during critical illness: applications in the trauma unit. Curr Opin Anaesthesiol 2011;24(2):195–201.

49. Siddiqi N, Stockdale R, Britton AM, et al. Interventions for preventing delirium in hospitalised patients. Cochrane Database Syst Rev 2007;(2):CD005563.

50. Inouye SK, van Dyck CH, Alessi CA, et al. Clarifying confusion: the confusion assessment method. A new method for detection of delirium. Ann Intern Med 1990;113(12):941–8.

51. Bergeron N, Dubois MJ, Dumont M, et al. Intensive care delirium screening checklist: evaluation of a new screening tool. Intensive Care Med 2001;27(5): 859–64.

52. Ely EW, Inouye SK, Bernard GR, et al. Delirium in mechanically ventilated patients: validity and reliability of the confusion assessment method for the intensive care unit (CAM-ICU). JAMA 2001;286(21):2703–10.

53. Ely EW, Margolin R, Francis J, et al. Evaluation of delirium in critically ill patients: validation of the Confusion Assessment Method for the Intensive Care Unit (CAM-ICU). Crit Care Med 2001;29(7):1370–9.

54. Plaschke K, von Haken R, Scholz M, et al. Comparison of the confusion assessment method for the intensive care unit (CAM-ICU) with the intensive care delirium screening checklist (ICDSC) for delirium in critical care patients gives high agreement rate(s). Intensive Care Med 2008;34(3):431–6.

55. Devlin JW, Fong JJ, Schumaker G, et al. Use of a validated delirium assessment tool improves the ability of physicians to identify delirium in medical intensive care unit patients. Crit Care Med 2007;35(12):2721–4 [quiz: 2725].
56. Fick DM, Cooper JW, Wade WE, et al. Updating the Beers criteria for potentially inappropriate medication use in older adults: results of a US consensus panel of experts. Arch Intern Med 2003;163(22):2716–24.
57. Inouye SK. Delirium in older persons. N Engl J Med 2006;354(11):1157–65.
58. Jano E, Aparasu RR. Healthcare outcomes associated with beers' criteria: a systematic review. Ann Pharmacother 2007;41(3):438–47.
59. Larsen KA, Kelly SE, Stern TA, et al. Administration of olanzapine to prevent postoperative delirium in elderly joint-replacement patients: a randomized, controlled trial. Psychosomatics 2010;51(5):409–18.
60. Prakanrattana U, Prapaitrakool S. Efficacy of risperidone for prevention of postoperative delirium in cardiac surgery. Anaesth Intensive Care 2007;35(5):714–9.
61. Kalisvaart KJ, de Jonghe JF, Bogaards MJ, et al. Haloperidol prophylaxis for elderly hip-surgery patients at risk for delirium: a randomized placebo-controlled study. J Am Geriatr Soc 2005;53(10):1658–66.
62. Wang W, Li HL, Wang DX, et al. Haloperidol prophylaxis decreases delirium incidence in elderly patients after noncardiac surgery: a randomized controlled trial*. Crit Care Med 2012;40(3):731–9.
63. Sampson EL, Raven PR, Ndhlovu PN, et al. A randomized, double-blind, placebo-controlled trial of donepezil hydrochloride (Aricept) for reducing the incidence of postoperative delirium after elective total hip replacement. Int J Geriatr Psychiatry 2007;22(4):343–9.
64. Gamberini M, Bolliger D, Lurati Buse GA, et al. Rivastigmine for the prevention of postoperative delirium in elderly patients undergoing elective cardiac surgery–a randomized controlled trial. Crit Care Med 2009;37(5):1762–8.
65. Tan JA, Ho KM. Use of dexmedetomidine as a sedative and analgesic agent in critically ill adult patients: a meta-analysis. Intensive Care Med 2010;36(6):926–39.
66. Bourne RS, Mills GH. Melatonin: possible implications for the postoperative and critically ill patient. Intensive Care Med 2006;32(3):371–9.
67. Aizawa K, Kanai T, Saikawa Y, et al. A novel approach to the prevention of postoperative delirium in the elderly after gastrointestinal surgery. Surg Today 2002;32(4):310–4.
68. Hudetz JA, Patterson KM, Iqbal Z, et al. Ketamine attenuates delirium after cardiac surgery with cardiopulmonary bypass. J Cardiothorac Vasc Anesth 2009;23(5):651–7.
69. Leung JM, Sands LP, Rico M, et al. Pilot clinical trial of gabapentin to decrease postoperative delirium in older patients. Neurology 2006;67(7):1251–3.
70. Breitbart W, Marotta R, Platt MM, et al. A double-blind trial of haloperidol, chlorpromazine, and lorazepam in the treatment of delirium in hospitalized AIDS patients. Am J Psychiatry 1996;153(2):231–7.
71. Riker RR, Fraser GL, Cox PM. Continuous infusion of haloperidol controls agitation in critically ill patients. Crit Care Med 1994;22(3):433–40.
72. Tesar GE, Murray GB, Cassem NH. Use of high-dose intravenous haloperidol in the treatment of agitated cardiac patients. J Clin psychopharmacol 1985;5(6):344–7.
73. Devlin JW, Roberts RJ, Fong JJ, et al. Efficacy and safety of quetiapine in critically ill patients with delirium: a prospective, multicenter, randomized, double-blind, placebo-controlled pilot study. Crit Care Med 2010;38(2):419–27.

74. Skrobik YK, Bergeron N, Dumont M, et al. Olanzapine vs haloperidol: treating delirium in a critical care setting. Intensive Care Med 2004;30(3):444–9.

75. Breitbart W, Tremblay A, Gibson C. An open trial of olanzapine for the treatment of delirium in hospitalized cancer patients. Psychosomatics 2002;43(3):175–82.

76. Kim SW, Yoo JA, Lee SY, et al. Risperidone versus olanzapine for the treatment of delirium. Hum Psychopharmacol 2010;25(4):298–302.

77. Han CS, Kim YK. A double-blind trial of risperidone and haloperidol for the treatment of delirium. Psychosomatics 2004;45(4):297–301.

78. Girard TD, Pandharipande PP, Carson SS, et al. Feasibility, efficacy, and safety of antipsychotics for intensive care unit delirium: the MIND randomized, placebo-controlled trial. Crit Care Med 2010;38(2):428–37.

79. Murray MJ, Cowen J, DeBlock H, et al. Clinical practice guidelines for sustained neuromuscular blockade in the adult critically ill patient. Crit Care Med 2002; 30(1):142–56.

80. Sagarin MJ, Barton ED, Chng YM, et al. Airway management by US and Canadian emergency medicine residents: a multicenter analysis of more than 6,000 endotracheal intubation attempts. Ann Emerg Med 2005;46(4):328–36.

81. Gronert GA. Cardiac arrest after succinylcholine: mortality greater with rhabdomyolysis than receptor upregulation. Anesthesiology 2001;94(3):523–9.

82. Weintraub HD, Heisterkamp DV, Cooperman LH. Changes in plasma potassium concentration after depolarizing blockers in anaesthetized man. Br J Anaesth 1969;41(12):1048–52.

83. List WF. Serum potassium changes during induction of anaesthesia. Br J Anaesth 1967;39(6):480–4.

84. Caro DA, Laurin EG. Neuromuscular blocking agents. In: Walls RM, Murphy MF, editors. Manual of emergency airway management. 3rd edition. Philadelphia: Williams & Wilkins; 2008. p. 248–62.

85. Watling SM, Dasta JF. Prolonged paralysis in intensive care unit patients after the use of neuromuscular blocking agents: a review of the literature. Crit Care Med 1994;22(5):884–93.

86. Raps EC, Bird SJ, Hansen-Flaschen J. Prolonged muscle weakness after neuromuscular blockade in the intensive care unit. Crit Care Clin 1994;10(4):799–813.

87. Lacomis D, Giuliani MJ, Van Cott A, et al. Acute myopathy of intensive care: clinical, electromyographic, and pathological aspects. Ann Neurol 1996;40(4): 645–54.

88. Naguib M, Lien CA. Pharmacology of muscle relaxants and their antagonists. In: Miller RD, editor. Miller's anesthesia. 7th edition. Philadelphia: Churchill Livingstone; 2009. p. 859–912.

89. Rudis MI, Sikora CA, Angus E, et al. A prospective, randomized, controlled evaluation of peripheral nerve stimulation versus standard clinical dosing of neuromuscular blocking agents in critically ill patients. Crit Care Med 1997;25(4):575–83.

90. Baumann MH, McAlpin BW, Brown K, et al. A prospective randomized comparison of train-of-four monitoring and clinical assessment during continuous ICU cisatracurium paralysis. Chest 2004;126(4):1267–73.

91. Overgaard CB, Dzavik V. Inotropes and vasopressors: review of physiology and clinical use in cardiovascular disease. Circulation 2008;118(10):1047–56.

92. Sperry JL, Minei JP, Frankel HL, et al. Early use of vasopressors after injury: caution before constriction. J Trauma 2008;64(1):9–14.

93. Biaggioni I, Robertson D. Adrenoceptor agonists & sympathmimetic drugs. In: Katzung BG, Masters SB, Trevor AJ, editors. Basic & clinical pharmacology. 11th edition. Ipswich (MA): McCraw-Hill Professional; 2009. p. 127–48.

94. Goodman LS, Gilman A, Brunton LL. Adrenergic agnoists and antagonists. Goodman & Gillman's manual of pharmacology and therpeutics. Ipswich (MA): McGraw-Hill Professional; 2008. p. 148–87.

95. Butterworth J. Do alpha agonists increase venous return? Anesthesiology 2004; 101(4):1038 [author reply: 1039].

96. Thiele RH, Nemergut EC, Lynch C 3rd. The clinical implications of isolated alpha(1) adrenergic stimulation. Anesth Analg 2011;113(2):297–304.

97. Antman EM, Anbe DT, Armstrong PW, et al. ACC/AHA guidelines for the management of patients with ST-elevation myocardial infarction: a report of the American college of cardiology/American heart association task force on practice guidelines (committee to revise the 1999 guidelines for the management of patients with acute myocardial infarction). Circulation 2004;110(9):e82–292.

98. Dellinger RP, Levy MM, Carlet JM, et al. Surviving Sepsis Campaign: international guidelines for management of severe sepsis and septic shock: 2008. Crit Care Med 2008;36(1):296–327.

99. Consortium for Spinal Cord Medicine. Early acute management in adults with spinal cord injury: a clinical practice guideline for health-care professionals. J Spinal Cord Med 2008;31(4):403–79.

100. Hollenberg SM. Vasoactive drugs in circulatory shock. Am J Respir Crit Care Med 2011;183(7):847–55.

101. Neumar RW, Otto CW, Link MS, et al. Part 8: adult advanced cardiovascular life support: 2010 American heart association guidelines for cardiopulmonary resuscitation and emergency cardiovascular care. Circulation 2010;122(18 Suppl 3):S729–67.

102. Hollenberg SM, Ahrens TS, Annane D, et al. Practice parameters for hemodynamic support of sepsis in adult patients: 2004 update. Crit Care Med 2004; 32(9):1928–48.

103. Martin C, Viviand X, Leone M, et al. Effect of norepinephrine on the outcome of septic shock. Crit Care Med 2000;28(8):2758–65.

104. De Backer D, Creteur J, Silva E, et al. Effects of dopamine, norepinephrine, and epinephrine on the splanchnic circulation in septic shock: which is best? Crit Care Med 2003;31(6):1659–67.

105. De Backer D, Biston P, Devriendt J, et al. Comparison of dopamine and norepinephrine in the treatment of shock. N Engl J Med 2010;362(9):779–89.

106. Bellomo R, Chapman M, Finfer S, et al. Low-dose dopamine in patients with early renal dysfunction: a placebo-controlled randomised trial. Australian and New Zealand Intensive Care Society (ANZICS) Clinical Trials Group. Lancet 2000;356(9248):2139–43.

107. Patel BM, Chittock DR, Russell JA, et al. Beneficial effects of short-term vasopressin infusion during severe septic shock. Anesthesiology 2002;96(3):576–82.

108. Dunser MW, Mayr AJ, Ulmer H, et al. Arginine vasopressin in advanced vasodilatory shock: a prospective, randomized, controlled study. Circulation 2003; 107(18):2313–9.

109. Russell JA, Walley KR, Singer J, et al. Vasopressin versus norepinephrine infusion in patients with septic shock. N Engl J Med 2008;358(9):877–87.

110. Dunser MW, Mayr AJ, Tur A, et al. Ischemic skin lesions as a complication of continuous vasopressin infusion in catecholamine-resistant vasodilatory shock: incidence and risk factors. Crit Care Med 2003;31(5):1394–8.

111. Awad AS, Goldberg ME. Role of clevidipine butyrate in the treatment of acute hypertension in the critical care setting: a review. Vasc Health Risk Manag 2010;6:457–64.

112. Chobanian AV, Bakris GL, Black HR, et al. Seventh report of the joint national committee on prevention, detection, evaluation, and treatment of high blood pressure. Hypertension 2003;42(6):1206–52.
113. Rhoney D, Peacock WF. Intravenous therapy for hypertensive emergencies, part 1. Am J Health Syst Pharm 2009;66(15):1343–52.
114. Rhoney D, Peacock WF. Intravenous therapy for hypertensive emergencies, part 2. Am J Health Syst Pharm 2009;66(16):1448–57.
115. Yang HJ, Kim JG, Lim YS, et al. Nicardipine versus nitroprusside infusion as antihypertensive therapy in hypertensive emergencies. J Int Med Res 2004; 32(2):118–23.
116. Marik PE, Varon J. Hypertensive crises: challenges and management. Chest 2007;131(6):1949–62.
117. Adams HP Jr, del Zoppo G, Alberts MJ, et al. Guidelines for the early management of adults with ischemic stroke: a guideline from the American heart association/American stroke association stroke council, clinical cardiology council, cardiovascular radiology and intervention council, and the atherosclerotic peripheral vascular disease and quality of care outcomes in research interdisciplinary working groups: the American academy of neurology affirms the value of this guideline as an educational tool for neurologists. Circulation 2007;115(20): e478–534.
118. Antihypertensive Treatment of Acute Cerebral Hemorrhage (ATACH) investigators. Antihypertensive treatment of acute cerebral hemorrhage. Crit Care Med 2010;38(2):637–48.
119. Liu-Deryke X, Janisse J, Coplin WM, et al. A comparison of nicardipine and labetalol for acute hypertension management following stroke. Neurocrit Care 2008;9(2):167–76.
120. Silke B, Verma SP, Hussain M, et al. Comparative haemodynamic effects of nicardipine and verapamil in coronary artery disease. Herz 1985;10(2):112–9.
121. Silke B, Verma SP, Nelson GI, et al. Haemodynamic dose-response effects of i.v. nicardipine in coronary artery disease. Br J Clin Pharmacol 1984;18(5):717–24.
122. Curran MP, Robinson DM, Keating GM. Intravenous nicardipine: its use in the short-term treatment of hypertension and various other indications. Drugs 2006;66(13):1755–82.
123. Neutel JM, Smith DH, Wallin D, et al. A comparison of intravenous nicardipine and sodium nitroprusside in the immediate treatment of severe hypertension. Am J Hypertens 1994;7(7 Pt 1):623–8.
124. Kwak YL, Oh YJ, Bang SO, et al. Comparison of the effects of nicardipine and sodium nitroprusside for control of increased blood pressure after coronary artery bypass graft surgery. J Int Med Res 2004;32(4):342–50.
125. Dorman T, Thompson DA, Breslow MJ, et al. Nicardipine versus nitroprusside for breakthrough hypertension following carotid endarterectomy. J Clin Anesth 2001;13(1):16–9.
126. Nordlander M, Sjoquist PO, Ericsson H, et al. Pharmacodynamic, pharmacokinetic and clinical effects of clevidipine, an ultrashort-acting calcium antagonist for rapid blood pressure control. Cardiovasc Drug Rev 2004;22(3):227–50.
127. Kieler-Jensen N, Jolin-Mellgard A, Nordlander M, et al. Coronary and systemic hemodynamic effects of clevidipine, an ultra-short-acting calcium antagonist, for treatment of hypertension after coronary artery surgery. Acta Anaesthesiol Scand 2000;44(2):186–93.
128. Pollack CV, Varon J, Garrison NA, et al. Peacock WFt. Clevidipine, an intravenous dihydropyridine calcium channel blocker, is safe and effective for the

treatment of patients with acute severe hypertension. Ann Emerg Med 2009; 53(3):329–38.

129. Powroznyk AV, Vuylsteke A, Naughton C, et al. Comparison of clevidipine with sodium nitroprusside in the control of blood pressure after coronary artery surgery. Eur J Anaesthesiol 2003;20(9):697–703.

130. Nguyen HM, Ma K, Pham DQ. Clevidipine for the treatment of severe hypertension in adults. Clin Ther 2010;32(1):11–23.

131. Kondo T, Brock M, Bach H. Effect of intra-arterial sodium nitroprusside on intracranial pressure and cerebral autoregulation. Jpn Heart J 1984;25(2):231–7.

132. Anile C, Zanghi F, Bracali A, et al. Sodium nitroprusside and intracranial pressure. Acta Neurochir (Wien) 1981;58(3–4):203–11.

133. Mann T, Cohn PF, Holman LB, et al. Effect of nitroprusside on regional myocardial blood flow in coronary artery disease. Results in 25 patients and comparison with nitroglycerin. Circulation 1978;57(4):732–8.

134. Ignarro LJ. After 130 years, the molecular mechanism of action of nitroglycerin is revealed. Proc Natl Acad Sci U S A 2002;99(12):7816–7.

135. Elkayam U, Kulick D, McIntosh N, et al. Incidence of early tolerance to hemodynamic effects of continuous infusion of nitroglycerin in patients with coronary artery disease and heart failure. Circulation 1987;76(3):577–84.

136. Varon J. Treatment of acute severe hypertension: current and newer agents. Drugs 2008;68(3):283–97.

137. Rhoney DH, Liu-DeRyke X. Effect of vasoactive therapy on cerebral circulation. Crit Care Clin 2006;22(2):221–43, vi.

138. Overgaard J, Skinhoj E. A paradoxical cerebral hemodynamic effect of hydralazine. Stroke 1975;6(4):402–10.

139. James DJ, Bedford RF. Hydralazine for controlled hypotension during neurosurgical operations. Anesth Analg 1982;61(12):1016–9.

140. Shepherd AM, Ludden TM, McNay JL, et al. Hydralazine kinetics after single and repeated oral doses. Clin Pharmacol Ther 1980;28(6):804–11.

141. Balser JR, Martinez EA, Winters BD, et al. Beta-adrenergic blockade accelerates conversion of postoperative supraventricular tachyarrhythmias. Anesthesiology 1998;89(5):1052–9.

142. Gray RJ, Bateman TM, Czer LS, et al. Use of esmolol in hypertension after cardiac surgery. Am J Cardiol 1985;56(11):49F–56F.

143. Gray RJ, Bateman TM, Czer LS, et al. Esmolol: a new ultrashort-acting beta-adrenergic blocking agent for rapid control of heart rate in postoperative supraventricular tachyarrhythmias. J Am Coll Cardiol 1985;5(6):1451–6.

144. Mooss AN, Hilleman DE, Mohiuddin SM, et al. Safety of esmolol in patients with acute myocardial infarction treated with thrombolytic therapy who had relative contraindications to beta-blocker therapy. Ann Pharmacother 1994;28(6): 701–3.

145. Kitiyakara C, Guzman NJ. Malignant hypertension and hypertensive emergencies. J Am Soc Nephrol 1998;9(1):133–42.

146. Pearce CJ, Wallin JD. Labetalol and other agents that block both alpha- and beta-adrenergic receptors. Cleve Clin J Med 1994;61(1):59–69 [quiz: 80–52].

147. Murphy MB, Murray C, Shorten GD. Fenoldopam: a selective peripheral dopamine-receptor agonist for the treatment of severe hypertension. N Engl J Med 2001;345(21):1548–57.

148. Landoni G, Biondi-Zoccai GG, Tumlin JA, et al. Beneficial impact of fenoldopam in critically ill patients with or at risk for acute renal failure: a meta-analysis of randomized clinical trials. Am J Kidney Dis 2007;49(1):56–68.

149. Ng TM, Shurmur SW, Silver M, et al. Comparison of N-acetylcysteine and fenoldopam for preventing contrast-induced nephropathy (CAFCIN). Int J Cardiol 2006;109(3):322–8.

150. Goodman S, Weiss Y, Weissman C. Update on cardiac arrhythmias in the ICU. Curr Opin Crit Care 2008;14(5):549–54.

151. Trappe HJ, Brandts B, Weismueller P. Arrhythmias in the intensive care patient. Curr Opin Crit Care 2003;9(5):345–55.

152. Fuster V, Ryden LE, Cannom DS, et al. ACC/AHA/ESC 2006 guidelines for the management of patients with atrial fibrillation: a report of the American college of cardiology/American heart association task force on practice guidelines and the European society of cardiology committee for practice guidelines (writing committee to revise the 2001 guidelines for the management of patients with atrial fibrillation): developed in collaboration with the European heart rhythm association and the heart rhythm society. Circulation 2006;114(7):e257–354.

153. Koh KK, Song JH, Kwon KS, et al. Comparative study of efficacy and safety of low-dose diltiazem or betaxolol in combination with digoxin to control ventricular rate in chronic atrial fibrillation: randomized crossover study. Int J Cardiol 1995; 52(2):167–74.

154. Segal JB, McNamara RL, Miller MR, et al. The evidence regarding the drugs used for ventricular rate control. J Fam Pract 2000;49(1):47–59.

155. Boudonas G, Lefkos N, Efthymiadis AP, et al. Intravenous administration of diltiazem in the treatment of supraventricular tachyarrhythmias. Acta Cardiol 1995;50(2):125–34.

156. Lundstrom T, Ryden L. Ventricular rate control and exercise performance in chronic atrial fibrillation: effects of diltiazem and verapamil. J Am Coll Cardiol 1990;16(1):86–90.

157. Phillips BG, Gandhi AJ, Sanoski CA, et al. Comparison of intravenous diltiazem and verapamil for the acute treatment of atrial fibrillation and atrial flutter. Pharmacotherapy 1997;17(6):1238–45.

158. Cheng JW, Rybak I. Use of digoxin for heart failure and atrial fibrillation in elderly patients. Am J Geriatr Pharmacother 2010;8(5):419–27.

159. Hume JR, Grant AO. Agents used in cardiac arrhythmias. In: Katzung B, Masters S, Trevor A, editors. Basic & clinical pharmacology. 11th edition. Ipswich (MA): McGraw-Hill Medical; 2009. p. 225–48.

160. Clemo HF, Wood MA, Gilligan DM, et al. Intravenous amiodarone for acute heart rate control in the critically ill patient with atrial tachyarrhythmias. Am J Cardiol 1998;81(5):594–8.

161. Marill KA, Wolfram S, Desouza IS, et al. Adenosine for wide-complex tachycardia: efficacy and safety. Crit Care Med 2009;37(9):2512–8.

162. Ilkhanipour K, Berrol R, Yealy DM. Therapeutic and diagnostic efficacy of adenosine in wide-complex tachycardia. Ann Emerg Med 1993;22(8):1360–4.

163. Gorgels AP, van den Dool A, Hofs A, et al. Comparison of procainamide and lidocaine in terminating sustained monomorphic ventricular tachycardia. Am J Cardiol 1996;78(1):43–6.

164. Ho DS, Zecchin RP, Richards DA, et al. Double-blind trial of lignocaine versus sotalol for acute termination of spontaneous sustained ventricular tachycardia. Lancet 1994;344(8914):18–23.

165. Garcia DA, Baglin TP, Weitz JI, et al. Parenteral anticoagulants: antithrombotic therapy and prevention of thrombosis, 9th ed: American college of chest physicians evidence-based clinical practice guidelines. Chest 2012;141(Suppl 2): e24S–43S.

166. Basu D, Gallus A, Hirsh J, et al. A prospective study of the value of monitoring heparin treatment with the activated partial thromboplastin time. N Engl J Med 1972;287(7):324–7.

167. Berkowitz SD. Treatment of established deep vein thrombosis: a review of the therapeutic armamentarium. Orthopedics 1995;18(Suppl):18–20.

168. Raschke RA, Reilly BM, Guidry JR, et al. The weight-based heparin dosing nomogram compared with a "standard care" nomogram. A randomized controlled trial. Ann Intern Med 1993;119(9):874–81.

169. Linkins LA, Dans AL, Moores LK, et al. Treatment and prevention of heparin-induced thrombocytopenia: antithrombotic therapy and prevention of thrombosis, 9th ed: American college of chest physicians evidence-based clinical practice guidelines. Chest 2012;141(Suppl 2):e495S–530S.

170. Lo GK, Juhl D, Warkentin TE, et al. Evaluation of pretest clinical score (4 T's) for the diagnosis of heparin-induced thrombocytopenia in two clinical settings. J Thromb Haemost 2006;4(4):759–65.

171. Pouplard C, Gueret P, Fouassier M, et al. Prospective evaluation of the '4Ts' score and particle gel immunoassay specific to heparin/PF4 for the diagnosis of heparin-induced thrombocytopenia. J Thromb Haemost 2007;5(7): 1373–9.

172. Abbate R, Gori AM, Farsi A, et al. Monitoring of low-molecular-weight heparins in cardiovascular disease. Am J Cardiol 1998;82(5B):33L–6L.

173. Francis CW, Pellegrini VD Jr, Totterman S, et al. Prevention of deep-vein thrombosis after total hip arthroplasty. Comparison of warfarin and dalteparin. J Bone Joint Surg Am 1997;79(9):1365–72.

174. Nieuwenhuis HK, Albada J, Banga JD, et al. Identification of risk factors for bleeding during treatment of acute venous thromboembolism with heparin or low molecular weight heparin. Blood 1991;78(9):2337–43.

175. Sanderink GJ, Guimart CG, Ozoux ML, et al. Pharmacokinetics and pharmacodynamics of the prophylactic dose of enoxaparin once daily over 4 days in patients with renal impairment. Thromb Res 2002;105(3):225–31.

176. Rabbat CG, Cook DJ, Crowther MA, et al. Dalteparin thromboprophylaxis for critically ill medical-surgical patients with renal insufficiency. J Crit Care 2005; 20(4):357–63.

177. Douketis J, Cook D, Meade M, et al. Prophylaxis against deep vein thrombosis in critically ill patients with severe renal insufficiency with the low-molecular-weight heparin dalteparin: an assessment of safety and pharmacodynamics: the direct study. Arch Intern Med 2008;168(16):1805–12.

178. Becker RC, Spencer FA, Gibson M, et al. Influence of patient characteristics and renal function on factor Xa inhibition pharmacokinetics and pharmacodynamics after enoxaparin administration in non-ST-segment elevation acute coronary syndromes. Am Heart J 2002;143(5):753–9.

179. Wilson SJ, Wilbur K, Burton E, et al. Effect of patient weight on the anticoagulant response to adjusted therapeutic dosage of low-molecular-weight heparin for the treatment of venous thromboembolism. Haemostasis 2001; 31(1):42–8.

180. Schulman S, Beyth RJ, Kearon C, et al. Hemorrhagic complications of anticoagulant and thrombolytic treatment: American college of chest physicians evidence-based clinical practice guidelines (8th Edition). Chest 2008;133(Suppl 6): 257S–98S.

181. Donat F, Duret JP, Santoni A, et al. The pharmacokinetics of fondaparinux sodium in healthy volunteers. Clin Pharmacokinet 2002;41(Suppl 2):1–9.

182. Bijsterveld NR, Moons AH, Boekholdt SM, et al. Ability of recombinant factor VIIa to reverse the anticoagulant effect of the pentasaccharide fondaparinux in healthy volunteers. Circulation 2002;106(20):2550–4.

183. Kuo KH, Kovacs MJ. Fondaparinux: a potential new therapy for HIT. Hematology 2005;10(4):271–5.

184. Lefevre G, Duval M, Gauron S, et al. Effect of renal impairment on the pharmacokinetics and pharmacodynamics of desirudin. Clin Pharmacol Ther 1997; 62(1):50–9.

185. Sorensen B, Ingerslev J. A direct thrombin inhibitor studied by dynamic whole blood clot formation. Haemostatic response to ex-vivo addition of recombinant factor VIIa or activated prothrombin complex concentrate. Thromb Haemost 2006;96(4):446–53.

186. Ageno W, Gallus AS, Wittkowsky A, et al. Oral anticoagulant therapy: antithrombotic therapy and prevention of thrombosis, 9th ed: American college of chest physicians evidence-based clinical practice guidelines. Chest 2012;141(Suppl 2):e44S–88S.

187. Garcia D, Ageno W, Bussey H, et al. Prevention and treatment of bleeding complications in patients receiving vitamin K antagonists, Part 1: prevention. Am J Hematol 2009;84(9):579–83.

188. Ageno W, Garcia D, Aguilar MI, et al. Prevention and treatment of bleeding complications in patients receiving vitamin K antagonists, part 2: treatment. Am J Hematol 2009;84(9):584–8.

189. Contreras M, Ala FA, Greaves M, et al. Guidelines for the use of fresh frozen plasma. British Committee for Standards in Haematology, Working Party of the Blood Transfusion Task Force. Transfus Med 1992;2(1):57–63.

190. van Ryn J, Stangier J, Haertter S, et al. Dabigatran etexilate–a novel, reversible, oral direct thrombin inhibitor: interpretation of coagulation assays and reversal of anticoagulant activity. Thromb Haemost 2010;103(6):1116–27.

191. Malherbe S, Tsui BC, Stobart K, et al. Argatroban as anticoagulant in cardiopulmonary bypass in an infant and attempted reversal with recombinant activated factor VII. Anesthesiology 2004;100(2):443–5.

192. Eerenberg ES, Kamphuisen PW, Sijpkens MK, et al. Reversal of rivaroxaban and dabigatran by prothrombin complex concentrate: a randomized, placebo-controlled, crossover study in healthy subjects. Circulation 2011;124(14): 1573–9.

193. Kubitza D, Becka M, Voith B, et al. Safety, pharmacodynamics, and pharmacokinetics of single doses of BAY 59-7939, an oral, direct factor Xa inhibitor. Clin Pharmacol Ther 2005;78(4):412–21.

194. Alvarez-Lerma F. Modification of empiric antibiotic treatment in patients with pneumonia acquired in the intensive care unit. ICU-Acquired Pneumonia Study Group. Intensive Care Med 1996;22(5):387–94.

195. Dupont H, Mentec H, Sollet JP, et al. Impact of appropriateness of initial antibiotic therapy on the outcome of ventilator-associated pneumonia. Intensive Care Med 2001;27(2):355–62.

196. Kollef MH, Sherman G, Ward S, et al. Inadequate antimicrobial treatment of infections: a risk factor for hospital mortality among critically ill patients. Chest 1999;115(2):462–74.

197. Luna CM, Vujacich P, Niederman MS, et al. Impact of BAL data on the therapy and outcome of ventilator-associated pneumonia. Chest 1997;111(3):676–85.

198. Rello J, Gallego M, Mariscal D, et al. The value of routine microbial investigation in ventilator-associated pneumonia. Am J Respir Crit Care Med 1997;156(1): 196–200.

199. Ruiz M, Torres A, Ewig S, et al. Noninvasive versus invasive microbial investigation in ventilator-associated pneumonia: evaluation of outcome. Am J Respir Crit Care Med 2000;162(1):119–25.

200. Kumar A, Roberts D, Wood KE, et al. Duration of hypotension before initiation of effective antimicrobial therapy is the critical determinant of survival in human septic shock. Crit Care Med 2006;34(6):1589–96.

201. Puskarich MA, Trzeciak S, Shapiro NI, et al. Association between timing of antibiotic administration and mortality from septic shock in patients treated with a quantitative resuscitation protocol. Crit Care Med 2011;39(9):2066–71.

202. Dellit TH, Owens RC, McGowan JE Jr, et al. Infectious diseases society of America and the society for healthcare epidemiology of America guidelines for developing an institutional program to enhance antimicrobial stewardship. Clin Infect Dis 2007;44(2):159–77.

203. Cooper MA, Shlaes D. Fix the antibiotics pipeline. Nature 2011;472(7341):32.

204. Chambers HF. Penicillins. In: Mandell GL, Bennett JE, Dolin R, editors. Principles and practice of infectious diseases, vol. 1, 5th edition. Philadelphia: Churchill Livingstone; 2000. p. 261–74.

205. Chambers HF. Other B-lactam antibiotics. In: Mandell GL, Bennett JE, Dolin R, editors. Principles and practice of infectious diseases, vol. 1, 5th edition. Philadelphia: Churchill Livingstone; 2000. p. 291–9.

206. Kelkar PS, Li JT. Cephalosporin allergy. N Engl J Med 2001;345(11):804–9.

207. Weiss ME, Adkinson NFJ. B-lactam allergy. In: Mandell GL, Bennett JE, Dolin R, editors. Principles and practice of infectious diseases, vol. 1, 5th edition. Philadelphia: Churchill Livingstone; 2000. p. 299–305.

208. Gruchalla RS, Pirmohamed M. Clinical practice. Antibiotic allergy. N Engl J Med 2006;354(6):601–9.

209. Karchmer AW. Cephalosporins. In: Mandell GL, Bennett JE, Dolin R, editors. Principles and practice of infectious diseases, vol. 1, 5th edition. Philadelphia: Churchill Livingstone; 2000. p. 274–91.

210. Solomkin JS, Mazuski JE, Bradley JS, et al. Diagnosis and management of complicated intra-abdominal infection in adults and children: guidelines by the surgical infection society and the infectious diseases society of America. Clin Infect Dis 2010;50(2):133–64.

211. Frumin J, Gallagher JC. Allergic cross-sensitivity between penicillin, carbapenem, and monobactam antibiotics: what are the chances? Ann Pharmacother 2009;43(2):304–15.

212. Hooper CD. Quinolones. In: Mandell GL, Bennett JE, Dolin R, editors. Principles and practice of infectious diseases, vol. 1, 5th edition. Philadelphia: Churchill Livingstone; 2000. p. 404–23.

213. Gilbert DN. Aminoglycosides. In: Mandell GL, Bennett JE, Dolin R, editors. Principles and practice of infectious diseases, vol. 1, 5th edition. Philadelphia: Churchill Livingstone; 2000. p. 307–36.

214. Moore RD, Lietman PS, Smith CR. Clinical response to aminoglycoside therapy: importance of the ratio of peak concentration to minimal inhibitory concentration. J Infect Dis 1987;155(1):93–9.

215. Nicolau DP, Belliveau PP, Nightingale CH, et al. Implementation of a once-daily aminoglycoside program in a large community-teaching hospital. Hosp Pharm 1995;30(8):674–6, 679–80.

216. Nicolau DP, Freeman CD, Belliveau PP, et al. Experience with a once-daily aminoglycoside program administered to 2,184 adult patients. Antimicrob Agents Chemother 1995;39(3):650–5.

217. Chuck SK, Raber SR, Rodvold KA, et al. National survey of extended-interval aminoglycoside dosing. Clin Infect Dis 2000;30(3):433–9.

218. Liu C, Bayer A, Cosgrove SE, et al. Clinical practice guidelines by the infectious diseases society of america for the treatment of methicillin-resistant Staphylococcus aureus infections in adults and children. Clin Infect Dis 2011;52(3):e18–55.

219. Fekety R. Vancomycin, teicoplanin, and the streptogramins: quinupristin and dalfopristin. In: Mandell GL, Bennett JE, Dolin R, editors. Principles and practice of infectious diseases, vol. 1, 5th edition. Philadelphia: Churchill Livingstone; 2000. p. 382–92.

220. Rybak M, Lomaestro B, Rotschafer JC, et al. Therapeutic monitoring of vancomycin in adult patients: a consensus review of the American society of health-system pharmacists, the infectious diseases society of America, and the society of infectious diseases pharmacists. Am J Health Syst Pharm 2009;66(1):82–98.

221. Herrmann DJ, Peppard WJ, Ledeboer NA, et al. Linezolid for the treatment of drug-resistant infections. Expert Rev Anti Infect Ther 2008;6(6):825–48.

222. Wunderink RG, Niederman MS, Kollef MH, et al. Linezolid in methicillin-resistant Staphylococcus aureus nosocomial pneumonia: a randomized, controlled study. Clin Infect Dis 2012;54(5):621–9.

223. Noskin GA. Tigecycline: a new glycylcycline for treatment of serious infections. Clin Infect Dis 2005;41(Suppl 5):S303–14.

224. Schriever CA, Fernandez C, Rodvold KA, et al. Daptomycin: a novel cyclic lipopeptide antimicrobial. Am J Health Syst Pharm 2005;62(11):1145–58.

225. Peppard WJ, Daniels A, Fehrenbacher L, et al. Evidence based approach to the treatment of community-associated methicillin-resistant Staphylococcus aureus. Infect Drug Resist 2009;2:27–40.

226. Cohen SH, Gerding DN, Johnson S, et al. Clinical practice guidelines for Clostridium difficile infection in adults: 2010 update by the society for healthcare epidemiology of America (SHEA) and the infectious diseases society of America (IDSA). Infect Control Hosp Epidemiol 2010;31(5):431–55.

227. Pappas PG, Kauffman CA, Andes D, et al. Clinical practice guidelines for the management of candidiasis: 2009 update by the Infectious Diseases Society of America. Clin Infect Dis 2009;48(5):503–35.

228. Walsh TJ, Anaissie EJ, Denning DW, et al. Treatment of aspergillosis: clinical practice guidelines of the Infectious Diseases Society of America. Clin Infect Dis 2008;46(3):327–60.

229. Lubetsky A, Yonath H, Olchovsky D, et al. Comparison of oral vs intravenous phytonadione (vitamin K1) in patients with excessive anticoagulation: a prospective randomized controlled study. Arch Intern Med 2003;163(20):2469–73.

230. Dentali F, Ageno W, Crowther M. Treatment of coumarin-associated coagulopathy: a systematic review and proposed treatment algorithms. J Thromb Haemost 2006;4(9):1853–63.

231. Steiner T, Rosand J, Diringer M. Intracerebral hemorrhage associated with oral anticoagulant therapy: current practices and unresolved questions. Stroke 2006;37(1):256–62.

232. Schulman S, Bijsterveld NR. Anticoagulants and their reversal. Transfus Med Rev 2007;21(1):37–48.

233. Luporsi P, Chopard R, Janin S, et al. Use of recombinant factor VIIa (NovoSeven((R))) in 8 patients with ongoing life-threatening bleeding treated with fondaparinux. Acute Card Care 2011;13(2):93–8.

234. Dager WE. Using prothrombin complex concentrates to rapidly reverse oral anticoagulant effects. Ann Pharmacother 2011;45(7–8):1016–20.

Pain Management in the ICU

Larry Lindenbaum, MD[b],*, David J. Milia, MD[a]

KEYWORDS

- Pain • Regional anesthesia • ICU • Trauma • Rib fractures

KEY POINTS

- There are many sources of pain in the ICU requiring different considerations for treatment.
- Uncontrolled pain is associated with other detrimental system physiologic responses.
- Pain scales, when used, can provide guidance in treatment effectiveness.
- As in other areas of ICU care, nursing protocols for pain management can help improve the overall care and therapy of patients.
- Opioid and nonopioid analgesic therapies, although generally effective, also can be associated with significant morbidity and mortality.
- Regional anesthesia techniques are quite effective on patients in the ICU, elderly patients especially, and are generally underutilized.

INTRODUCTION

For the intensive care unit (ICU) practitioner, pain management has many unique considerations and challenges. Critically ill patients often have multiple systemic disease processes requiring rapid evaluations and changes in treatment plans. Further, many patients in the ICU are incapable of communicating clearly, either as a direct result of their injuries or illness or because of intubation and sedation requirements. Together, these circumstances make the assessment and treatment of potentially painful conditions difficult. In the ICU setting, there are myriad sources of pain, both disease related as well as from many of the therapies and treatments used to sustain and restore life. Sources of pain range from invasive procedures, surgeries, and placement of monitoring devices, to direct nociceptive stimuli from injury, inflammation, and immobility.[1–3]

There are systemic effects produced by pain, and these may add to the physiologic insult of the patient in the ICU. Comprehensive treatment of pain can lessen these effects substantially.[4–6] Pain affects all body systems through neurohormonal

Disclosures: Neither author has any affiliation with any company with direct financial interest in the subject matter or materials discussed herein.

[a] Division of Surgery and Trauma Critical Care, Medical College of Wisconsin, 9200 West Wisconsin Avenue, Milwaukee, WI 53226, USA; [b] Department of Anesthesiology, Medical College of Wisconsin, 9200 Wisconsin Avenue, Milwaukee, WI 53226, USA
* Corresponding author.
E-mail address: llindenb@mcw.edu

mechanisms, catecholamine release, sympathetic outpouring, and the general stress response (Table 1).[7–9] Physiologic responses to pain include anxiety, tachycardia, diaphoresis, and catabolism. This results in increased myocardial oxygen demand, increased bowel motility, tachypnea, activation of the renin-angiotensin-aldosterone axis, and the production of a large number of cytokines. Further, it is also believed that pain may result in immune system dysfunction, hypercoagulable states, altered glucose control, patient-ventilator dyssynchrony, acute restrictive respiratory physiology, and disrupted sleep quality.[4–7,10]

Consequent to these deep interactions between pain and other physiologic processes, it is critical that clinicians caring for these patients be knowledgeable in the assessment and management of pain. Despite the known issues relating to the lack of pain treatment, there exists a paucity of evidence-based data supporting treatment principles. Most data are extrapolated from other settings and transferred directly to the ICU, further complicating the care of these patients. This underscores the need for ICU clinicians to be facile in the understanding and management of pain in this setting.

PATHOPHYSIOLOGY OF PAIN
Definitions and Types of Pain

Pain is variably defined by different investigators and organizations over the past 100 years, although most recently the International Association for the Study of Pain has adopted what is now the most widely held definition: "Pain is an unpleasant sensory and emotional experience associated with actual or potential tissue damage, or described in terms of such damage."[11] Although this definition serves to describe pain as a whole, it is helpful to classify pain based on its characteristics, both to better direct treatment and to assist research into specific pain states. To this end, the International Association for the Study of Pain has classified pain according to (1) region of

| Table 1 |
| Systemic and physiologic consequences of pain |

System	Effect
Immune/Inflammatory	Downregulated immunomodulation through cytokine release and leukocyte dysfunction (especially natural killer cells). Increased prostaglandin production from high cell turnover, muscle breakdown.
Cardiovascular	Increases in Vo_2 (oxygen consumption) through increased adrenergic tone.
Gastrointestinal	Decreased motility.
Renal	Anasarca through activation of the Renin-Angiotensin system.
Endocrine	Hyperglycemia and hypotension through dysregulation of cortisol and insulin. Increased catabolism.
Respiratory	Hyperventilation, ventilator dyssynchrony, lowered functional residual capacity, hypoxia.
Psychological	Depression, fatigue, psychosis, sleep deprivation, and anxiety through altered neurohumeral responses.
Hematological	Alterations in platelet function resulting in thromboembolic disease and gastrointestinal bleeding. Decreased mobility leading to increased risk of venous thromboembolism.

Adapted from Fishman SM, Ballantyne JC, Rathmell JP, editors. Bonica's management of pain. 4th edition. Philadelphia: Lippincott, Williams and Wilkins; 2010. p. 1589; with permission.

the body involved, (2) system experiencing the dysfunction, (3) duration and pattern of occurrence, (4) intensity and time since onset, and (5) etiology.[12] An additional category based on neurochemical mechanism has been proposed to augment this classification scheme for the purposes of guiding research and treatment.[13] These definitions and classifications of pain are distinct from that of *nociception*, a term that refers merely to the sensory process that is triggered by the inciting event (although it may be maintained by different, distinct processes). From a clinical standpoint, it is useful to characterize the major subdivisions of pain as somatic, visceral, neuropathic, or mixed, as this is what is frequently used to help guide specific therapy.[4,7]

In the ICU, pain originates primarily as a result of short-duration stimuli with or without some degree of chronicity. This pathophysiologic mechanism can simply be described as activation of the neural afferent (nociceptive) signals that have arisen from tissue damage. It is important to remember that the acute pain experienced by the patient in the ICU can be a manifestation of both the underlying illness or injury as well as iatrogenically derived pain from therapies, such as monitor placement, surgery, and immobility.[1,2] Turning, in fact, is one of the most painful and distressing procedures endured by patients in routine ICU care.[14] Further, patients can acquire chronic pain syndromes during an ICU stay, presumably from inadequately treated prolonged and/or repeated pain experiences.[3,8]

For the ICU clinician, it is particularly helpful to divide pain into the subtypes most commonly seen in this setting: (1) acute postoperative or posttraumatic pain, and (2) neuropathic pain. This simple classification can serve to guide therapeutic approaches and is effective enough for use in the acute management of these patients. In the ICU, the subjective experience of pain by the patient is often limited by the patient's capacity to communicate. ICU pain is predominantly in the somatic domain. This type of pain is often described as dull and aching, is typically well localized, and is well suited to therapies including opiates and nonsteroidal anti-inflammatory agents (NSAIDs); medications that form the mainstay of ICU pain management. Visceral pain is often seen in the ICU setting and can arise from poor bowel care or from underlying gastrointestinal pathology. Opiates and NSAIDs typically do not work well for this subtype and anticholinergics should be considered if patients are not responding well to traditional somatic pain therapies. Neuropathic pain is less well documented in the ICU but deserves consideration, especially in those with prolonged stays or injuries directly involving neurovascular structures.

PAIN ASSESSMENT

Acute pain, when unrecognized and undertreated, has both physiologic and psychological implications affecting patient outcomes.[15–17] Adequate and appropriate treatment and management of pain relies on a standardized, systematic approach to guide initiation and titration of therapy. Provider assessments (at both the physician and nurse level) of pain are typically underestimated[18] and it is accepted that patient assessment of pain should guide therapy. In verbal, communicative patients, traditional pain scales can be used.[19,20] In the ICU, however, patients are often unable to verbalize their pain or participate in traditional pain-assessment techniques. This may be because of respiratory status, mental status, iatrogenic sedation, multiple procedures, or a combination of all.[21]

Physiology-Based Scales

Although physiologic indicators can correlate with pain levels,[22] caution should be taken with a physiologic-based treatment algorithm. Heart rate and blood pressure increase with increasing levels of pain, but it should be recognized that these changes might occur for other physiologic (or pathophysiologic) reasons. Conversely, such changes in physiologic disturbances may be absent during periods of undertreated pain as well. Based on prior studies, it is recommended that the changes in vital signs described previously should be used to alert providers to the possibility of untreated or undertreated pain and further investigation is warranted.[23]

Behavioral-Based Scales

With physiologic parameters proving unreliable for the assessment and treatment of pain in sedated or unresponsive patients, a large study was undertaken to describe behavioral abnormalities exhibited by patients in pain. The study examined behaviors in conscious patients with the assumption these same behaviors would likely be noted in unconscious patients.[24] The most commonly noted behaviors were grimacing, muscle rigidity, wincing, eye shutting, and fist clenching.

It was noted that nurses frequently used these behaviors to assess and treat pain, but in a nonsystematic approach that was difficult to study. Consequently, multiple pain scales have been developed incorporating these behavioral changes. These scales can be grouped into unidimensional and multidimensional. An unidimensional approach uses only 1 dimension (eg, behavioral, physiologic) but may use one or more domains (eg, wincing, eye shutting, grimacing) within that dimension. A multidimensional approach uses more than 1 dimension and any number of domains within those dimensions.[25] Studies have noted that self-reported pain measures correlate better with multidomain scales and that no single domain correlates well with self-reported pain scores.[26]

Unidimensional Assessment Tools

The most common unidimensional assessment tools are the Behavioral Pain Scale (BPS), Pain Behavior Assessment Tool (PBAT), and the Critical-care Pain Observation Tool (CPOT). The BPS, the earliest and most widely tested pain assessment tool, uses 3 behavioral domains, each one graded on a 1 to 4 scale.[27] The validity of the BPS was shown with patients undergoing painful procedures scoring higher than those undergoing nonpainful procedures.[28] As such, it is a reliable, valid tool for pain assessment, but critics have cautioned that including movement as a behavioral domain may underestimate pain, as sedated patients may not exhibit excessive movement with painful stimuli.[22] The PBAT includes 3 behavioral domains with several descriptors each. The CPOT is a unidimensional tool for both intubated and nonintubated patients. It relies on 4 behavioral domains with a point scale devoted to each.[29] Its notable strengths are its ease of use and dedication of descriptors to both intubated and nonintubated patients.

Multidimensional Assessment Tools

The most common multidimensional assessment tools are the Pain Assessment and Intervention Notation (PAIN) Algorithm, and the Nonverbal Pain Scale (NVPS). The PAIN Algorithm, originally designed for research, relies on 3 parts. It includes a pain assessment, an assessment of opioid tolerance, and a guideline for treatment decision and documentation.[30] Assessment uses 6 behavioral domains and 3 physiologic parameters. After consideration of these 9 fields, the severity is recorded on a 0 to 10 scale. This tool is criticized as being too long and cumbersome for clinical utility and has a lack of reliability testing in the literature.[22] NVPS, originally designed for intubated, sedated burn victims, builds on the FLACC (Face, Legs, Activity, Cry, Consolability) platform constructed for children.[31] Included in this assessment are both physiologic and behavioral domains. The validity and reliability have been demonstrated in the literature.[32]

Although feasibility, validity, and reliability were examined in most of these assessment tools, rigorous outcomes-based research is lacking. Further testing is required before any one of the tools can be considered preferred. Thus, no one of these methods is considered superior to any other and none should be regarded as the gold standard.

Outcomes of Algorithm-Based Analgesia Administration

Most current studies presented in the literature pertaining to algorithm-based analgesia administration are presented in combination with sedation. Separation of pain assessment from anxiety and delirium is difficult and not always clinically feasible. A formal discussion of sedation and delirium is beyond the scope of this article.

Gelinas and colleagues[33] studied preimplementation and postimplementation of the CPOT assessment tool examining the feasibility of nurse training, documentation, and an amount of pain medication administered. Improved documentation with an overall increase in the number of pain assessments was shown, whereas a decrease in the overall amount of analgesia administered was noted. An explanation for the decreased analgesia administration was that the providers in the study were able to use this tool to discriminate pain from other symptoms (eg, anxiety, delirium). This study was not designed to show differences in patient outcomes.

The first step in the Analgesia-Delirium-Sedation (ADS) Protocol was to assess injured patients' level of pain before administration of sedatives. Following titration of pain medications to a predetermined goal, delirium and anxiety were then assessed and treated. Nursing staff were trained and assessments were repeated on a 4-hour schedule. Patients in the protocol group had decreased ventilator days as well as an overall shorter hospitalization.[34] Other studies have shown similar results.[35] In a randomized study performed by Brook and colleagues,[36] a protocol involving fentanyl for pain and lorazepam for anxiety resulted in decreased hospital and ICU length of stay over a nonprotocolized regimen. Although no one protocol is better than another, there appears to be no harm in its introduction. Sessler and Pedram[37] summarized these protocols with the following simple questions: Is the patient comfortable? Is the patient in pain? Is the patient anxious? Different assessment strategies may be used to answer these questions. Directing treatment toward the answers is the foundation of analgesia-sedation treatment protocols.

INTRAVENOUS AGENTS
Traditional Opioids

Intravenous opioids have been the mainstay of pain medications in the ICU for years. Recently, more data have become available on agents such as remifentanil and ketamine. Most patients are currently maintained on a regimen built on a foundation of traditional opioids.[38,39] The sedating side effect of these medications has been used to assist with compliance with mechanical ventilation. NSAIDs, such as ketorolac, although used frequently in the general surgical population, will not be discussed, as there are few data in the ICU population and use should be limited given the side-effect profile.

Much of the pharmacokinetic data for opioids come from single-dose studies from healthy volunteers.[40] Caution is required in the critically ill population receiving continuous infusions, as these patients have altered volume status, protein-binding capability, and end-organ (renal and hepatic) function. Morphine, fentanyl, and hydromorphone are the most commonly used opioids in the ICU setting.[41] They exhibit stimulation of the μ-opioid, κ-opioid, and o-opioid receptors with the primary site being the u-receptor.[42] Opioids are divided into 3 classes and are broken down by chemical structure: (1) morphine-like agents (morphine and hydromorphone); (2) meperidine-like agents (meperidine, fentanyl, and remifentanil); and (3) diphenylheptanes, which include methadone.[42]

The intravenous route is preferred in the ICU,[40] as this affords a faster onset, higher bioavailability, and better dose titration. Of the 3, fentanyl has the fastest onset because of its high lipophilicity. It should be noted that this characteristic allows fentanyl to accumulate in patients after frequent dosing or continuous infusion.[43] Opioids are metabolized in the liver and excreted renally. Morphine undergoes glucuronidation to active metabolites that can accumulate in patients with decreased renal function. Although fentanyl does not have an active metabolite, the parent compound may accumulate in patients with renal insufficiency, and should be dosed cautiously.[44] Hydromorphone-3-glucuronide (the metabolite of hydromorphone) is inactive and therefore hydromorphone should be considered the drug of choice in patients exhibiting decreased renal function.[19]

Tolerance, the decrease in a drug's efficacy over time despite constant plasma concentrations, is exhibited with all opioids.[45] Synthetic opioids, such as fentanyl, may exhibit tolerance earlier than their nonsynthetic counterparts. This is likely because of the higher receptor affinity.[46] Tolerance may develop in as quickly as one week of continuous or high-dose infusion. Rapid discontinuation or de-escalation may lead to withdrawal symptoms and may be confused for other sources of delirium. Methadone reduces the occurrence of these effects.[47]

Remifentanil

The side-effect profile of morphine (pruritis, histamine release, and accumulation of active metabolites) may at times prohibit its use.[48] Although the synthetic agents (fentanyl, alfentanil, and sufentanil) have better adverse-effect profiles, they can still accumulate in critically ill patients, leading to prolonged drug effects.[19] Remifentanil has been evaluated as a superior alternative. Chemically, it is in the same class as fentanyl; however, its clearance is quite different. Remifentanil is broken down by nonspecific esterases and it's metabolism is unaffected by critical illness.[49] The metabolite, remifentanil acid, is an inactive carboxylic acid with a low affinity for the μ-receptor.[50] The efficacy of remifentanil for prolonged mechanical ventilation was evaluated by Evans and Park.[51] They maintained patients from 3 to 33 days on doses ranging from 0.08 μg/kg to 0.43 μg/kg with all patients showing signs of recovery within 10 minutes of discontinuing the medication. In a blinded, randomized trial evaluating remifentanil versus morphine for mechanically ventilated patients, Dahaba and colleagues[52] noted a decreased need for dose adjustment, increased time spent in optimal sedation, and decreased ventilator hours (14.1 vs 18.1). A similar study in cardiac patients noted similar results with significantly shorter interval from ICU admission to extubation as well as time to ICU discharge.[53] This study also evaluated cost, noting no difference between the 2 groups.[54]

Remifentanil was evaluated in neurologic patients in the ICU, including patients suffering traumatic brain injury. There was no difference in time to extubation between remifentanil and fentanyl, but neurologic function assessment was improved in the remifentanil.[55] A retrospective study by Bauer and colleagues[56] evaluating remifentanil in patients undergoing supratentorial brain tumor surgery noted decreased ventilator days in the remifentanil group (1.8 vs 3.7 days). Interestingly, 3 patients in the fentanyl group required computed tomography scans of the head, as they did not awaken for neurologic assessments; a situation not encountered in the remifentanil group.

Ketamine

Ketamine is a phencyclidine derivative causing disorganization between thalamono-cortical and limbic systems leading to a dissociative state. The anesthetic properties of ketamine work primarily through the central nervous system (CNS) on the N-methyl-D-aspartate receptors, whereas the analgesia effects are obtained with stimulation of the μ-opioid and κ-opioid receptors.[57] Ketamine, at subanesthetic infusion rates, delivers effective analgesia while exhibiting qualities favorable in the critically ill patient. Unlike high-dose opioid infusions, patients on a ketamine infusion will maintain pharyngeal and laryngeal reflexes while preserving respiratory effort.[58] Ketamine reduces airway resistance and can treat severe bronchospasm refractory to traditional bronchodilators. Increases in Pao_2 associated with decreases in $Paco_2$ are noted in ventilated patients with severe bronchospasm when given ketamine.[59] Studies evaluating dynamic compliance (as a surrogate for bronchospasm) have noted relative increases in patients undergoing ketamine infusions.[60]

Ketamine, in addition to its favorable effects on respiratory physiology, has hemodynamic effects desired in a critically ill patient.[61] Studies show no significant changes in systolic, diastolic, or mean arterial pressures when given in standard doses.[62] There is no significant change in peripheral vascular resistance, a favorable property in many critically ill states. Vasopressor requirements in patients on ketamine are unchanged or decreased as compared with patients on fentanyl infusions.[63] This finding, along with the need for decreased volume resuscitation, was also noted in traumatic brain injury.[64]

Caution should be exhibited in patients with decompensated heart failure or cardiogenic shock.[65] Patients with pulmonary hypertension should likely not receive ketamine, as there may be some elevation of pulmonary pressures.[66] Despite the positive effects seen in traumatic brain injury (as well as literature supporting the absence intracranial pressure elevation with infusion) ketamine is a both a proconvulsant and anticonvulsant and should be avoided in patients with seizure disorders.

REGIONAL ANALGESIA
Overview

For most patients in the ICU, pain management with systemic opioids is both effective and appropriate. There are times, however, when this method is less than ideal, either because of excessive/uncontrolled side effects or simple inability to adequate obtain pain control. For some of these patients, pain management through a more targeted technique can be ideal. Consider an elderly patient with multiple rib fractures unable to breathe well secondary to pain, but too sedate or obtunded from opioids. Placement of a continuous epidural or paravertebral block may enable this patient to maintain spontaneous ventilation and allow the patient to participate in respiratory and physical therapy.

Effective use of regional analgesia in the ICU has its share of barriers. Practitioners must be skilled in the placement of varied blocks. They must be knowledgeable of the various techniques to know what is possible. Practitioners must be aware of complications unique to the placement of these blocks and catheters. Nursing must be comfortable with the management of the devices used for continuous infusion. It is unlikely that all of these requirements are met in many hospitals, which limits the utility of many of these anesthetic techniques. Further, at present there is a relative dearth of evidence supporting the use of many available techniques in the ICU as a means of improving outcomes.

Indications and Contraindications

Analgesic management with regional techniques should be considered whenever the risk of system use of narcotics is high or when the pain itself is reasonably well localized to one or more anatomic areas. Large surgical incisions, such as a thoracotomy or laparotomy, upper and lower extremity orthopedic procedures, and rib fractures from trauma, are examples of this type of pain. These sources of pain can frequently be managed by the placement of a continuous epidural (thoracic or lumbar) or extremity block, such as a femoral or sciatic nerve. Further, the use of regional techniques for short-term control of pain for procedural benefits can be of great benefit, especially in a morbidly obese patient with obstructive sleep apnea and hypersensitivity to the respiratory depression associated with opioids. Benefits associated with regional analgesia are somewhat contradictory and do not always seem to show improvements in outcome variables.[67–70] There is good evidence that, at least in the case of neuraxial techniques, use of regional analgesia can both shorten the duration of mechanical ventilation and reduce the incidence of pneumonia.[71] Additionally and potentially more compelling, there is a growing body of evidence linking the use of narcotics and sedatives to the development of delirium and cognitive dysfunction,[38,72,73] which might be reduced or avoided altogether by the successful use of these techniques.

Not all patients in the ICU can be considered candidates for regional pain management; even should they meet the considerations noted previously. For example, the patient with multiple trauma, for whom adequate positioning cannot be performed, patients with severe scoliosis or other anatomic deformities, patients in whom the location of the block is obscured by either infection or their underlying injuries, and those with coagulopathies all may be ineligible for placement of a regional block. With regard to patients receiving anticoagulation therapy or otherwise at increased risk of bleeding, there are consensus guidelines available from the American Society of Regional Anesthesia delineating risk factors, complications, and recommendations, which are regularly updated.[74]

Continuous techniques require the presence of an indwelling catheter through which local anesthetic is infused. Infection related to placement of the catheter or to the patient's underlying illness (eg, sepsis) is a consideration before undertaking a regional technique. Overall, there are a variety of factors to be considered before using a regional technique in the ICU.

Epidural, Intrathecal, and Paravertebral Analgesia

Thoracic, vascular, and orthopedic procedures have long benefited from postoperative pain control with epidural analgesia. Data suggest that thoracic epidural analgesia with bupivacaine and morphine can provide superior analgesia with fewer opioid-related side effects than intravenous narcotic therapy, at least in some populations.[67] Further, epidural analgesia can improve some measures of postoperative outcomes in high-risk patients, including a reduced incidence of thromboembolism and myocardial infarction, as well as improvements in bowel and pulmonary function.[75] Additionally, a Cochrane review comparing epidural to systemic opioid techniques in elective abdominal surgery concluded that the use of a regional technique reduced time on ventilator, cardiovascular and gastrointestinal complications, and the incidence of acute renal failure, in addition to providing superior pain control.[68] Finally, a study using the National Trauma Data Bank (NTDB) noted increasing numbers of rib fractures correlated with increasing extrapulmonary complications. Patients sustaining more than 6 fractures were at a significantly increased risk of mortality compared with those injuring fewer. Epidural analgesia lowered morbidity and mortality and was especially helpful in patients with more than 4 fractures; however, most studies have failed to demonstrate that other outcome variables (eg, length of ICU or hospital stay, mortality) are affected.

Intrathecal techniques, both single dose and continuous, have the most data supporting their use for operative (and immediate postoperative) pain control. Nonsurgical patients in the ICU are rarely treated with these techniques secondary to their increased complication risk.[76] Further, the risk of undesirable side effects from intrathecal administration of opioid is much higher than that seen with epidural administration secondary to cerebrospinal fluid concentrations reaching an order of magnitude higher than that seen with epidural administration. Some of these side effects include respiratory depression, somnolence, and pruritis.

Paravertebral blockade is in many respects very similar to traditional epidural techniques. The primary advantages to a paravertebral block are its one-sided nature and its limited spread to only 1 or 2 dermatomes from the site of needle placement. A catheter can be placed to enhance the degree of spread somewhat and to provide continuous analgesia. It is also possible to place multiple catheters to enable wide coverage of the thoracic cage unilaterally. A unique risk associated with the placement of a paravertebral block, as opposed to an epidural or intrathecal technique, is the development of a pneumothorax. A comparison of block techniques, and their indications and associated risks, can be found in **Table 2**.[75]

Table 2
Techniques, indications, and considerations for regional blocks in the intensive care unit

Type of Block	Block Indication	Special Considerations
Thoracic epidural	Thoracic surgery, chronic pancreatitis, upper abdominal surgery, rib fractures	Epidural hematoma or abscess, hypotension from sympathetic blockade, accidental intrathecal puncture/administration.
Lumbar epidural	Trauma, lower extremity surgery	Same as thoracic epidural.
Paravertebral block	Unilateral thoracic surgery, trauma, or pain	Pneumothorax.
Intercostal block	Chest tube placement, rib fracture	Pneumothorax, high potential for intravascular injection, highest systemic concentrations of local anesthetic even without intravascular injection.
Femoral or sciatic block	Thigh, knee, leg pain	Positioning challenges with sciatic block. Fewer hemodynamic derangements than neuraxial techniques.
Interscalene, supraclavicular, infraclavicular, or axillary block	Arm, shoulder, or hand pain, trauma, or surgery	Technique dependent. Variable spread. Intravascular or intrathecal injection, phrenic nerve block (100% with interscalene).

Adapted from Fishman SM, Ballantyne JC, Rathmell JP, editors. Bonica's management of pain. 4th edition. Philadelphia: Lippincott, Williams and Wilkins; 2010. p. 1589; with permission; and *Data from* Fishman SM, Ballantyne JC, Rathmell JP, editors. Bonica's management of pain. 4th edition. Philadelphia; Lippincott, Williams and Wilkins; 2010. p. 1596.

Intercostal Nerve and Interpleural Blocks

For patients with limited chest trauma, or patients experiencing pain secondary to chest tubes, epidural analgesia is frequently either simply not considered or considered unnecessary by some. However, the pain associated with even singular rib fracture can cause pulmonary complications secondary to decreased respiratory effort and the frequent need for large doses of opioids to ameliorate the pain associated with movement. For these patients, especially if epidural analgesia is contraindicated, it is prudent to consider intercostal nerve blocks. Data on the utility of intercostal blocks in the ICU are limited. One study comparing the effectiveness of intercostal blockade with that of an epidural found the epidural to be superior in providing analgesia; however, improvements in other parameters, such as respiratory performance and ICU length of stay, only trended to be in favor of the epidural.[77] Disadvantages to the intercostal technique include the need for multiple injections, even at single levels of injury, as adequate pain control typically requires anesthesia covering the injured rib as well as one level above and below. Additionally, duration of analgesia is typically in the range of 4 to 8 hours maximally and continuous techniques cannot be recommended secondary to complication rates. Further, serum levels of local anesthetic are highest after intercostal blockade, as compared with any other form of peripheral or neuraxial nerve block, thereby increasing the risk of local anesthetic toxicity when considering more than just 1 or 2 ribs.

Related to the intercostal nerve block is the interpleural block. This type of block is not recommended for several reasons, including the loss of local anesthetic via chest drains, dilution of local anesthetic in the pleural space by blood or pus, and the highly variable nature of the nerve blockade secondary to substantial changes in local anesthetic concentrations from positional effects.

Peripheral Nerve Blocks

There are few data available specifically on the use of peripheral nerve blockade in the ICU setting. Exclusively, all randomized controlled trials involving peripheral nerve blockade are in the perioperative setting and include patients both in and out of the ICU without outcomes comparisons. As with other regional techniques, however, the use of systemic opioids and the complications associated with those medications is reduced when peripheral blockade is available and the patient's anatomic pain is amenable to this type of intervention.

CONSIDERATIONS IN THE GERIATRIC POPULATION

The geriatric population (patient age >65) deserves special consideration, as treatment of surgical and traumatic pain differs from that of their younger counterparts. This population exhibits differences in sensitivity to painful stimuli, has increased sensitivity of the CNS, and suffers from pharmacodynamic and pharmacokinetic changes affecting medication doses and side effects.[78] As the excess catecholamine release from pain in the elderly can have cardiac side effects, undertreatment may be as dangerous as the side effects from overtreatment.[79]

Pain Threshold

Research suggests that as age increases, pain threshold increases as well. There appears, however, to be a concomitant decrease in pain tolerance.[80] Given these opposed changes, elderly patients experience postoperative pain in the same fashion as younger patients. Although the elderly may have a lack of the sense of pain with arteriolar occlusion, myocardial ischemia, and bowel distension, there is no evidence that advanced age dulls the "sense" of pain.[81,82]

Delirium and CNS Effects

Delirium, as discussed elsewhere in this issue, is recognized as a significant cause of morbidity and mortality in critically ill patients. Elderly patients are more subject to CNS disturbances especially during times of severe physiologic stress.[83] Pain itself can lead to delirium, thereby complicating assessment of pain.[84] This cycle is exacerbated in patients with preexisting dementia or delirium.[78] It is well recognized that most traditional pain medications can lead to delirium as well. Finding a balance between adequate pain control while limiting CNS impairment can be a challenge, but doing so should not interfere with treating the patient's pain.

Alterations in Drug Metabolism

Pharmacodynamics change very little with increasing age.[85,86] The dose required to achieve the same end-point may be decreased and the therapeutic window may be narrowed. Conversely, pharmacokinetics can be greatly affected by advanced age.[87] Increasing age yields decreased lean body mass, decreased total body water, and an increased proportion of body fat. These changes combine to alter the volume of distribution of medications, affecting clearance and elimination.[88] Elderly patients will exhibit decreased renal and hepatic drug clearance. The renal blood flow decreases approximately 10% per decade of life after the age of 50. Liver mass decreases with age, as does hepatic blood flow.[89] The combined affect is to decrease drug metabolism.[90] Decreased circulating albumin interferes with drug binding, as well.[91] Also, cardiac, pulmonary, and neurologic depression seen in aging make hypotension, hypoxia, hypercarbia, acidosis, and altered fluid regulation more common. This depressed basal organ function may not be present at rest, only presenting itself during times of physiologic stress.[88]

Rib Fractures in the Elderly

Elderly trauma patients with rib fractures exhibit an observed mortality higher than expected for a given injury severity scale. It is likely a combination of the underlying lung injury, as well as other extrathoracic injuries. In one study, this patient population had twice the mortality of similarly injured younger patients. Each injured rib increased mortality by nearly 20% with a concomitant 30% increase in the risk of pneumonia.[92] Adequate pain control is necessary to avoid delayed pulmonary complications. Respiratory depression associated with narcotic analgesia, however, may instead contribute to such complications. Regional and local analgesia in this population has very favorable data.

A retrospective study by Bulger and colleagues analyzed elderly patients receiving epidural analgesia compared with those receiving traditional pain medications.[92] In that study, the epidural group was more severely injured and had higher rates of pulmonary complications, total length of stay, and length of ICU stay. Despite the higher chest abbreviated injury score and increased complication rates, this group had a significantly lower mortality (11% vs 25%).[93] In the absence of contraindications, regional analgesia should be offered to elderly patients with 4 or more rib fractures, or those with respiratory compromise secondary to injured ribs.[94]

REFERENCES

1. Desbiens NA, Wu AW. Pain and suffering in seriously ill hospitalized patients. J Am Geriatr Soc 2000;48(Suppl 5):S183–6.

2. Stanik-Hutt JA, Soeken KL, Belcher AE, et al. Pain experiences of traumatically injured patients in a critical care setting. Am J Crit Care 2001;10(4):252–9.
3. Desbiens NA, Wu AW, Broste SK, et al. Pain and satisfaction with pain control in seriously ill hospitalized adults: findings from the SUPPORT research investigations. For the SUPPORT investigators. Study to Understand Prognoses and Preferences for Outcomes and Risks of Treatment. Crit Care Med 1996;24(12):1943–4.
4. Doyle D, Hanks GW, MacDonald N, editors. Oxford textbook of palliative medicine. 2nd ed. Oxford (England): Oxford University Press; 1998.
5. Epstein J, Breslow MJ. The stress response of critical illness. Crit Care Clin 1999; 15(1):17–33.
6. Lewis KS, Whipple JK, Michael KA, et al. Effect of analgesic treatment on the physiological consequences of acute pain. Am J Hosp Pharm 1994;51(12):1539–54.
7. Jacox A, Carr D, Payne R, et al. Clinical practice guideline number 9: management of cancer pain. Rockville (MD): Agency for Health Care Policy and Research, US Dept of Health and Human Services; 1994. AHCPR Publication No. 94–0592.
8. Cross SA. Pathophysiology of pain. Mayo Clin Proc 1994;69(4):375–83.
9. Willis WD, Westlund KN. Neuroanatomy of the pain system and of the pathways that modulate pain. J Clin Neurophysiol 1997;14(1):2–31.
10. Curtiss CP, Haylock PJ. Managing cancer and noncancer chronic pain in critical care settings. Knowledge and skills every nurse needs to know. Crit Care Nurs Clin North Am 2001;13(2):271–80.
11. Merskey H, Bogduk N, editors. Classification of chronic pain. IASP task force on taxonomy. 2nd edition. Seattle (WA): IASP Press; 2011. p. 209–14.
12. Merskey H, Bogduk N. Classification of chronic pain. 2nd edition. Seattle (WA): International Association for the Study of Pain; 1994. p. 3–4.
13. Turk DC, Okifuji A. Pain terms and taxonomies of pain. In: Bonica JJ, Loeser JD, Chapman CR, et al, editors. Bonica's management of pain. Hagerstown (MD): Lippincott Williams & Wilkins; 2001. p. 18–21.
14. Pasero C, McCaffery M. Pain in the critically ill. Am J Nurs 2002;102(1):59–60.
15. Granja C, Lopes A, Moreira S, et al. Patients' recollections of experiences in the intensive care unit may affect their quality of life. Crit Care 2005;9:96–109.
16. Puntillo K, Miaskowski C, Summer G. Pain. In: Carrieri-Kohlman C, Lindsey A, West C, editors. Pathophysiolgical phenomena in nursing: human responses to illness. St Louis (MO): Saunders; 2003. p. 235–54.
17. Schelling G, Richter M, Roozendaal B, et al. Exposure to high stress in the intensive care unit may have negative effects on health-related quality-of-life outcomes after cardiac surgery. Crit Care Med 2003;31:1971–80.
18. Hall-Lord ML, Larsson G, Steen B. Pain and distress among elderly intensive care patients: comparison of patients' experiences and nurses' assessments. Heart Lung 1998;27:123–32.
19. Jacobi J, Fraser GL, Coursin DB, et al. Clinical practice guidelines for the sustained use of sedatives and analgesics in the critically ill adult. Crit Care Med 2002;30(1):119–41.
20. Sessler CN, Jo Grap M, Ramsay MA. Evaluating and monitoring analgesia and sedation in the intensive care unit. Crit Care 2008;12(Suppl 3):S2.
21. Kwekkeboom KL, Herr K. Assessment of pain in the critically ill. Crit Care Nurs Clin North Am 2001;13:181–94.
22. Puntillo K, Miaskowski C, Kehrle K, et al. Relationship between behavioral and physiological indicators of pain, critical care patients' self-reports of pain, and opioid administration. Crit Care Med 1997;25:1159–66.

23. Herr K, Coyne PJ, Key T, et al. Pain assessment in nonverbal patients: position statement with clinical practice recommendations. Pain Manag Nurs 2006;7: 44–52.

24. Puntillo KA, Morris AB, Thompson CL, et al. Pain behaviors observed during six common procedures: results from Thunder Project II. Crit Care Med 2004;32: 421–7.

25. Li D, Puntillo K, Miaskowski C. A review of objective pain measures for use with critical care adult patients unable to self-report. J Pain 2008;9(1):2–10.

26. Labus J, Keefe F, Jensen M. Self-reports of pain intensity and direct observations of pain behavior: when are they correlated? J Pain 2003;102:109–24.

27. Payen JF, Bru O, Bosson JL, et al. Assessing pain in critically ill sedated patients by using a behavioral pain scale. Crit Care Med 2001;29(12):2258–63.

28. Aissaoui Y, Zeggwagh A, Zekraoui A, et al. Validation of a behavioral pain scale in critically ill, sedated, and mechanically ventilated patients. Anesth Analg 2005; 101:1470–6.

29. Gelinas C, Fillion L, Puntillo KA, et al. Validation of the critical-care pain observation tool in adult patients. Am J Crit Care 2006;15(4):420–7.

30. Pudas-Tahka S, Axelin A, Antaa R, et al. Pain assessment tools for unconscious or sedated intensive care patients: a systematic review. J Adv Nurs 2008;65(5): 946–56.

31. Merkel S, Shayevitz J, Voepel-Lewis T, et al. The FLACC: a behavioral scale for scoring postoperative pain in young children. Pediatr Nurs 1997;23:293–7.

32. Odhner M, Wegman D, Freeland N, et al. Assessing pain control in nonverbal critically ill adults. Dimens Crit Care Nurs 2003;22:260–7.

33. Gelinas C, Arbour C, Michaud C, et al. A pre and post evaluation of the implementation of the Critical-Care Pain Observation Tool on pain assessment/ management nursing practices in the intensive care unit with nonverbal critically ill adults. Int J Nurs Stud 2011. http://dx.doi.org/10.1016/j.ijnurstu.2011.03.012.

34. Robinson B, Mueller E, Henson K, et al. An analgesia-delirium-sedation protocol for critically ill trauma patients reduces ventilator days and hospital length of stay. J Trauma 2008;65(3):517–26.

35. Chanques G, Jaber S, Barbotte E, et al. Impact of systematic evaluation of pain and agitation in an intensive care unit. Crit Care Med 2006;34(6):1691–9.

36. Brook AD, Ahrens TS, Schaiff R, et al. Effect of a nursing-implemented sedation protocol on the duration of mechanical ventilation. Crit Care Med 1999;27(12): 2609–15.

37. Sessler C, Pedram S. Protocolized and target-based sedation and analgesia in the ICU. Crit Care Clin 2009;25:489–513.

38. Pandharipande PP, Pun BT, Herr DL, et al. Effect of sedation with dexmedetomidine vs lorazepam on acute brain dysfunction in mechanically ventilated patients: the MENDS randomized controlled trial. JAMA 2007;298(22):2644–53.

39. Mehta S, Burry L, Fischer S, et al. Canadian survey of the use of sedatives, analgesics, and neuromuscular blocking agents in critically ill patients. Crit Care Med 2006;34(2):374–80.

40. Hall LG, Oyen LJ, Murray MJ. Analgesic agents. Pharmacology and application in critical care. Crit Care Clin 2001;17(4):899–923, viii.

41. Martin J, Franck M, Sigel S, et al. Changes in sedation management in German intensive care units between 2002 and 2006: a national follow-up survey. Crit Care 2007;11(6):R124.

42. Trescot AM, Datta S, Lee M, et al. Opioid pharmacology. Pain Physician 2008; 11(Suppl 2):S133–53.

43. Sessler CN, Varney K. Patient-focused sedation and analgesia in the ICU. Chest 2008;133(2):552–65.
44. Davies G, Kingswood C, Street M. Pharmacokinetics of opioids in renal dysfunction. Clin Pharmacokinet 1996;31(6):410–22.
45. Dumas EO, Pollack GM. Opioid tolerance development: a pharmacokinetic/pharmacodynamic perspective. AAPS J 2008;10:537–51.
46. Hofbauer R, Tesinsky P, Hammerschmidt V, et al. No reduction in the sufentanil requirement of elderly patients undergoing ventilatory support in the medical intensive care unit. Eur J Anaesthesiol 1999;16(10):702–7.
47. Tobias JD. Tolerance, withdrawal, and physical dependency after long-term sedation and analgesia of children in the pediatric intensive care unit. Crit Care Med 2000;28(6):2122–32.
48. Mazoit JX, Butscher K, Samii K. Morphine in postoperative patients: pharmacokinetics and pharmacodynamics of metabolites. Anesth Analg 2007;105:70–8.
49. Wilhelm W, Kreuer S. The place for short-acting opioids: special emphasis on remifentanil. Critical Care 2008;12(3):S5.
50. Egan TD, Lemmens HJ, Fiset P, et al. The pharmacokinetics of the new short-acting opioid remifentanil (GI87084B) in healthy adult male volunteers. Anesthesiology 1993;79:881–92.
51. Evans TN, Park GR. Remifentanil in the critically ill. Anaesthesia 1997;52:800–1.
52. Dahaba AA, Grabner T, Rehak PH, et al. Remifentanil versus morphine analgesia and sedation for mechanically ventilated critically ill patients: a randomized double blind study. Anesthesiology 2004;101:640–6.
53. Müllejans B, López A, Cross MH, et al. Remifentanil versus fentanyl for analgesia based sedation to provide patient comfort in the intensive care unit: a randomized, double-blind controlled trial. Crit Care 2004;8:R1–11.
54. Müllejans B, Matthey T, Scholpp J, et al. Sedation in the intensive care unit with remifentanil/propofol versus midazolam/fentanyl: a randomised, open-label, pharmacoeconomic trial. Critical Care 2006;10:R91.
55. Karabinis A, Mandragos K, Stergiopoulos S, et al. Safety and efficacy of analgesia-based sedation using remifentanil versus standard hypnotic-based regimens in intensive care unit patients with brain injuries: a randomised, controlled trial [ISRCTN50308308]. Crit Care 2004;8:R268–80.
56. Bauer C, Kreuer S, Ketter R, et al. Remifentanil-propofol versus fentanyl-midazolam combinations for intracranial surgery: influence of anaesthesia technique and intensive sedation on ventilation times and duration of stay in the ICU. Anaesthesist 2007;56:128–32.
57. Craven R. Ketamine. Anaesthesia 2007;62(Suppl 1):48–53.
58. Green SM, Krauss B. The semantics of ketamine. Ann Emerg Med 2000;36:480–2.
59. Nehama J, Pass R, Bechtler-Karsch A, et al. Continuous ketamine infusion for the treatment of refractory asthma in a mechanically ventilated infant: case report and review of the pediatric literature. Pediatr Emerg Care 1996;12:294–7.
60. Youssef-Ahmed MZ, Silver P, Nimkoff L, et al. Continuous infusion of ketamine in mechanically ventilated children with refractory bronchospasm. Intensive Care Med 1996;22:972–6.
61. Indvall J, Ahlgren I, Aronsen KF, et al. Ketamine infusions: pharmacokinetics and clinical effects. Br J Anaesth 1979;51:1167–72.
62. Hijazi Y, Bodonian C, Bolon M, et al. Pharmacokinetics and haemodynamics of ketamine in intensive care patients with brain or spinal cord injury. Br J Anaesth 2003;90:155–60.

63. Tobias JD, Martin LD, Wetzel RC. Ketamine by continuous infusion for sedation in the pediatric intensive care unit. Crit Care Med 1990;18:819–21.

64. Schmittner MD, Vajkoczy SL, Horn P, et al. Effects of fentanyl and S(+)-ketamine on cerebral hemodynamics, gastrointestinal motility, and need of vasopressors in patients with intracranial pathologies: a pilot study. J Neurosurg Anesthesiol 2007;19:257–62.

65. Bovill JG. Intravenous anesthesia for the patient with left ventricular dysfunction. Semin Cardiothorac Vasc Anesth 2006;10:43–8.

66. Hedenstierna G. Pulmonary perfusion during anesthesia and mechanical ventilation. Minerva Anestesiol 2005;71:319–24.

67. Rudin A, Flisberg P, Johansson J, et al. Thoracic epidural analgesia or intravenous morphine analgesia after thoracoabdominal esophagectomy: a prospective follow-up of 201 patients. J Cardiothorac Vasc Anesth 2005;19(3): 350–7.

68. Nishimori M, Ballantyne JC, Low JH. Epidural pain relief versus systemic opioid-based pain relief for abdominal aortic surgery. Cochrane Database Syst Rev 2006;(3):CD005059.

69. Park WY, Thompson JS, Lee KK. Effect of epidural anesthesia and analgesia on perioperative outcome: a randomized, controlled Veterans Affairs cooperative study. Ann Surg 2001;234(4):560–659.

70. Tziavrangos E, Schug SA. Regional anaesthesia and perioperative outcome. Curr Opin Anaesthesiol 2006;19(5):521–5.

71. Bulger EM, Edwards T, Klotz P, et al. Epidural analgesia improves outcome after multiple rib fractures. Surgery 2004;136(2):426–30.

72. Lloyd DG, Ma D, Vizcaychipi MP. Cognitive decline after anaesthesia and critical care. Cont Educ Anaesth Crit Care Pain 2012;12(3):105–9.

73. Rudolph JL, Marcantonio ER. Postoperative delirium: acute change with long-term implications. Anesth Analg 2011;112(5):1202–11.

74. Horlocker TT, Wedel DJ. Regional anesthesia in the anticoagulated patient: defining the risks (the third ASRA Consensus Conference on Neuraxial Anesthesia and Anticoagulation). Reg Anesth Pain Med 2010;28(3):172–97.

75. Liu S, Carpenter RL, Neal JM. Epidural anesthesia and analgesia. Their role in postoperative outcome. Anesthesiology 1995;82:1474–506.

76. Clark F, Gilbert HC. Regional analgesia in the intensive care unit. Principles and practice. Crit Care Clin 2001;17:943–66.

77. Hashemzadeh S, Hashemzadeh K. Comparison thoracic epidural and intercostal block to improve ventilation parameters and reduce pain in patients with multiple rib fractures. J Cardiovasc Thorac Res 2011;3(3):87–91.

78. McCleane G. Pain and the elderly patient. In: McCleane G, Smith H, editors. Clinical management of the elderly patient in pain. New York: The Haworth Medical press; 2006. p. 1–6,

79. Sinatra R. Role of Cox-2 inhibitors in the evolution of acute pain management. J Pain Symptom Manage 2002;24(Suppl 1):S18–27.

80. Gibson SJ. Pain and aging: the pain experiences over the adult lifespan. In: Dostrovsky JO, Carr DB, Koltzenburg M, editors. Proceedings of the 10th World Congress on Pain. Seattle, WA: IASP Press; 2003. p. 767–90.

81. Cleeland C. Undertreatment of cancer pain in elderly patients. JAMA 1998; 279(23):1914–5.

82. Gibson S, Farrell M. A review of age differences in the neurophysiology of nociception and the perceptual experience of pain. Clin J Pain 2004;20(4): 227–39.

83. Rohan D, Buggy D, Crowley S, et al. Increased incidence of postoperative cognitive dysfunction 24 hours after minor surgery in the elderly. Can J Anaesth 2005; 52:137–42.
84. Lynch EP, Lazor MH, Gellis JE, et al. The impact of postoperative pain on the development of postoperative delirium. Anesth Analg 1998;86:781–5.
85. Auburn F, Monsel S, Langeron O, et al. Postoperative titration of intravenous morphine in the elderly patient. Anesthesiology 2002;96:17–23.
86. Daykin A, Bowen D, Daunders D, et al. Respiratory depression after morphine in the elderly. Anaesthesia 1986;41(9):910–4.
87. Shafer SL, Flood P. The pharmacology of opioids. In: Silverstein JH, Rooke GA, Reves JG, et al (editors). Geriatric anesthesiology. 2nd edition. New York: Springer; 2009. p. 209–28, Chapter 15.
88. Cook DJ, Rooke GA. Priorities in perioperative geriatrics. Anesth Analg 2003;96: 1823–36.
89. Silverstein J, Bloom H, Cassel C. New challenges in anesthesia: new practice opportunities. Anaesthiol Clin 2003;17:453–65.
90. Benet L, Kroetz D, Sheiner L. Pharmacokinetics: the dynamics of drug absorption, distribution, and elimination. In: Hardman J, Limbird L, editors. Goodman and Gilman's the pharmacological basis of therapeutics. 9th edition. New York: McGraw-Hill; 1996. p. 3–28, Chapter 1.
91. Henry C. Mechanisms of changes in basal metabolism during aging. Eur J Clin Nutr 2000;54:77–91.
92. Bulger E, Arneson M, Mock C, et al. Rib fractures in the elderly. J Trauma 2000; 48(6):1040–7.
93. Flagel B, Luchette F, Reed L, et al. Half-a-dozen ribs: the breakpoint for mortality. Surgery 2005;138(4):717–25.
94. Ho A, Karmaker M, Critchley L. Acute pain management of patients with multiple fractured ribs: a focus on regional techniques. Curr Opin Crit Care 2011;17: 323–7.

Family Engagement Regarding the Critically Ill Patient

Jessica L. Weaver, MD[a], Ciarán T. Bradley, MD, MA[b],
Karen J. Brasel, MD, MPH[c,d],*

KEYWORDS

- Critically ill patients • Family-centered care • End-of-life care • Intensive care unit

KEY POINTS

- Nowhere is the need for family-centered care greater than among critically ill patients.
- Families in the Study to Understand Prognoses and Preferences for Outcomes and Risks of Treatments trial reported that 50% of patients able to communicate spent over half of their final days in moderate or severe pain.
- Scheduled, time-based meetings are an effective strategy to improve communication about all aspects of care, and increase the likelihood for successful discussions about goal-directed care.
- Clear, thorough documentation of meetings is a critical part of communication to allow all health care providers to understand important discussions.
- Family-centered care is an extension of patient-centered care, as the family will likely be the primary support system when the patient survives critical illness.

The Institute of Medicine strongly recommends a health care system that supports family members.[1] Nowhere is the need for family-centered care greater than with critically ill patients. Simplistically, family-centered care is primarily about communication. Unfortunately, family perception of communication in the intensive care unit (ICU) is quite poor.[2–5] This article reviews some strategies to improve communication, including family meetings and family presence at resuscitation. It also highlights some of the areas within the realm of ICU care in which family engagement is particularly important, including advance directives, end-of-life care, brain death, and organ donation.

FAMILY MEETINGS

Family meetings are an opportunity for a patient's family and care team to discuss patient prognosis and goals of care, and allow the family to voice any questions or

[a] Department of Surgery, School of Medicine, University of Louisville, Louisville, KY 40292, USA;
[b] Department of Surgery, Memorial Sloan-Kettering Cancer Center, Box 435, 1275 York Avenue, New York, NY 10065, USA; [c] Department of Surgery, Medical College of Wisconsin, Milwaukee, WI 53226, USA; [d] Department of Bioethics and Medical Humanities, Medical College of Wisconsin, Milwaukee, WI 53226, USA
* Corresponding author.
E-mail address: kbrasel@mcw.edu

Surg Clin N Am 92 (2012) 1637–1647
http://dx.doi.org/10.1016/j.suc.2012.08.004
0039-6109/12/$ – see front matter © 2012 Published by Elsevier Inc.

surgical.theclinics.com

concerns. Communication between the medical team and the family during these meetings is vitally important, and yet is often inadequate. The ICU Working Group, convened to develop an ICU end-of-life research and education agenda, identified communication as a necessary area of improvement.[6] Numerous studies, including the Study to Understand Prognoses and Preferences for Outcomes and Risks of Treatments (SUPPORT), have found serious shortcomings in physician-family communication.[2–5]

Open communication benefits both patients and their families. Families in the SUPPORT trial reported that 50% of patients able to communicate spent more than half of their final days in moderate or severe pain. Reduced family participation in the decision-making process is associated with increased unnecessary treatments as well as physician-family conflicts.[4] The French FAMIREA group showed that a lack of regular meetings with the medical team increases anxiety in the patient's family members, and perceived contradictions in the information received is associated with an increased rate of depression in these families.[7] A similar study showed that posttraumatic stress disorder, a common finding among family members of patients who are dying in the hospital, can be lessened by increasing the length of family meetings as well as by allowing the family members more time to talk.[8]

Although there are several studies looking at the quality of communication during family meetings, few examine the documentation of these meetings, despite its importance in communication between care providers. Sharing information through the medical record reduces risk, reduces duplication and waste, and improves decision making. This written record also supports other functions, such as billing.[9] Documentation can be addressed by a standard form for physicians to use during family meetings, but the outcomes of such an intervention have not been studied.[10]

This increased emphasis on communication may not be enough; there is ample evidence that family members do not understand everything discussed during these meetings. Azoulay and colleagues[3] found that 54% of patient representatives failed to comprehend the patient's diagnosis, prognosis, or treatment. Another study found that only 19% of primary patient surrogates reported poor understanding, but 47% of surrogates surveyed met the study's criteria for poor understanding. Better understanding was not associated with more time spent with the medical team.[11] Given this pervasive poor understanding, it is important that multiple members of the patient's care team help the patient's family by consistently reemphasizing the most important aspects of the patient's condition and treatment, and that this information is consistent across specialties. One way of ensuring the consistency of communication is with thorough documentation of family meetings in the patient's medical record.

Having a written record of what occurs in family meetings is important from a legal standpoint. Decisions to sign a do-not-resuscitate (DNR) order or withdrawal/withhold treatment are routinely made in these meetings, and there should be a record of not only when the decision was reached, but why the decision was made and who was there when it happened. If this information detailing this discussion is not documented in the medical record, then there is no proof that it actually occurred. Without proper documentation of how decisions were made, decisions can be challenged. Such challenges undermine family and provider trust and can result in family complaints or dissatisfaction, and even legal action.

Family meetings can easily consume 30 minutes or more of a physician's time, multiple times per week. These meetings are integral to patient care, and proper documentation of the meetings and time spent are still an important component of physician billing practices. Notes should document who attended the meeting, how long it lasted, what decisions were made, and any conflicts that might have been voiced.

ADVANCE DIRECTIVES

According to federal law, an advance directive is defined as a written instruction, such as a living will or durable power of attorney for health care, that is recognized under state law (whether statutory or as recognized by the courts of the state), relating to the provision of health care when the individual is incapacitated. The 2 most common examples are living wills and health care powers of attorney. A living will is a legal document in which the patient describes and defines what life-sustaining treatments he or she would want in the event of incapacity and terminal illness. Patients may also designate a power of attorney for health care; this person has the legal authority to make health care decisions on behalf of the patient should he or she lose decision-making capacity. Decision-making capacity refers to the capacity to make medical decisions and to provide informed consent to treatment. This is different from competence, a legal term. Competence is determined by a court, not by a physician. With or without this legal document, the surrogate, or proxy, is expected to use substituted judgment—to reconstruct what the patient would have wanted in a particular situation using formal and informal statements the patient may have made previously. DNR status is often included under this heading, although DNR orders represent the specific order written in a medical record that is intended to carry out the patient's wishes outlined in an advanced directive.

The Patient Self-Determination Act, passed in 1990, requires any institution receiving Medicare or Medicaid funds to inform patients in writing of their right to accept or refuse treatment and their right to an advance directive. The act itself does not help guide subsequent care in any way. Unfortunately, advance directive completion rates remain low, with population-based studies reporting their use in only 15% to 25% of adult patients.[12]

Buy-In

Lack of formal advanced directives is not the only barrier to patient-directed care in the surgical ICU. There is a general consensus by intensivists and nonsurgical providers that surgeons hesitate to withdraw life-sustaining therapy on their operative patients despite a competent patient's or surrogate's request to do so. One reason may be the phenomenon of surgical buy-in.[13]

Surgeons' preoperative discussions with patients cover the risk of the operation as well as a long list of therapies that patients might need to undertake in the postoperative setting, such as ventilatory support or hemodialysis. Consent for surgery is often taken as consent for these postoperative therapies—"buy-in." Conflicts about buy-in may arise in the postoperative setting as patient preferences change, depending on the clinical picture and the potential for recovery. Surgeons may refuse entirely to withdraw life-sustaining procedures or argue demonstrably for continuation of life-sustaining therapy based on the surgeon's vision of the patient's potential for meaningful recovery and interpretation of the preoperative discussion surrounding operative consent.

PALLIATIVE AND END-OF-LIFE CARE

Half of all patients who die in the hospital have been in the ICU within the last 3 days of their lives. Up to 90% of these deaths involve withdrawing or withholding treatment.[14] In the ICU, many patients suffer uncontrolled pain,[5] and their families experience severe depression and anxiety.[15] A palliative care team can aid the attending physician with symptom control, with an emphasis on controlling pain as well as providing spiritual and psychosocial support.

One possible next step to increase palliative services for patients would be the institution of a palliative care bundle.[16] This approach has been used by Mosenthal and colleagues[17] and has been shown to decrease time to signing a DNR or withdrawing life support, as well as shorten the length of ICU and hospital stay in patients who die within that year, without any overall change in mortality. A palliative care bundle is a standardized set of procedures used by critical care physicians to assess the palliative care needs of all of their patients. This assists critical care physicians in providing palliative care services to their own patients, identifies other aspects of care, such as social work or spiritual support that may be necessary, and identifies patients most likely to benefit from an increased level of expertise in palliative care. Bundle elements include:

- Identification of a medical decision maker
- Determination of advance directive status
- Investigation of resuscitation preference
- Distribution of family information leaflet
- Regular pain assessment
- Optimal pain management
- Offer of social work support
- Offer of spiritual support
- Interdisciplinary family meeting

Good palliative and end-of-life care for patients with an unexpected illness has some significant differences compared with patients with a known terminal illness. Some differences include young age, unknown goals of care, and lack of an established relationship. Families of these patients who die are at high risk of a complicated grief response. Part of caring for these patients is caring for their families, and doing what one can to minimize the risk of complicated grief. Advocating family presence during resuscitation and ensuring that families can visit after death is an important part of decreasing risk, as is clear communication and time spent when giving bad news.

Specific Protocols

Specific activities at or near the end of life requiring either protocols or guidelines include terminal weaning, pain management, and palliative sedation. Known protocols help all caregivers to understand these treatments as accepted components of care, and provide a reference for new or unfamiliar providers as well as family members. Although palliative care consultants are intimately familiar with these activities, they should also be familiar to all who practice in an ICU setting. An example of a terminal weaning protocol is shown in **Fig. 1**.

Sedation

A sedation protocol uses any number of different medications to achieve the desired effect. If the desired effect is ordinary symptom management, relief without altering consciousness is the goal. However, when sedating medicines, along with other measures of symptom relief, are titrated to effect, this could result in increased levels of sedation. This concept is sometimes referred to as proportionate palliative sedation. It is understood that although proportionate palliative sedation occasionally results in sedation to unconsciousness, this is not its intent.

Palliative sedation, on the other hand, is the controlled administration of sedative medications to reduce patient consciousness to the minimum extent necessary to render intolerable and refractory suffering tolerable.[18] Although not intended, this

Terminal weaning

An example of a protocol for terminal weaning is below:

1. Notify chaplain; ask family/surrogates if they wish chaplain or other clergy present before or during remove from mechanical ventilation
2. Discontinue paralytics and test for return of neuromuscular function.
3. Ensure adequate sedation and pain management.
4. Prepare space at the bedside for family members.
5. Ask Respiratory Therapist to silence all ventilator alarms; set FIO_2 to 21% and remove PEEP. Observe for signs of respiratory distress, adjust medication
6. Reduce IMV rate to 4 and/or pressure support to 6 over 5-15 minutes. Observe for signs of respiratory distress and adjust medications to optimize patient comfort.
7. Deflate endotrachial tube cuff, extubate and suction (if necessary) once comfort is achieved and the family consent to extubation. Remove ventilator from bedside.
8. In some situations, it may be desirable to leave the endotracheal tube in for patient comfort. In these rare cases, have T-piece available at bedside. Observe for signs of respiratory distress, adjust medication

Fig. 1. Terminal weaning protocol. PEEP, positive end-expiratory pressure; RMV, removal from mechanical ventilation.

may result in respiratory depression. This scenario is an illustration of the principle of double effect, a bioethical term that refers to 2 types of consequences (the intended consequences and the unintended side effects) that may be produced by a single action.

When palliative sedation is planned, it should be done with a fully informed patient (if the patient has decision-making capacity) and family, along with involvement of the multidisciplinary care team. An advance directive should be completed along with a DNR order. Specific documentation is imperative. The documentation should address the reasons for the decision, the legal agent making the decision, individuals who participated in the decision, expectations of the decision, and any alternatives to the decision that were discussed.

Family presence during resuscitation

Family presence during resuscitation (FPDR) means that the family is present in a location that affords visual and/or physical contact with the patient during resuscitation.[19-21] This locale may be the emergency department, trauma bay, hospital ward, or ICU. Resuscitation is a sequence of events initiated to sustain life or prevent further deterioration of the patient's condition during an acute health episode. Benefits for families who witness the resuscitation of a family member include knowing that everything possible was being done for the patient, reducing anxiety, feeling of being supportive and helpful to the patient and staff, sharing critical information about the patient's condition, maintaining family-patient relationships, closure on a life shared together, and fostering grieving.[19-28]

There are a variety of concerns expressed by health care professionals with respect to FPDR: That the event may be too traumatic for the family; that clinical care might be impeded; that family members may become too emotional or out of control; that staff may experience increased stress; that staff are focused on the patient and may not be available to assist the family; and the risk of legal action.[19-24,26,29-31]

Despite the concerns of health care providers, family members who experience FPDR report that they would agree to be present again if a similar event occurred.[24,25,32-35] Family members not only emphatically asserted the right to be present but stated that FPDR was important and helpful to them.[32,33,36] In addition, prior research indicates no adverse psychological effects for family members and the operations of the critical care providers was not disrupted by the family presence.[21,25,32,33,36] Although anecdotal reports of legal action exist, the legal action does not appear to be due to the actual presence of a family member but a result of actions of health care providers that could (and likely would) be ascertained from the medical record.

There are several important steps in a family presence program, including the protocol itself, in addition to the preparation, education, and culture change necessary in many institutions before implementation. Successful programs require a designated support staff (family facilitator) available at all times, ideally with no other clinical responsibilities. This support staff can be a medical social worker, chaplain, or nurse, but must be specifically trained in the amount of medical information to relay and in recognizing the family response to the resuscitation events. This person first assesses the family to determine whether they would be appropriate candidates for family presence. Sometimes this involves an independent decision; sometimes the family is asked. Providers are then asked whether family presence is appropriate; a "no" decision is absolute. If family, support staff, and provider are in agreement, the family is prepared for what they might see, are told where to stand/sit, what to do if they feel faint, and that they might be asked to leave at any time. During the resuscitation, the support staff member explains interventions, interprets jargon, provides information about expected outcomes, supplies comfort measures, gives opportunities to ask questions, and grants an opportunity to see, touch, and speak to the patient. Given the medical background of the support staff, they might or might not be able to fulfill all of these responsibilities. Once the resuscitation is over, the support person remains with the family, providing support and another opportunity to ask questions. If appropriate, a bereavement protocol is implemented. An abbreviated example of a family presence protocol is shown in **Fig. 2**.

Brain death
An individual with irreversible cessation of all functions of the entire brain, including the brain stem, is dead. This is both a medical and legal definition. It does not require consent or participation by family or surrogate decision makers. However, appropriate efforts should be made to discuss the patient's medical condition in the process of determining brain death with family or surrogate decision makers before evaluating the patient for brain death.

In accordance with the Uniform Determination of Death Act, passed in 1980, which replaced the Uniform Brain Death Act of 1978, guidelines for determination of brain death are developed at an institutional level. Unfortunately, guidelines for determining brain death vary widely across institutions, and in many cases do not conform with current guidelines established by the American Academy of Neurology.[37,38] These include:

- Establishing a known cause of brain death
- Ensuring normothermia, normotension, absence of toxic substances
- Performing a clinical neurologic examination (**Fig. 3**)
- Performing an apnea test

If a certain period of time has passed since the onset of the brain insult that excludes the possibility of recovery (in practice, usually several hours), 1 neurologic examination should be sufficient to pronounce brain death. However, in the United States some state statutes require 2 examinations. Legally, all physicians are allowed to determine

Starting Point: The Physician/Team Decision

- The physician/team is informed that family is present
- Physician/team agrees to offer family presence option
- Physician/team determines positioning of the family within the treatment area
1.   Patient Assessment (proceed to Step 2 if patient not alert)
  - If patient is alert and oriented, FF or other staff asks patient if he or she would like to have family present provided team or other circumstances allow
2.   Family Assessment
  - FF assesses family for appropriateness of family presence
  - **Exclusion criteria:**
    - Combativeness
    - Agitation
    - Extreme emotional instability
    - Altered mental status
    - Intoxication
3.   FF prepares family for actual presence at resuscitation
  - FF explains/describes the setting and the circumstances
  - FF explains ground rules for family presence
4.   Procedure for Actual Family Presence
  - FF announces family's presence to the team
  - FF provides comfort measures to family – chairs, tissues
  - *FF remains physically present (within arm's length or closer of family members) throughout resuscitation*
  - FF provides general description of events without offering diagnosis or prognosis
  - When feasible, team invites family members to bedside to touch patient or for other contact
5.   FF assesses advisability of continued family presence and directs break as indicated
6.   Completion of Family Presence Option
  - Address family concerns
  - Help family process what they saw
  - Provide additional resources
  - Arrange for further medical update/conference
  - Address other psychological/social needs
7.   Documentation in Medical Record

Fig. 2. Abbreviated protocol to guide family presence during resuscitation. FF, family facilitator.

brain death in most states. Neurologists, neurosurgeons, and intensive care specialists may have specialized expertise.

Confirmatory testing is not mandatory in most clinical situations. In adults, confirmatory testing cannot supersede (such as transcranial doppler ultrasound) clinical observations that are not consistent with brain death, because establishing death by brain criteria is a clinical diagnosis. The interpretation of each of these tests requires expertise.

ORGAN DONATION

Under United States law, the regulation of organ donation is left to states within the limitations of the Uniform Determination of Death Act, the National Organ Transplant Act of 1984, and the United Network for Organ Sharing. Each state's Uniform Anatomic Gift Act seeks to streamline the process and standardize the rules among the various states.

The demand for organs significantly surpasses the number of donors everywhere in the world. In the United States about 108,000 people are on the waiting list. As one way of addressing this shortage, in 2003 the Department of Health and Human Services collaborated with leading transplantation organizations to launch the

CLINICAL CRITERIA FOR BRAIN DEATH:
A. Cerebral unresponsiveness
  1. Deep coma
  2. No motor response to painful stimuli in all extremities, determined by nail bed pressure stimulus
  3. No motor response to supraorbital or temporomandibular pressure
B. Absence of brain stem reflexes
  1. Pupils must be 4mm or greater in size. There must be no response to bright light
  2. Ocular movement
    a. Absence of spontaneous eye movement
    b. No oculocephalic reflex. Testing should only be performed when no fracture or instability of the cervical spine is apparent
    c. No oculovestibular reflex. (movement of the eyes to cold caloric stimulation)
  3. Facial sensation and facial motor response
    a. No corneal reflex to touch with a cotton swab
    b. No jaw reflex
    c. No grimacing to noxious stimuli, including pressure of the nail beds, supraorbital ridge, or temporomandibular joint region
  4. No gag response to posterior pharynx stimulation with tongue blade
  5. No cough response to bronchial stimulation with suctioning catheter or irrigation
  6. No spontaneous swallowing or yawning
C.   No evidence of respiratory effort with formal apnea test

Fig. 3. Clinical criteria necessary for the determination of brain death.

Breakthrough Collaborative, calling on all hospitals to increase their organ donation rates to 75% or higher.

Most organ donation for organ transplantation is done in the setting of brain death. As another strategy to address the ever-increasing demand, transplantation has returned to its roots; as of July 2007, all transplantation hospitals are required by the United Network for Organ Sharing to develop and follow protocols that facilitate organ donation after cardiac death.[39] There has been a subsequent order-of-magnitude increase of donation after cardiac death.

Regulations from the Centers for Medicare and Medicaid Services require hospitals to notify the local Organ Procurement Organization (OPO) of individuals whose death is imminent or who have died in the hospital. One way to achieve this threshold is to establish specific triggers for notification of the local OPO. All health care providers are trained to recognize these triggers and initiate contact with the OPO; this does not require physician or family consent or notification. Examples of such clinical triggers include:

- Any discussion of withdrawal of life-sustaining therapies by the physician or family
- Glasgow Coma Score of less than or equal to 4
- Patients with a neurologic insult
- Absence of 2 or more cranial nerve reflexes
- First indication of brain death or brain death testing
- Cardiac death

Regulations from the Centers for Medicare and Medicaid Services require that the person who initiates the request to the family is a representative of the OPO or a trained, designated requestor. Although it is theoretically possible for hospital clinicians to be trained as designated requestors, in practice this person is almost always an OPO representative.

The Uniform Anatomic Gift Act of 2006 legally bars others from revoking the consent of a donor after death who legally registered as a donor during his or her lifetime (without an indication that the consent was no longer valid). This rule has led to the increasing adoption of "first-person registries," whereby a patient registers his or her wishes via a driver's license or Web site. Although legally valid, many OPOs choose to obtain either assent or consent from next of kin as well. Occasional conflict arises when the wishes of the family are not congruent with the expressed wishes of the patient.

The Uniform Anatomic Gift Act also requires that the OPO determine whether all organs are suitable for transplantation, even if the patient had an advance directive in place stating that such treatment was not wanted. A 2007 amendment emphasizes that the attending physician should consult with the patient or surrogate as early as possible to determine and follow the patient's wishes, even if doing so results in the loss of potentially transplantable organs.[35]

SUMMARY

Much of what has been discussed revolves around communication. Communication is a crucial part of intensive care, yet it often falls short of expectations. Because of the nature of the illness requiring intensive care, much of the communication involves families without the benefit of patient interaction; many times, caregivers and family members have never met. Clear communication can be difficult when there is no prior relationship, the event requiring intensive care is unexpected, the outcome is unknown, and there is little information to guide prognostication. Scheduled, time-based meetings are an effective strategy to improve communication about all aspects of care, and increase the likelihood for successful discussions about goal-directed care. Clear, thorough documentation of these meetings is a critical part of this communication to allow all health care providers to understand these important discussions. Family-centered care is an extension of patient-centered care, because the family will likely be the primary support system when the patient survives a critical illness. Should the patient not survive, enhanced communication with family through scheduled meetings and FPDR lessens the risk of complicated grief.

REFERENCES

1. Institute of Medicine. Crossing the quality chasm: a new health system for the 21st century. Washington, DC: National Academy Press; 2001.
2. Barr J, Ghandi R, Hirsch G, et al. Clinical practice guidelines for support of the family in the patient-centered intensive care unit: American College of Critical Care Medicine Task Force 2004-2005. Crit Care Med 2007;35:605–22.
3. Azoulay E, Chevret S, Leleu G, et al. Half the families of intensive care unit patients experience inadequate communication with physicians. Crit Care Med 2000;28:3044–9.
4. Azoulay É, Pouchard F. Communication with family members of patients dying in the intensive care unit. Curr Opin Crit Care 2003;9:545–50.
5. The SUPPORT principal investigators: a controlled trial to improve care for seriously ill hospitalized patients: the study to understand prognoses and preferences for outcomes and risks of treatments (SUPPORT). JAMA 1995;274:1591–8.
6. Rubenfeld GD, Randall CJ. End-of-life in the intensive care unit: a research agenda. Crit Care Med 2001;29:2001–6.
7. The FAMIREA group. Symptoms of anxiety and depression in family members of intensive care unit patients: ethical hypothesis regarding decision-making capacity. Crit Care Med 2001;29:1893–7.

8. Lautrette A, Darmon M, Megarbane B, et al. A communication strategy and brochure for relatives of patients dying in the ICU. N Engl J Med 2007;356:469–78.
9. Roderick N. Creating an infrastructure for the productive sharing of clinical information. Top Health Inf Manage 2000;20:85–91.
10. Whitmer M, Hughes B, Hurst SM, et al. Innovative solutions: family conference progress note. Dimens Crit Care Nurs 2005;24:83–8.
11. Rodriguez RM, Navarette E, Schwaber J, et al. A prospective study of primary surrogate decision makers' knowledge of intensive care. Crit Care Med 2008; 36:1633–6.
12. Salmond SW, David E. Attitudes toward advance directives and advance directive completion rates. Orthop Nurs 2005;24:117–27.
13. Schwarze ML, Bradley CT, Brasel KJ. Surgical "buy-in": the contractual relationship between surgeons and patients that influences decisions regarding life-supporting therapy. Crit Care Med 2010;38:843–8.
14. Curtis JR, Patrick DL, Shannon SE, et al. The family conference as a focus to improve communication about end-of-life care in the intensive care unit: opportunities for improvement. Crit Care Med 2001;29(Suppl 2):N26–33.
15. Pochard F, Azoulay E, Chevret S, et al. Symptoms of anxiety and depression in family members of intensive care unit patients: ethical hypothesis regarding decision-making capacity. Crit Care Med 2001;29:1893–7.
16. Nelson JE, Mulkerin CM, Adams LL, et al. Improving comfort and communication in the ICU: a practical new tool for palliative care performance measurement and feedback. Qual Saf Health Care 2006;15:264–71.
17. Mosenthal AC, Murphy PA, Barker LK, et al. Changing the culture around end-of-life care in the trauma intensive care unit. J Trauma 2008;64:1587–93.
18. Kirk TW, Mahon MM, Palliative Sedation Task Force of the National Hospice and Palliative Care Organization Ethics Committee. National Hospice and Palliative Care Organization (NHPCO) position statement and commentary on the use of palliative sedation in imminently dying terminally ill patients. J Pain Symptom Manage 2010;39:914–23.
19. York NL. Implementing a family presence protocol option. Dimens Crit Care Nurs 2004;23:84–8.
20. Maclean SL, Guzzetta CE, White C, et al. Family presence during cardiopulmonary resuscitation and invasive procedures: practices of critical care and emergency nurses. J Emerg Nurs 2003;29:208–21.
21. Compton S, Madgy A, Goldstein M, et al. Emergency medical service providers' experience with family presence during cardiopulmonary resuscitation. Resuscitation 2006;70:223–8.
22. Halm MA. Family presence during resuscitation: a critical review of the literature. Am J Crit Care 2005;14:494–511.
23. Terzi AB, Aggelidou D. Witnessed resuscitation: beneficial or detrimental? J Cardiovasc Nurs 2008;23:74–8.
24. Meyers TA, Eichhorn DJ, Guzzetta CE, et al. Family presence during invasive procedures and resuscitation. Am J Nurs 2000;100:32–42.
25. Robinson SM, Mackenzie-Ross S, Campbell Hewson GL, et al. Psychological effect of witnessed resuscitation on bereaved relatives. Lancet 1998;352:614–7.
26. Knott A, Kee CC. Nurses' beliefs about family presence during resuscitation. Appl Nurs Res 2005;18:192–8.
27. Mian P, Warchal S, Whitney S, et al. Impact of a multifaceted intervention on nurses' and physicians' attitudes and behaviors toward family presence during resuscitation. Crit Care Nurse 2007;27:52–61.

28. Tucker TL. Family presence during resuscitation. Crit Care Nurs Clin North Am 2002;14:177–85.
29. Eichhorn DJ, Meyers TA, Mitchell TG, et al. Opening the doors: family presence during resuscitation. J Cardiovasc Nurs 1996;10:59–70.
30. Kirchhoff C, Stegmaier J, Buhmann S, et al. Trauma surgeons' attitude towards family presence during trauma resuscitation: a nationwide survey. Resuscitation 2007;75:267–75.
31. Rosenczweig C. Should relatives witness resuscitation? ethical issues and practical considerations. CMAJ 1998;158:617–20.
32. Duran CR, Oman KS, Abel JJ, et al. Attitudes toward and beliefs about family presence: a survey of healthcare providers, patients' families, and patients. Am J Crit Care 2007;16:270–82.
33. Belanger MA, Reed S. A rural community hospital's experience with family-witnessed resuscitation. J Emerg Nurs 1997;23:238–9.
34. Mangurten J, Scott SH, Guzzetta CE, et al. Effects of family presence during resuscitation and invasive procedures in a pediatric emergency department. J Emerg Nurs 2006;32:225–33.
35. US Department of Health and Human Services. Donate: give the gift of life. Available at: www.organdonor.gov. Accessed April 1, 2012.
36. Doyle CJ, Post H, Burney RE, et al. Family participation during resuscitation: an option. Ann Emerg Med 1987;16:673–5.
37. Greer DM, Varelas PN, Haque S, et al. Variability of brain death determination guidelines in leading US neurologic institutions. Neurology 2008;70:284–9.
38. Wijdicks EF, Varelas PN, Gronseth GS, et al. Evidence-based guideline update: determining brain death in adults. Report of the quality standards subcommittee of the American Academy of Neurology. Neurology 2010;74:1911–8.
39. Steinbrook R. Organ donation after cardiac death. N Engl J Med 2007;357:209–13.

A Case Study of a Multiply Injured Patient

Jennifer Roberts, MD, John A. Weigelt, MD, DVM, MMA*

KEYWORDS

- Multiples injuries • Evaluation • Pain control • Management • Case studies

KEY POINTS

- The initial evaluation of severely injured patients requires an organized, rapid, and thorough evaluation of the patient where life-threatening injuries are identified and treated simultaneously.
- Epidural analgesia is the preferred technique for pain control in adults with severe chest wall injury unless contraindicated. Early use of rib blocks for all rib fractures is another technique to control pain until an epidural catheter can be placed.
- Improving tissue perfusion and correction of acidosis in a trauma patient with hemorrhagic shock is achieved via volume restoration initially with balanced salt solutions and blood as necessary.
- In the hemodynamically normal patient, nonoperative management of splenic injury is successful 90% to 95% of the time. This strategy should be the initial treatment modality of choice, irrespective of the degree of injury.
- All critically injured patients with associated risk factors should receive some form of stress ulcer chemical prophylaxis. There is no difference in efficacy between histamine 2 blockers, proton pump inhibitor, or mucosal protectant agents.
- The multiply injured trauma patient is at high risk for venous thromboembolism. Prophylaxis requires chemical and mechanical methods that should be started as soon as possible after admission. When a brain injury is present but stable based on computed tomography, chemical prophylaxis is safe.

Mr. T is a 50-year-old man who was the unrestrained driver in a motor vehicle crash. He was traveling approximately 65 mph when he lost control, drifted into a ditch, and struck a tree head on. The vehicle had sustained significant intrusion damage into the driver's compartment, with a fractured windshield and airbag deployment. Mr. T was found unconscious in the field several meters from the vehicle with labored breathing and an obvious lower extremity deformity. His initial vital signs included a heart rate of

Department of Surgery, Division of Trauma and Surgical Critical Care, Medical College of Wisconsin, 9200 West Wisconsin Avenue, Milwaukee, WI 53226, USA
* Corresponding author.
E-mail address: jweigelt@mcw.edu

Surg Clin N Am 92 (2012) 1649–1660
http://dx.doi.org/10.1016/j.suc.2012.08.016
0039-6109/12/$ – see front matter © 2012 Published by Elsevier Inc.

137 bpm, blood pressure of 98/62 mm Hg, a respiratory rate of 40 breaths per minute with oxygen saturations at 96%. He arrives to your trauma bay in full spine precautions, a semi-rigid C-collar, a 20-gauge IV in his left hand with 500 mL of 0.9 normal saline hanging, and oxygen via face mask at 10 L/min.

The initial evaluation of severely injured patients requires an organized, rapid, and thorough evaluation of the patient where life-threatening injuries are identified and treated simultaneously.

THE ABCDEs OF TRAUMA EVALUATION

The American College of Surgeons Committee on Trauma devised a systematic approach that recognizes that life threatening injuries must be identified and treated before definitive workup. This approach is outlined in the Advanced Trauma and Life Support course, and has become the gold standard for the evaluation of the injured patient.[1] Principles from the Advanced Trauma and Life Support course emphasize that initial management must focus on 5 initial assessments:

1. Airway maintenance with cervical spine protection;
2. Breathing and ventilation;
3. Circulation with hemorrhage control;
4. Disability and neurologic status; and
5. Exposure/environment: Completely undress the patient and prevent hypothermia.

Our patient is breathing 40 times a minute. The question is whether the patient has an airway or breathing problem. Getting the patient to speak is a quick way to ascertain if his airway is adequate or not. Our patient can speak, although is short of breath. On further inspection he is not expanding his left hemothorax and a clinical diagnosis is made of a left pneumothorax or hemothorax.

This is a decision point regarding interventions. If the patient is normotensive and not hypoxic, a chest x-ray can confirm the clinical suspicion. Alternatively, if blood pressure or oxygenation is abnormal, then immediate placement of the chest tube is appropriate. Based on this patient's pulse, blood pressure, and falling oxygen saturation, a decision is made to place a left chest tube.

A chest tube is placed in a posterior lateral position and 500 mL of blood returns. A chest x-ray is obtained, which shows the chest tube to be in good position and the lung expanded. It also demonstrates multiple left-sided rib fractures. The patient is noted to have a flail chest on the left and his oxygen saturation is only 90%. Flail chest is defined as segmental fractures of 3 or more adjacent ribs resulting in an unstable segment of chest wall that moves paradoxically during respiration. Another decision now is whether intubation is required or not. Current protocols employ selective intubation along with adequate pain control for most patients with a flail chest.

Management of Rib Fractures and Flail Chest

Chest wall injuries vary significantly in terms of injury severity. Rib fractures represent high-energy trauma to the chest wall and increasing numbers of rib fractures are associated with increasing pulmonary morbidity and mortality. Flail chest is associated with mortality rates between 10% and 20%. Flail chest occurs when at least 3 contiguous ribs are fractured in multiple segments. Paradoxic movement of the chest wall occurs as the patient generates negative intrapleural pressure during inspiration. Although flail chest increases the work of breathing, the greatest source of ventilatory dysfunction occurs from the underlying pulmonary contusion.[2,3] Contused segments of lung have decreased compliance, increased pulmonary vascular resistance, and increased capillary leak resulting in hypoxia from ventilation-perfusion mismatch.[4] As a result, current treatment strategies are aimed at reducing pain secondary to the rib fractures, which should allow improved ventilation and oxygenation.

Principles of pain management

Immobility of the chest wall as a result of patient splinting is thought to be a major contributor to hypoventilation, atelectasis, pneumonia, and ventilatory failure after severe injury.[5] The mainstay of pain control in trauma patients has been parental narcotics. A patient-controlled analgesia regimen with a fast-acting opioid is an appropriate starting point. Nonsteroidal anti-inflammatory drugs, such as ketorolac and muscle relaxants, are also effective adjuncts for patients with mild to moderate injuries. The doses of pain control agents, particularly opioids, vary among individuals depending on prior narcotic use, injury severity, and patient's perception of pain. As a result, optimal pain control requires careful monitoring and titration according to individual patient response. Intercostal nerve block using a combination local anesthetic with or without epinephrine involves the administration of 2 to 3 mL of solution into the inferior margin of the rib is also an employed for pain control. A benefit of rib blocks is that they can be given early in the patient's course and require no special administration techniques. A drawback of rib blocks is that pain control is short limited, lasting up to only 6 hours, and only technically feasible for mid to lower rib fractures.

For patients with severe chest wall injuries ($\leq$4 rib fractures), epidural analgesia (EA) demonstrates promising results for pain control and decreased morbidity and mortality from respiratory complications. The Eastern Association for the Surgery of Trauma has stated that EA is the optimal modality of pain relief for severe, blunt, thoracic trauma. They recommend that all patients over the age of 65 be provided EA unless contraindicated and that younger patients with severe blunt chest injury should also be considered for EA.[6] EA can be administered at the thoracic or lumbar level and analgesic agents are delivered via a bolus, continuous infusion, or a patient-controlled demand system. EA has been shown to increase functional residual capacity and vital capacity, and decrease chest wall paradox in flail segments.[6–8] Perhaps the biggest advantage of EA is the ability to accomplish this without the sedative effects of parental narcotics, allowing patients to participate with pulmonary toilet.[6,9]

EA is the preferred technique for pain control in adults with severe chest wall injury unless contraindicated. Early use of rib blocks for all rib fractures is another technique to control pain until an epidural catheter can be placed. Further evaluation of Mr. T shows him to be alert, yet confused and anxious. He has weak and thready pulses in his upper extremities and lower extremities bilaterally and an open femur fracture. His skin is pale and cool to the touch and his vital signs now read: pulse, 138 bpm; blood pressure, 88/68 mm Hg; respiratory rate, 34 breaths per minute; and oxygen saturation, 99% via facemask. Although his oxygenation problems have been solved, he remains hypotensive with a tachycardia. A diagnosis of hypovolemic shock is most likely.

Treatment of this patient's shock begins with placement of 2 large-bore IVs and infusion of crystalloid. An infusion of 2 L of a balanced salt solution, such as lactated Ringers, is an appropriate starting point. If he continues to show signs of poor tissue perfusion or shock, blood is indicated. Any external blood loss should be controlled at this time. His femur fracture is an obvious source of blood loss and, unless external bleeding is obvious, placing the injured leg in a traction splint prevents further blood loss and relieves pain associated with any patient movement during the rest of the evaluation. Pulse assessment before and after splint application is necessary. Open fractures should be covered with a sterile wet dressing and antibiotics should be given. Early fracture fixation improves patient outcomes.

Improving tissue perfusion and correction of acidosis in a trauma patient with hemorrhagic shock is achieved via volume restoration, initially with balanced salt solutions and blood as necessary. Vasopressors, steroids, and sodium bicarbonate are not indicated in the initial resuscitation.[10]

After infusion of 2 L of lactated Ringers solution and 2 U of packed red blood cells (PRBCs), the patients pulse slows to 106 bpm and his blood pressure improves to 110/72 mm Hg. He remains confused, but seems calmer and is able to cooperate with the remainder of the examination. The pulse in his left lower extremity remains palpable after gentle reduction of his femur fracture as preparations are made for a hare traction splint.

Mr. T opens his eyes to speech, localizes to pain, and is confused when answering questions about his crash. Papillary examination reveals 3-mm, symmetric, and reactive pupils bilaterally. A Glasgow Coma Scale (GCS) score is calculated at 12, which indicates a moderate head injury. Exposure does not reveal any further external injuries.

Because the patient is now hemodynamically normal with adequate oxygenation. A complete history and physical is completed without any new findings. A decision regarding imaging studies is needed.

Imaging

Hemodynamically abnormal patients should not be sent for computed tomography (CT) because of the chance that their clinical condition can rapidly deteriorate despite adequate monitoring. Focused Assessment Sonography in Trauma (FAST) and diagnostic peritoneal lavage are important adjuncts used to identify sources of blood loss in hemodynamically abnormal patients and are not discussed further here. Before determining necessary diagnostic studies, it is important to categorize all injuries requiring further evaluation. Our patient's depressed level of consciousness and possible skull fracture warrant evaluation with a noncontrast head CT.[11] Alert and awake patients without neurologic or distracting injuries who have no neck pain or tenderness on active range of motion can have their C-collars cleared without the need for cervical spine imagine. Because of this patient's distracting injuries (GCS 12, femur fracture) a noncontrast cervical spine CT is the screening test of choice. Cervical collars should be removed as soon as possible; this can be safely done after a normal helical cervical CT. Patients with persistent posterior neck pain can be further evaluated with flexion/extension films or magnetic resonance imaging based on physician judgment.[12,13] A thoracic CT scan is appropriate given his sudden deceleration mechanism and lack of a seatbelt use; there is a 2% chance that he may have a missed great vessel injury despite a normal appearing mediastinum on chest x-ray.[14,15] Finally, Mr. T's initial presentation in hypovolemic shock, presence of left upper quadrant abdominal tenderness, and potential need for operative intervention for a lower extremity fracture support the need for abdominal CT.[16] Our patient also requires imaging of his left wrist, femur, knee, and ankle.

CT of the head, cervical spine, chest, abdomen, and pelvis demonstrate a subdural hematoma without evidence of midline shift, 8 left-sided rib fractures associated with a flail segment, and a pulmonary contusion. The left chest tube is in correct position, with resolution of pneumothorax and minimal residual left pleural blood. Last, a grade III splenic laceration and a comminuted midshaft fracture of the left femur are identified.

Management of his various injuries requires a number of critical care skills to be used. Each injury is discussed separately.

Management of Closed Head Injuries

Motor vehicle collisions account for 25% of annual hospitalizations and 34% of annual deaths from traumatic brain injury (TBI). The most common mass lesion identified in these crashes is a subdural hematoma, occurring in 20% to 40% of severely head injured patients. This injury results from sheering of the bridging veins that course between the brain parenchyma to the dural layers. Major morbidity comes from the mass effect of the lesion on the brain as well as the associated cerebral contusion beneath the subdural. However, secondary injury is a major source of both morbidity and mortality, and as such the mainstay of treatment is directed at preventing secondary damage. It is well-established that hypoxia and ischemia are the responsible mechanisms for secondary brain injury. Prospective data collected in the National Trauma Brain Injury data bank demonstrate that mortality is doubled in patients who have a single episode of systolic blood pressure below 90 mm Hg and when combined with oxygen saturations below 90%, have poorer neurologic outcomes.[17–19]

Our patient requires intensive care unit (ICU) admission without invasive intracranial pressure (ICP) monitoring. Current recommendations for ICP monitoring include a severe brain injury defined as a GCS of 8 or lower and evidence of hematomas, swelling, herniation, or compression of the basal cisterns on axial imaging. Optimization of hemoglobin and hematocrit is important for adequate oxygen delivery. However, increased red cell volume results in greater blood viscosity and potentially decreased microvascular cerebral blood flow. The point at which the benefits of hemodilution outweigh reduced oxygen-carrying capacity is unknown. This is supported by Salim et al,[20] who performed a retrospective review of 1,150 patients with TBI after blunt injury. Authors found that anemic patients who were transfused had higher mortality rates (odds ratio [OR], 2.19) and more complications (OR, 3.67) than anemic patients who were not transfused.[20] Current recommendations indicate traditional goals of a hematocrit of 30% and a hemoglobin of 10 mg/dL are likely optimal. In the index patient, one can reasonably expect 2 U of blood loss each from the splenic laceration, femur fracture, and rib fractures. Having only received 2 U PRBCs thus far makes close hemodynamic monitoring and a need for future transfusion likely. Correction of coagulopathy with fresh frozen plasma should also coincide with PRBC administration.

Hypertonic saline and mannitol

Hyperosmolar therapy works to reduce ICP by 2 mechanisms. First, both therapies create an osmolar gradient that causes water to flow from cells within the brain into the systemic circulation. Second, rapid plasma expansion reduces whole blood viscosity, which in turn results in improved cerebral blood flow.[17] Hypertonic saline comes in varying concentrations from 3% to 23.4%, and there is no consensus on a standard concentration that should be used for treatment of increased ICP.[17,21] Regardless of the solution used, resuscitating hypovolemia to a normal blood pressure and serum sodium concentration between 155 and 160 mEq/L is appropriate. Mannitol is effective at reducing ICP; however, there is sufficient evidence that administration exacerbates hypotension in an under-resuscitated patient. It is therefore contraindicated in this patient.

Management of Solid Organ Injury

In the past, most traumatic splenic injuries were treated with celiotomy and splenectomy regardless of the degree of injury based on the fear of mortality from exsanguination. Originally attempted in children, nonoperative management (NOM) of splenic injury has become more common in adults and is now the treatment of choice in hemodynamically normal patients.

Several grading systems exist describing splenic injury. Most commonly referenced is the American Association for the Surgery of Trauma scale. Ranging from 0 to 5, this scale uses a CT and intraoperative appearance of splenic injury based on degree of hematoma or laceration and proximity to the splenic hilum. Concern that more severe injuries (grades III–V) are not amendable to NOM has been largely disproved. Multiple retrospective and more recently prospective, noncomparative studies have shown that injury grade, and degree of hemoperitoneum is not predictive of NOM failure.[22,23] NOM is also possible in the presence of multisystem injuries, including those with neurologic impairment; NOM is safe and effective in pediatric and adult populations.[24,25] The presence of a blush on CT scan indicates ongoing bleeding and is associated with an increased need for operative intervention. Depending on institutional capability, this scenario may represent an area where angiography and embolization may improve NOM success.[26,27]

In the hemodynamically normal patient, NOM of splenic injury is successful 90% to 95% of the time. This strategy should be the initial treatment modality of choice, irrespective of the degree of injury.[26,27]

Serial hematocrits, re-imaging, and activity restrictions

Patients undergoing NOM of grade III or higher splenic injuries likely require observation in an ICU setting. A common practice of measuring serial hematocrits and setting a "cutoff" value that triggers either transfusion or operation is not supported in the literature. Careful hemodynamic monitoring, serial physical examinations, and assessment of endpoints of resuscitation (urine output, base deficit) is likely more effective than relying on any 1 laboratory value in determining need for operation. The presence of hypotension despite adequate resuscitation represents a situation in which celiotomy and splenectomy is appropriate. After successful NOM, follow-up CT is controversial and findings rarely alter management. Potential indications for repeat CT include persistent symptoms 1 week after injury or rare instances when a patient may want to resume contact sports or other high-risk activities.[28,29] Limited evidence exists on the amount of time required for an injured spleen to recover its normal integrity. Bed rest for longer than 24 hours is not associated with decreased rates of delayed splenic rupture and may be detrimental in terms of the risks of thromboembolic complications and immobility. Best evidence supports avoidance of contact sports or activities that involve contact to the torso for at least 2 to 3 months.

Ventilatory Support

All patients with major blunt chest trauma have some degree of respiratory dysfunction. The use of noninvasive methods of assistance, such as continuous positive airway pressure has been shown to decrease mechanical ventilation rates, infectious complications such as nosocomial pneumonia, and overall mortality. As a result, such methods may now be used as a means to avoid mechanical ventilation. When supplemental oxygen, aggressive pulmonary toilet, and noninvasive means of support fail to provide adequate assistance, mechanical ventilation is necessary. Historically, all patients with an unstable chest wall were treated with mechanical ventilation for "internal support" of the flail segment until the chest wall demonstrated evidence of healing. In the 1980s, this concept was challenged. Shackford et al[30] found that survival was worse in the obligatory mechanical ventilation group owing to complications from mechanical ventilation. They concluded that mechanical ventilation should be used to correct abnormalities of gas exchange rather than to treat chest wall instability. Overall use of mechanical ventilation decreased from 74% to 38% and mortality decreased from 14% to 8%.

Once the decision to use mechanical ventilation is made, there are no modes of ventilation that are superior to others. In general, volume-controlled modes, such as synchronized intermittent mechanical ventilation, with traditional tidal volumes of 10 to 12 mL/kg are appropriate starting points. Severe pulmonary contusion can result in noncompliant lungs and ventilator-induced lung injury. In these instances, low tidal volume ventilation (6 mL/kg) reduces iatrogenic injury and improve mortality.[31,32] The use of positive end-expiratory pressure in acute respiratory distress syndrome serves to improve oxygenation by increasing functional residual capacity and is a useful adjunct for patients with progressive hypoxemia on traditional ventilation. In severe hypoxia, reverse ratio ventilation (I/E ratio) may improve oxygenation by increasing the time spent in inhalation, recruiting alveoli, and decreasing intrapulmonary shunting. A known side effect of reverse ratio ventilation is hypercarbia, which results from insufficient expiratory times. The resulting respiratory acidosis is generally accepted until an arterial pH of 7.25, where a buffer can be added to prevent worsening acid–base status.

Stress Ulcer Prophylaxis

Pathogenesis of stress ulceration and indications for treatment

Stress ulcers are superficial erosions in the gastric mucosa that are common to patients with acute, life-threatening injuries. Unlike the majority of peptic ulcers, the pathophysiology behind the development of stress ulceration is not related to acid hypersecretion or *Helicobacter pylori* infection. Systemic hypotension resulting in catecholamine release and inflammatory cytokines results in splanchnic vasoconstriction and resulting hypoperfusion of the gastrointestinal tract. Consequently, stress ulcerations result from impaired blood flow, not decreased gastric pH. Our patient has a moderate head injury requiring ICU observation along with multisystem trauma, and as such requires prophylaxis. The initiation of prophylaxis should commence at the onset of risk factors, typically admission to the ICU. Duration of prophylaxis is somewhat controversial. Studies evaluating at least 7 days of prophylaxis have not demonstrated a difference in gastrointestinal bleeding rates or mortality. Most studies now recommend discontinuation of stress ulcer prophylaxis after discharge from the ICU setting.[33] Our approach is usually to stop the stress ulcer prophylaxis once feeding is started.

Pharmacologic approach to prophylaxis

Once the decision to start prophylaxis is made, the clinician must choose between proton pump inhibitors, histamine-2 blockers, and mucosal protection agents. There are multiple meta-analyses and randomized, controlled trials comparing pharmaceutical regimens for the prevention of stress ulceration. All agents are effective relative to no prophylaxis in the prevention of clinically significant mucosal ulceration. There is no consensus that a single agent is more effective than another with similar rates of side effects, such as the development of nosocomial pneumonia.[34–36] Histamine-2 antagonists and proton pump inhibitors can be given orally or intravenously with a goal of maintaining the gastric pH to greater than 4. Sucralfate is an aluminum salt of sucrose that works by maintaining the structural integrity of gastric mucosa. For maximum efficacy, 5 to 10 mL must be administered orally or via nasogastric tube every 4 to 6 hours. A potential drawback to the use of sucralfate is that it binds and blocks absorption of many common drugs used in an ICU setting. Also, sucralfate should not be used in patients with renal failure, owing to accumulation of aluminum.

All critically injured patients with associated risk factors should receive some form of stress ulcer chemical prophylaxis. There is no difference in efficacy between histamine-2 blockers, proton pump inhibitors, or mucosal protectant agents.

Venous Thromboembolism

Scope of the problem and associated risk factors

The trauma patient population is at highest risk for developing venous thromboembolic (VTE) complications. Without prophylaxis, up to 60% of trauma patients will develop a deep vein thrombosis. With prophylaxis, the risk of symptomatic VTE ranges from 1% to 7.6%.[37–39] In fact, pulmonary embolism is the third most common cause of death in trauma patients who survive beyond hospital day 3.[40] Major trauma often precipitates Virchow's triad: Hypercoagulability, stasis, and endothelial injury. Long bone fractures, pelvic fractures, head injury, prolonged immobilization, and spinal cord injury are the most commonly identified risk factors.[37–39,41]

Methods of prophylaxis

There are multiple mechanical and chemical modalities available for the prevention of VTE. In the general trauma patient population, chemical prophylaxis with low-dose unfractionated heparin or low molecular weight heparin in conjunction with mechanical prophylaxis is started on admission to the hospital or as soon as bleeding risk is acceptable.[39] Mechanical methods of prophylaxis including sequential compression devices or intermittent pneumatic compression devices are effective relative to no prophylaxis or if chemical methods are contraindicated. However, best practice is to use them in conjunction with chemical prophylaxis when not contraindicated by the presence of a lower extremity injury.

The index case presents an additional consideration in the timing of chemical prophylaxis: Intracranial bleeding. Evidence suggests that among patients with TBI, symptomatic VTE rates may be as high as 15% if prophylaxis is delayed longer than 48 hours.[39,42,43] Unfortunately, few studies have examined bleeding risk associated with thromboprophylaxis in the presence of a brain injury. In a prospective study of 525 brain-injured patients who received prophylaxis within 48 hours of admission, 18 had progressive hemorrhagic changes on head CT, resulting in 6 in whom there was a change in management.[44] These findings were echoed in a similar retrospective study in which 402 patients received chemical prophylaxis 24 hours after repeat head CT imaging and did not show evidence of progression of intracranial bleeding. A nonsignificant 11 of 402 patients demonstrated progression of their head bleed versus 26 of 410 patients who did not receive prophylaxis.[45] The conclusion was that VTE prophylaxis can be safely started in this population after 24 hours if CT of the brain shows no further bleeding. This clearly represents an area where further prospective research regarding all modalities of VTE prophylaxis is warranted. Our approach uses these data in a multidisciplinary approach with neurosurgical consultation in determining optimal timing of VTE prophylaxis in TBI patients.

The multiply injured trauma patient is at high risk for VTE. Prophylaxis requires chemical and mechanical methods that should be started as soon as possible after admission. When a brain injury is present but stable based on CT scanning, chemical prophylaxis is safe.

Chest Tube Management

Pneumothorax or hemothorax after an injury is sufficiently managed by chest tube drainage in 85% of patients. Most chest tubes are removed within 3 to 7 days. Prolonged drainage or re-accumulation of blood in the pleural space is an indication for further drainage. Many approaches are used to resolve this retained hemothorax. A recent study compared many different methods and concluded no method is best, but video-assisted thoracoscopic surgery is commonly used with good success. No timing was identified as best either, but it is usually done within 7 days of injury.[46] CT is done preoperatively to help guide this minimal invasive technique.

Early Rehabilitation Assessment

As the patient recovers in the hospital, early referral to a physician specializing in physical medicine and rehabilitation is important. Acute rehabilitation centers provide up to 5 hours of coordinated therapy whereby injured patients work on mobility, speech, activities of daily living, and vocational training with the ultimate goal of returning to work as a productive member of the community. The rehabilitation team commonly consists of occupational, physical, and speech therapists; psychologists; orthotists; rehabilitation nurses; and social workers and case managers. The coordination of care is lead by a physiatrist who determines a patient's disability and then prescribes the appropriate treatments. For patients who do not progress during their hospitalization, or for those with limited functional reserve who cannot participate in intensive inpatient rehabilitation, subacute rehabilitation centers may be useful. These centers offer less rigorous therapies, generally for up to 2 hours each day. For patients with decreased endurance, multiple serious medical comorbidities and deconditioning, nursing homes with limited therapies may be the appropriate option for recovery until the patient can participate in more demanding therapy. Case managers and social workers should be involved early in a patient's hospitalization to optimize resources, and help with financial issues commonly affecting placement decisions.

The majority of multisystem injured patients return to work after injury rehabilitation; however, up to 80% have some level of impairment. For patients with a prolonged stay in the ICU, only 40% return to their former employment and 23% retire or require prolonged sick leave.[47,48] Interestingly, injury severity is a poor predictor of return to work. The presence of specific injuries including, TBI, spinal cord, and multiple extremity fractures, are more predictive of functional outcome after trauma.[49]

SUMMARY

Traumatic injury remains a significant cause of morbidity and mortality for patients worldwide. The initial assessment and management is a sequential process in which all life-threatening injuries are identified and treated systematically. For patients who present in hemorrhagic shock, improving tissue perfusion and correction of acidosis is essential and is achieved via volume restoration with balanced salt solutions and blood as necessary. Once the initial resuscitation is complete, careful categorization of each injury and management pitfalls anticipated when treating them is crucial to providing optimal patient care. Commonly, in a polytrauma situation, 1 injured system directly affects the physiology of another. The prevention of hypotension and hypoxia are critical for best outcomes in patients with TBI. Selective intubation, early pain control, and aggressive pulmonary toilet in patients with severe chest trauma are important management techniques. NOM of blunt solid organ injuries is now the standard of care and should be considered in all patients who respond to initial resuscitative efforts. The prevention of common complications, such as VTE and stress ulceration of the gastrointestinal track, should not be overlooked. The final step to recovery is early involvement of a case manager to evaluate the patient's support system and a rehabilitation specialist. The ultimate goal in rehabilitation of a multiply injured patient is to return each patient to as much independent function and ability to contribute to society as possible.

REFERENCES

1. American College of Surgeons. Advanced trauma and life support. Chicago: Author; 2008.
2. Cappello M, Legrand A, De Troyer A. Determinants of rib motion in flail chest. Am J Respir Crit Care Med 1999;159(3):886–91.
3. Craven KD, Oppenheimer L, Wood LD. Effects of contusion and flail chest on pulmonary perfusion and oxygen exchange. J Appl Physiol 1979;47(4):729–37.
4. Pulmonary contusion and flail chest management: practice management guideline. Boston: ARDSNet Publications | NHLBI ARDS Network; 2012.
5. Desai PM. Pain management and pulmonary dysfunction. Crit Care Clin 1999; 15(1):151–66.
6. Simon BJ, Cushman J, Barraco R, et al. Pain management guidelines for blunt thoracic trauma. J Trauma 2005;59(5):1256–67.
7. Mackersie RC, Karagianes TG, Hoyt DB, et al. Prospective evaluation of epidural and intravenous administration of fentanyl for pain control and restoration of ventilatory function following multiple rib fractures. J Trauma 1991;31(4):443–9.
8. Karmakar MK, Ho AM. Acute pain management of patients with multiple fractured ribs. J Trauma 2003;54(3):615–25.
9. Worthley LI. Thoracic epidural in the management of chest trauma. A study of 161 cases. Intensive Care Med 1985;11(6):312–5.
10. Kaufmann C. Initial assessment and management. In: Moore EJ, Feliciano DV, Mattox KL, editors. New York: McGraw-Hill; 2008. p. 169–80.
11. Mower WR, Hoffman JR, Herbert M, et al. Developing a decision instrument to guide computed tomographic imaging of blunt head injury patients. J Trauma 2005;59(4):954–9.
12. Como JJ, Diaz JJ, Dunham CM, et al. Practice management guidelines for identification of cervical spine injuries following trauma: update from the eastern association for the surgery of trauma practice management guidelines committee. J Trauma 2009;67(3):651–9.
13. Hoffman JR, Wolfson AB, Todd K, et al. Selective cervical spine radiography in blunt trauma: methodology of the National Emergency X-Radiography Utilization Study (NEXUS). Ann Emerg Med 1998;32(4):461–9.
14. Nagy K, Fabian T, Rodman G, et al. Guidelines for the diagnosis and management of blunt aortic injury: an EAST Practice Management Guidelines Work Group. J Trauma 2000;48(6):1128–43.
15. Blackmore CC, Zweibel A, Mann FA. Determining risk of traumatic aortic injury: how to optimize imaging strategy. AJR Am J Roentgenol 2000;174(2):343–7.
16. Stanescu L, Linnau K, Burdick T, et al. Diagnostic and interventional radiology. In: Moore EJ, Feliciano DV, Mattox KL, editors. New York: McGraw-Hill; 2008. p. 261–319.
17. The Brain Trauma Foundation; 2012. Available at: http://tbiguidelines.org/glHome.aspx?gl=1. Accessed 2012.
18. Chesnut RM, Marshall LF, Klauber MR, et al. The role of secondary brain injury in determining outcome from severe head injury. J Trauma 1993;34(2):216–22.
19. Marmarou A, Saad A, Aygok G, et al. Contribution of raised ICP and hypotension to CPP reduction in severe brain injury: correlation to outcome. Acta Neurochir Suppl 2005;95:277–80.
20. Salim A, Hadjizacharia P, DuBose J, et al. Role of anemia in traumatic brain injury. J Am Coll Surg 2008;207(3):398–406.
21. Doyle JA, Davis DP, Hoyt DB. The use of hypertonic saline in the treatment of traumatic brain injury. J Trauma 2001;50(2):367–83.

22. Kohn JS, Clark DE, Isler RJ, et al. Is computed tomographic grading of splenic injury useful in the nonsurgical management of blunt trauma? J Trauma 1994; 36(3):385–9.

23. Sartorelli KH, Frumiento C, Rogers FB, et al. Nonoperative management of hepatic, splenic, and renal injuries in adults with multiple injuries. J Trauma 2000;49(1):56–61.

24. Archer LP, Rogers FB, Shackford SR. Selective nonoperative management of liver and spleen injuries in neurologically impaired adult patients. Arch Surg 1996; 131(3):309–15.

25. Keller MS, Sartorelli KH, Vane DW. Associated head injury should not prevent nonoperative management of spleen or liver injury in children. J Trauma 1996; 41(3):471–5.

26. Schurr MJ, Fabian TC, Gavant M, et al. Management of blunt splenic trauma: computed tomographic contrast blush predicts failure of nonoperative management. J Trauma 1995;39(3):507–12.

27. Davis KA, Fabian TC, Croce MA, et al. Improved success in nonoperative management of blunt splenic injuries: embolization of splenic artery pseudoaneurysms. J Trauma 1998;44(6):1008–13.

28. Uecker J, Pickett C, Dunn E. The role of follow-up radiographic studies in nonoperative management of spleen trauma. Am Surg 2001;67(1):22–5.

29. Allins A, Ho T, Nguyen TH, et al. Limited value of routine followup CT scans in nonoperative management of blunt liver and splenic injuries. Am Surg 1996; 62(11):883–6.

30. Shackford SR, Virgilio RW, Peters RM. Selective use of ventilator therapy in flail chest injury. J Thorac Cardiovasc Surg 1981;81(2):194–201.

31. ARDSNet Publications | NHLBI ARDS Network; 2012. Available at: http://www. ardsnet.org/ardsnet_publications_public. Accessed 2012.

32. Petrucci N, Iacovelli W. Ventilation with lower tidal volumes versus traditional tidal volumes in adults for acute lung injury and acute respiratory distress syndrome. Cochrane Database Syst Rev 2003;(3):CD003844.

33. Martin LF, Booth FV, Reines HD, et al. Stress ulcers and organ failure in intubated patients in surgical intensive care units. Ann Surg 1992;215(4):332–7.

34. Lin PC, Chang CH, Hsu PI, et al. The efficacy and safety of proton pump inhibitors vs histamine-2 receptor antagonists for stress ulcer bleeding prophylaxis among critical care patients: a meta-analysis. Crit Care Med 2010;38(4): 1197–205.

35. Lasky MR, Metzler MH, Phillips JO. A prospective study of omeprazole suspension to prevent clinically significant gastrointestinal bleeding from stress ulcers in mechanically ventilated trauma patients. J Trauma Inj Infect Crit Care 1998;44(3): 527–33.

36. Cook DJ, Reeve BK, Guyatt GH, et al. Stress ulcer prophylaxis in critically ill patients. Resolving discordant meta-analyses. JAMA 1996;275(4):308–14.

37. Geerts W, Cook D, Selby R, et al. Venous thromboembolism and its prevention in critical care. J Crit Care 2002;17(2):95–104.

38. Knudson MM, Ikossi DG, Khaw L, et al. Thromboembolism after trauma: an analysis of 1602 episodes from the American College of Surgeons National Trauma Data Bank. Ann Surg 2004;240(3):490–6.

39. Gould MK, Garcia DA, Wren SM, et al. Prevention of VTE in nonorthopedic surgical patients: antithrombotic therapy and prevention of thrombosis, 9th ed: American College of Chest Physicians Evidence-Based Clinical Practice Guidelines. Chest 2012;141(Suppl 2):e227S–77S.

40. Geerts WH, Code KI, Jay RM, et al. A prospective study of venous thromboembolism after major trauma. N Engl J Med 1994;331(24):1601–6.
41. Dennis JW, Menawat S, Von Thron J, et al. Efficacy of deep venous thrombosis prophylaxis in trauma patients and identification of high-risk groups. J Trauma 1993;35(1):132–8.
42. Kim KS, Brophy GM. Symptomatic venous thromboembolism: incidence and risk factors in patients with spontaneous or traumatic intracranial hemorrhage. Neurocrit Care 2009;11(1):28–33.
43. Reiff DA, Haricharan RN, Bullington NM, et al. Traumatic brain injury is associated with the development of deep vein thrombosis independent of pharmacological prophylaxis. J Trauma 2009;66(5):1436–40.
44. Norwood SH, Berne JD, Rowe SA, et al. Early venous thromboembolism prophylaxis with enoxaparin in patients with blunt traumatic brain injury. J Trauma 2008; 65(5):1021–6.
45. Scudday T, Brasel K, Webb T, et al. Safety and efficacy of prophylactic anticoagulation in patients with traumatic brain injury. J Am Coll Surg 2011;213(1): 148–53.
46. DuBose J, Inaba K, Demetriades D, et al. Management of post-traumatic retained hemothorax: a prospective, observational, multicenter AAST study. J Trauma Acute Care Surg 2012;72(1):11–22.
47. Holbrook TL, Anderson JP, Sieber WJ, et al. Outcome after major trauma: 12-month and 18-month follow-up results from the Trauma Recovery Project. J Trauma 1999; 46(5):765–71.
48. Anke AG, Stanghelle JK, Finset A, et al. Long-term prevalence of impairments and disabilities after multiple trauma. J Trauma 1997;42(1):54–61.
49. MacKenzie EJ, Shapiro S, Smith RT, et al. Factors influencing return to work following hospitalization for traumatic injury. Am J Public Health 1987;77(3): 329–34.

A Case Study in Intra-abdominal Sepsis

Jasmeet S. Paul, MD[a],*, Timothy J. Ridolfi, MD[b]

KEYWORDS

- Intra-abdominal infections • Management • Diverticulitis • Reconstruction • Sepsis

KEY POINTS

- Intra-abdominal infections are a common problem for the general surgeon and can be a major source of morbidity and mortality in the intensive care unit if the patient presents with septic shock.
- The basic principles of care include prompt resuscitation, antibiotics, and source control.
- Principles of Damage Control Laparotomy can provide a framework for operative management of intra-abdominal infections.

Intra-abdominal infections (IAIs) are a common problem for the general surgeon and a major source of morbidity and mortality in the intensive care unit (ICU). Some of these patients present with peritonitis and can rapidly progress to septic shock and need prompt resuscitation, antibiotics, and source control. The management of these patients can be complex, requiring skill in ICU management, operative source control, damage control techniques, and reconstruction. This article will use a detailed case study to outline the management of a patient with severe IAI from diverticulitis with these issues in mind.

A 67-year-old woman presented to the emergency department after a fall at home. She reported several days of abdominal pain and diarrhea. On physical examination she was febrile to 103.7°F. Pulse rate was 110 beats per minute, and blood pressure was 74/40 mm Hg with a mean arterial pressure (MAP) of 51 mm Hg. The woman was diaphoretic and lethargic but able to give a history. Abdominal examination revealed tenderness and a palpable fullness in the left lower quadrant. Rectal examination was normal. Laboratory evaluation showed a white blood cell count of 21,300 with 90% neutrophils, hematocrit of 38%, creatinine of 2.5 mg/dL, lactate of 6 mmol/L, hypokalemia, and hypophosphatemia.

[a] Division of Trauma and Critical Care, Department of Surgery, Medical College of Wisconsin, 9200 West Wisconsin Avenue, Milwaukee, WI 53226, USA
[b] Department of Surgery, Medical College of Wisconsin, 9200 West Wisconsin Avenue, Milwaukee, WI 53226, USA
* Corresponding author.
E-mail address: jpaul@mcw.edu

Surg Clin N Am 92 (2012) 1661–1677
http://dx.doi.org/10.1016/j.suc.2012.08.014
0039-6109/12/$ – see front matter © 2012 Published by Elsevier Inc.

The patient was determined to be in septic shock, and goal-directed, protocol-driven resuscitation was initiated in the emergency department. A right subclavian central venous catheter was placed, and the central venous pressure (CVP) was 4 mm Hg. A 1000 cc bolus of Lactated Ringers (LR) solution was given, which increased MAP to 60 mm Hg and CVP to 6 mm Hg. A right radial artery catheter was placed, and a norepinephrine continuous infusion was initiated and titrated to a goal MAP of 65 mm Hg. The woman received another 1000 cc bolus of LR, which brought the CVP up to 9 mm Hg; LR was then continued at 150 cc/h infusion. An indwelling urinary catheter was placed to monitor urine output (UOP). During the resuscitation, she became progressively lethargic and was electively intubated. A venous blood gas was obtained, and the central venous oxygen saturation (ScvO2) was 74%. Two sets of blood cultures were drawn, and the woman received intravenous metronidazole and ciprofloxacin for presumed diverticulitis. She was then transferred to the surgical ICU (SICU) for further resuscitation.

INITIAL RESUSCITATION

Septic shock is defined as severe sepsis with hypotension that is minimally responsive to fluid administration.[1] The initial goals of management of this group of patients are resuscitation using early goal-directed therapy (EGDT), prompt antibiotic administration, and source control. The Surviving Sepsis Campaign (SSC) delineates the steps and protocols for the management of septic shock.[2]

EGDT was shown to decrease in-hospital mortality in a study by Rivers and colleagues.[3] Patients identified to be in either septic shock or having signs of severe sepsis were aggressively resuscitated via a protocol-driven treatment regimen for the first 6 hours after presentation to the emergency department. Goals of resuscitation were defined as CVP of 8 to 12 mm Hg, MAP greater than 65 mm Hg, UOP greater than 0.5 cc/kg/h, and ScvO2 greater than 70%. Patients progress through the protocol in a step-wise fashion (**Fig. 1**).

Patients in septic shock have a large fluid requirement to overcome the effects of vasodilation, ranging between 7 to 20 L within the first 72 hours.[3] The goal CVP is 8 mm Hg (12 mm Hg in ventilated patients), and fluid boluses should be used to reach and maintain this level of preload.[2] Two broad groups of fluids have been used for resuscitation, crystalloids and colloids. The most commonly used crystalloid solutions are LR solution and normal saline (NS) solution. Both are readily available and inexpensive. Caution should be used with large-volume administration of NS, as a hypercholremic metabolic acidosis can occur due to a large chloride load (154 mEq/L). LR contains less chloride but also contains 4 mEq/L of potassium, which may not be well tolerated in patients with renal failure. Although both of these fluids are isotonic, a significant volume will migrate into the extravascular space due to increased capillary permeability and changes in oncotic pressure.[4] Given the capillary leak, albumin is often used as a primary resuscitative fluid with the assumption that it will remain in the intravascular space.[5] There are numerous single-institution series and meta analyses comparing crystalloids and albumin for resuscitation that have had mixed results.[6,7] A large randomized–controlled trial was undertaken enrolling 7000 hypotensive patients admitted to the ICU, 1200 of whom had severe sepsis.[8] They were randomized to either NS or 4% albumin as the primary resuscitative fluid. Overall there was no difference in morbidity or mortality in either group. In the subset of patients with severe sepsis, the mortality rate was 30.7% versus 35.3%, which did not reach statistical significance. Although the conclusion of the authors was that both 4% albumin and NS were clinically equivalent treatments, many have suggested crystalloid be used due to its decreased cost.[5]

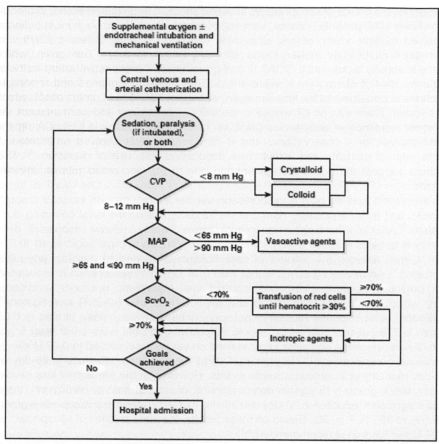

Fig. 1. Protocol for early goal-directed therapy. (*From* Rivers E, Nguyen B, Havstad S, et al. Early goal-directed therapy in the treatment of severe sepsis and septic shock. N Engl J Med 2001;345(19):1396; with permission.)

VASOPRESSORS

Persistent hypoperfusion can lead to end organ damage and death in patients suffering from septic shock. A MAP of greater than 65 mm Hg has been suggested as a target to maintain perfusion based on animal studies, but there is little experimental evidence for this goal in humans.[9] Patients with baseline comorbidities may in fact require a higher goal MAP, and standard measures of perfusion should be used to titrate the MAP to higher level. Adequate fluid resuscitation as measured by a CVP of 8 to 10 mm Hg should be achieved before the administration of vasopressors; however, patients in severe hypoperfusion states may require early administration of vasopressors. The SSC recommends either norepinephrine or dopamine be started as a first-line agent. Norepinephrine has mainly alpha-adrenergic agonist effects with some beta-adrenergic activity. Dopamine has dose-dependent effects, with moderate doses having a predominant beta-adrenergic activity and higher doses exhibiting potent alpha-adrenergic activity. However, this dose-dependent response is unreliable in critically ill patients.[10] Until recently, there had been no large-scale trial comparing the choice of vasopressors in septic shock. A large observational trial evaluated over 1000 patients in shock, with 462 in septic shock.[11] Although most patients received multiple vasopressors, dopamine use was an independent predictor of mortality in multivariate analysis (odds ratio [OR] 2.05 (1.25–3.37)). The sepsis occurrence in acutely Ill patients II (SOAP II) trial group study[12] prospectively studied 1679 patients, 1044 of whom were in septic shock. They were randomized to either norepinephrine or dopamine as the first-line agent with open-label use of other vasopressors as needed. There was no difference in mortality or secondary end points except for a higher incidence of arrhythmias (24% vs 12%) in the dopamine group. A recent meta-analysis of 4 observational and 6 randomized trials showed an increased odds ratio of mortality and arrhythmias associated with use of dopamine.[13] The authors suggest the use of norepinephrine due to the decreased rate of adverse events.

Vasopressin acts as both a vasopressor, via the V1 receptor on vascular smooth muscle, and as an antidiuretic hormone via V2 receptors on the renal collecting duct system.[14] After an initial surge in vasopressin levels, there is a relative vasopressin deficiency in patients in septic shock. Infusion of vasopressin at physiologic levels (0.01–0.04 U/min) reduces the amount of catecholamines needed to maintain adequate perfusion.[15] Administering doses higher than 0.04 U/min of vasopressin is associated with potentially deleterious vasoconstriction of renal, mesenteric, pulmonary, and coronary vasculature.[14] The vasopressin and septic shock trial (VASST) investigators[16] compared norepinephrine infusion to norepinephrine with vasopressin titrated to 0.03 U/min in 778 patients with septic shock. All patients enrolled were on at least 5 μg/min of norepinephrine and were either started on vasopressin titrated to 0.03 U/min or additional norepinephrine (5–15 μg/min). Overall there was no difference in 28-day or 90-day mortality or in serious adverse events. However, in the predefined less severe septic shock group (>15 μg/min norepinephrine infusion at time of enrollment), there was a significant reduction in 28-day and 90-day mortality rates in the vasopressin group (26.5% vs 35.7% $P = .05$). Based on these results, the early addition of vasopressin at 0.04 U/min infusion is recommended.[5,17]

END POINTS OF RESUSCITATION AND MONITORING

The goal of therapy is to maintain adequate end organ perfusion and function. As there are few direct measures of perfusion, the effectiveness of fluid resuscitation and vasopressor use is measured by end points of resuscitation. Although there is controversy regarding their validity, the most commonly used end points are MAP, CVP, UOP, ScvO2, serum lactate clearance, and correction of a base deficit.[18]

Although varying targets of MAP have not been directly studied in septic shock, levels of greater than 65 mm Hg are thought to preserve tissue perfusion.[9,19] Patients with underlying comorbidites will likely require a higher MAP to maintain autoregulation and tissue perfusion. CVP is used as a surrogate for preload with a goal pressure of 8 to 12 mm Hg.[2,3] However, the validity of CVP is often called into question as it is affected by numerous factors.[20] According to the Surviving Sepsis Guidelines CVP of 8 mm Hg indicates adequate preload; however, in practice, patients with a lower CVP may actually be volume overloaded. A practical approach to a hypotensive patient with low CVP is to administer a fluid challenge and monitor change in CVP and MAP. If there is no concomitant rise in both values, further volume resuscitation may be harmful to the patient.

Given the potential unreliability of the CVP measurement, pulse pressure variation may predict those patients who are potentially fluid responsive.[21] Briefly, a calculation is performed using the maximal pulse pressure during inspiration and the minimal pulse pressure measured in expiration. A percentage difference of 13% is suggestive of patients who would be responsive to fluid.[22] There are commercially available devices that will measure pulse pressure variation as well as determine stroke volume and cardiac output from an arterial catheter.[23] A full discussion of pulse pressure variation and these devices is beyond the scope of this article.

Lactic acidemia is associated with hypoperfusion and may be a prognositic marker in patients in septic shock.[18] A single lactate level is likely of low clinical utility; however, the clearance of serum lactate levels over time can predict mortality in patients with severe sepsis. Serial lactate levels are drawn, and then lactate clearance is calculated by the equation $[(\text{lactate}_{initial} - \text{lactate}_{delayed})/\text{lactate}_{initial}] \times 100\%$. Nguyen and colleagues[24] studied lactate clearance in 111 patients initially undergoing EGDT in the emergency department. Those patients who had a lactate clearance greater than 10% over the first 6 hours had a lower in-hospital, 30-day and 60-day mortality rates. Jones and colleagues[25] prospectively compared lactate clearance to monitoring ScvO2 as the method to measure total body oxygen metabolism. Two hundred forty-seven patients were randomized and underwent EDGT as outlined by Rivers and colleagues[3] (**Table 1**), except lactate clearance of greater than 10% was used instead of ScvO2 of greater than 70% as the goal in the last step of the protocol in 1 group. There was no difference in mortality in the 2 groups, and they concluded a protocol targeting lactate clearance was not inferior to a protocol that used ScvO2.

EMPIRIC ANTIBIOTICS

Prompt administration of empiric intravenous antibiotics likely to cover pathogens causing sepsis is recommended by the SSC.[2] It is suggested that an important portion of a sepsis bundle is the rapid administration of antibiotics.[26] In a retrospective study of over 2000 patients in septic shock, Kumar and colleagues[27] noted a decrease in survival by 7.6% for each hour of delay in administering antibiotics. Patients who received antibiotics within the first 30 minutes of hypotension had a survival of 82.7% versus 42% if treatment was delayed to 6 hours. Gaieski and colleagues[28] prospectively studied 261 patients undergoing EGDT and reported a lower mortality when antibiotics were given within 1 hour of arrival to the emergency department (19.5% vs 33.2%).

Table 1 Antimicrobial choices for acute diverticulitis		
	Monotherapy	Combination
Low Risk	Ampicillin/sulbactam Ticarcillin/clavulanate Cefoxitin Cefotetan Moxifloxacin	Quinolone[a] + metronidazole Cefazolin + metronidazole
High Risk	Imipenum/cilastatin Meropenum Piperacillin/tazobactam	Aztreonam + metronidazole Aminoglycoside[b] + metronidazole Third or fourth generation cephalosporin[c] + metronidazole

See text for definition of low- and high-risk patients.
[a] Ciprofloxacin, levofloxacin, or gatifloxacin.
[b] Gentamicin or tobramycin.
[c] Cefepime, cefotaxime, ceftazidime, ceftizoxime, or ceftriaxone.
Adapted from Weigelt JA. Empiric treatment options in the management of complicated intra-abdominal infections. Cleve Clin J Med 2007;74(Suppl 4):S34; with permission.

Patients with IAIs should be administered empiric antibiotics that cover enteric gram-negative aerobic and facultative bacilli and entericgram-positive streptococci. The most commonly isolated organisms in diverticulitis mirror those in other IAis. A majority of patients will have mixed aerobic and anaerobic bacteria, with *Escherichia coli* and *Bacteroides fragilis* as the most common isolates,[29] and antimicrobial therapy should be directed toward those organisms. Although there are not recommendations for specific antibiotic regimens, guidelines for IAIs were recently updated.[30] There is little level 1 evidence on antibiotic selection, and most often recommendations are made based on expert consensus.[31] However, stratifying patients as low risk or high risk can help the clinician navigate guidelines. Low-risk patients generally present with a community acquired infection and have few preexisting comorbid conditions. Conversely, high-risk patients present with malnutrition, liver or kidney dysfunction, higher Acute Physiology and Chronic Health Evaluation (APACHE) II scores, and hospital-acquired infections.[32] Specific regimens for treatment of complicated diverticulitis can either be single-agent or combination therapy, with regimens recommended for both low-risk and high-risk patients (**Table 1**).[31–33] Community-specific factors such as the presence of multidrug-resistant organisms (*Pseudomonas*, extended-spectrum β-lactamase producing *Enterobacteriaceae,* and methicillin-resistant *Staphylococcus aureus)* will affect choice of antibiotic. Antifungal therapy is not recommended in low-risk patients unless *Candida* is grown from intra-abdominal cultures. Antifungal use in high-risk patients should be considered on a case-by-case basis.[32] Fluconazole is the antifungal of choice; however, in patients with resistance or in those critically ill, therapy with an echinocandin (caspofungin, micafungin, or anidulafungin) is acceptable.[30]

The optimal duration of antimicrobial therapy is an unanswered question. The Surgical Infection Society (SIS)/Infectious Diseases Society of America (IDSA) guidelines[30] recommend limiting therapy to 4 to 7 days unless there is inadequate source control. Patients undergoing therapy for greater than 7 days are at risk for toxicities and superinfection with *Clostridium difficile,* with no decrease in treatment failures. Patients who have adequate source control will show signs of resolution of infection (afebrile, normal white blood cell counts, resumption of an oral diet) within the 7 days of antimicrobial treatment.

Source Control

Source control is a cornerstone in the management of the patient with septic shock. The core elements of source control include rapid diagnosis and control of the infection via drainage of an abscess, debridement of devitalized or infected tissue, or removal of an infected medical device.[34] The SSC guidelines recommend all patients with severe sepsis be "evaluated for the presence of a focus of infection amenable to source control measures...."[2] Indwelling urinary catheters or vascular catheters are obvious examples of infected medical devices that can be removed or replaced with minimal morbidity. Orthopedic hardware, prosthetic mesh and prosthetic heart valves need to be evaluated on a case-by-case basis.

Source control is an integral component of the management of patients with IAIs.[32] The most common etiologies of IAI include pancreatic necrosis, biliary tract or gastrointestinal perforation, or inflammation. Failure to achieve source control in patients with IAI is associated with increased postoperative infections and morbidity.[35] Although there are no randomized trials regarding the optimal management of IAI, current recommendations suggest using the method that causes the least physiologic upset possible, minimizing anatomic and physiologic trauma.[34] Image-guided percutaneous drainage is often the mode of choice in patients with well-localized and contained intra-abdominal abscess or in those who are poor surgical candidates. However, in the case of ongoing contamination from gastrointestinal ischemia or perforation, open surgical drainage and debridement are necessary for appropriate source control. In these cases, wide drainage of purulence, resection of necrotic or ischemic bowel, and debridement of fecal matter, hematoma, and necrotic tissue are required.[36]

ADJUNCTIVE MEASURES

The recommendations regarding the use of corticosteroids have changed overtime based on 2 major studies in patients with septic shock. Annane and colleagues[37] demonstrated a decreased need for vasopressors in patients with refractory septic shock and a survival advantage in those with relative adrenal insufficiency. The corticosteroid therapy of septic shock (CORTICUS)[38] trial studied patients with less severe septic shock and noted a decreased duration of shock in those treated with corticosteroids but no mortality difference. They did not assess patients for relative adrenal insufficiency. The SCC guidelines recommend corticosteroids be used in patients with refractory septic shock (poorly responsive to fluids and vasopressor therapy) and do not recommend routine assessment for relative adrenal insufficiency.[2]

Recombinant human activated protein C (rhAPC), also known as drotrecogin alfa, was included in the SSC guidelines based on the prospective recombinant human activated protein C worldwide evaluation in severe sepsis (PROWESS) study group[39] and administration of drotrecogin alfa (Activated) in early stage severe sepsis (ADDRESS) study group[40] studies. The PROWESS trial examined patients with severe sepsis and an average APACHE II score of 25 and demonstrated a lower risk of 28-day mortality in those treated with rhAPC (24.7% vs 30.8%). Based on the results of a subsequent subgroup analysis,[41] the ADDRESS trial enrolled patients with an APACHE II score less than 25 and showed no difference in mortality. The final SSC recommendation was that administering rhAPC to patients with sepsis-induced multiple organ dysfunction and a high risk of death or an APACHE II score greater than 25. The prospective recombinant human activated protein C worldwide evaluation in severe sepsis and septic shock (PROWESS-SHOCK) study[42] enrolled adults with severe sepsis and high risk of death in an attempt to provide further validation of the previous studies. The study has been completed, but the results have not been published as of yet. However, preliminary results showed a 28-day all-cause mortality rate of 26.4% in patients treated with rhAPC compared with 24.4% in those given placebo. Based on these preliminary data, the US Food and Drug Administration (FDA) withdrew drotrecogin alfa from the market.[43] At this time, rhAPC should not be used in any patients with septic shock.

Diagnosis and Nonoperative Management of Diverticulitis

While in the SICU, the patient's resuscitation continued; the CVP was maintained between 8 and 10 mm Hg with LR administration, and her norepinephrine requirements diminished. The patient's UOP improved to 0.6 cc/kg/h. Serial lactate levels were drawn and were down trending throughout the initial 12 hours. The following morning, her serum creatinine improved to 1.3 mg/dL, and she underwent a noncontrast computed tomography (CT) scan of the abdomen and pelvis. There was extensive diverticulosis in the sigmoid and descending colon as well as thickening of the wall of the sigmoid colon. There was also a 7 × 10 cm fluid collection in the left paracolic gutter with surrounding inflammation. This was felt to be consistent with a Hinchey stage 3/4 perforation. The following morning, she returned to the radiology department for a percutaneous drainage of the abscess. The cavity was accessed, and feculent material and pus were aspirated. A 10 French pigtail catheter was placed and connected to a drainage bag. She returned to the SICU and continued to require norepinephrine, and a vasopressin infusion at 0.04 U/min was started.

The diagnosis of acute diverticulitis can often be made based on history and physical findings, especially in patients who have had previously confirmed diverticulitis. However, in many cases of abdominal pain, it may be uncertain whether acute diverticulitis is present, and adjunctive studies are helpful and warranted.[44] Alternative diagnoses include irritable bowel syndrome, gastroenteritis, bowel obstruction, inflammatory bowel disease, appendicitis, ischemic colitis, colorectal cancer, urinary tract infection, kidney stones, and gynecologic disorders. An elevated white blood cell count often is helpful in confirming the presence of an inflammatory process.

Although several different modalities have been used to evaluate patients with suspected diverticular disease, CT has emerged as the study of choice. Advantages of CT scanning include the ability to make an accurate diagnosis and stage the severity of disease, and the therapeutic ability to drain an abscess with CT guidance. Disadvantages of CT scan include radiation exposure and the cost of the examinations.

CT findings consistent with diverticulitis were first described more than 25 years ago. These signs included the presence of diverticula, pericolic fat stranding, colonic wall thickening more than 4 mm, and abscess formation.[45]

CT has the added advantage of detecting other intraperitoneal findings, including hepatic abscesses, pyelophlebitis, small bowel obstruction, colonic strictures/ obstruction, and colovesical fistulas. A prospective study found a sensitivity of 97%, specificity of 98%, and global accuracy of 98%. It identified localized perforation and abscesses with a sensitivity of 100% and specificity of 91%.[46]

Multiple classification systems for diverticulitis exist. Prior to the routine use of CT scan, Hinchey and colleagues[47] published their classification for acute diverticulitis. The Hinchey classification is used in international literature to distinguish 4 stages of perforated disease identified at the time of surgery. There are many modifications to the Hinchey classification that incorporate CT scan findings. One such modification was made by Kaiser and colleagues[48] (stage 0 mild clinical diverticulitis, stage 1a confined pericolic inflammation, stage 1b confined pericolic abscess, stage 2 pelvic or distant intraabdominal abscess, stage 3 generalized purulent peritonitis, stage 4 fecal peritonitis), which was based on clinical, CT, or operative findings. Other classifications are based solely on CT scan with the argument that CT findings are the most valuable indication as to the likelihood that medical treatment with antibiotics will fail. Ambrosetti and colleagues[49] have proposed such a classification of sigmoid diverticulitis. Diverticulitis is subdivided into moderate disease or mild disease in the case of localized sigmoid wall thickening (>5 mm) and inflammation of the pericolic fat. The term severe disease is used instead in the case of abscess, extraluminal air or extraluminal contrast extravasation. Irrespective of the classification system used CT scan findings are an important aspect of developing a treatment plan.

Acute diverticulitis can be divided into complicated and uncomplicated diverticulitis. Complicated diverticulitis refers to acute diverticulitis accompanied by abscess, fistula, obstruction, or free intra-abdominal perforation. Most patients with uncomplicated sigmoid diverticulitis respond to medical treatment with broad-spectrum antibiotics. Hospital admission is dependent on systemic illness, age, and comorbidities. Even when hospital admission is necessary, an initial conservative approach has been validated.[50–53] Patients with uncomplicated diverticulitis generally experience significant decreases in their abdominal pain, temperature and white blood cell count within the first 48 hours after initiation of antibiotic therapy.[54,55]

Diverticular abscesses are a common complication of acute diverticulitis, occurring in 15% to 20% of cases.[46,56,57] According to the American Society of Colon and Rectal Surgeons practice parameters for sigmoid diverticulitis, "Radiologically guided percutaneous drainage is usually the most appropriate treatment for patients with a large diverticular abscess." Recommendations also include hospitalization, intravenous antibiotics, and medical treatment alone for abscesses less than 2 cm.[44] Other studies have advocated the routine percutaneous drainage of abscess larger then 3 to 5 cm or all pelvic abscesses.[58,59]

Operative Management of Diverticulitis

The next day, the patient was taken to the operating room for failure of nonoperative management. She underwent a sigmoid colectomy with Hartmann pouch. Prior to creation of the end colostomy and abdominal closure, she became hypothermic, hypotensive, and acidotic. The procedure was terminated, and the woman's abdomen was temporarily closed with an abdominal vacuum pack.

Emergency surgery is indicated in patients with diffuse peritonitis or for those who fail nonoperative management of acute diverticulitis. This is usually seen in the setting of Hinchey 3 or 4 diverticulitis. The standard of care in most cases is a sigmoid resection, closure of the rectal stump, and creation of an end-descending colostomy, also known as a Hartmann procedure. Widespread use of the Hartmann procedure has replaced delayed sigmoid resection, known as the 3-staged technique, which was commonly practiced before the 1980s, and involved proximal diversion, subsequent resection and primary anastomosis with maintenance of stoma, and finally colostomy closure.[60] The aggregate mortality in a total of 1051 patients reported in 54 combined studies between 1966 and 2003 was almost 19% and was associated with a 24% incidence of wound infection and a 10% incidence of stoma complications.[61] Unfortunately, bowel reconstruction after Hartmann procedure requires a new laparotomy, and a high percentage of patients will not undergo further surgery due to other medical problems, and therefore remain with a permanent stoma.[62]

A single-staged technique of sigmoid resection with primary anastomosis is becoming a recognized alternative to Hartmann procedure for the treatment of acute diverticulitis. Primary resection and anastomosis have gained popularity after their successful application in the repair of penetrating traumatic colon injuries.[63,64] A subsequent case series using primary resection and anastomosis with or without protective stoma and intraoperative lavage has been reported in the treatment of acute diverticulitis, and several advantages of this approach have been recognized. Creation of an anastomosis during the initial resection avoids the technical difficulty of colostomy reversal and the additional cost and length of hospital stay, and improves the likelihood for maintaining intestinal continuity.[65,66] This approach is an acceptable alternative to treating patients with low-grade Hinchey 1 and 2 disease who undergo laparotomy for diverticular peritonitis, and it is supported by the European Association of Endoscopic Surgeons as a treatment option in perforation with purulent peritonitis (Hinchey 3) when used with protective stoma.[67] Recent comparative reviews of the literature reflect favorably on the use of primary resection and anastomosis compared with Hartmann procedure in advanced staged diverticulitis, but they must be interpreted with caution due to considerable selection bias, lack of prospective randomized trials, and heterogeneity of patient disease.[68] Primary anastomosis is contraindicated in fecal peritonitis, septic shock, hemodynamic instability, chronic steroid therapy, and poor condition of the patient.

Laparoscopic peritoneal lavage is an alternative in the management of Hinchey grade 2 pelvic abscesses and perforated diverticulitis with diffuse purulent perito-nitis.[69] There are case series published and prospective studies showing benefits compared with conventional management.[70–73] Proponents suggest it achieves a lower mortality rate and stoma formation rate, less wound infections, and shorter operating time. No significant differences were found with respect to recurrence rates compared with resection and primary anastomosis. But even though there is some available evidence, the lack of prospective clinical trials, with the exception of the study published by Myers and colleagues,[72] has limited the widespread use of lapa-roscopic lavage.

Damage Control for Intra-Abdominal Sepsis

The patient was brought back to the SICU and underwent continued resuscitation. A lithium indicator dilution cardiac output monitor device (LiDCO) was used to determine she had fluid-responsive hypotension. At this point her hematocrit had fallen to 25, and international normalized ratio (INR) was 1.4; she was transfused 2 units pRBC and 2 units fresh frozen plasma (FFP). Over the next 12 hours, her vasopressor requirements were eliminated, and her acidosis improved. On postoperative day (POD) 2, she was taken back to the operating room for a planned relaparotomy. Her abdomen was washed out, and there were no signs of ongoing contamination or peritonitis. Her small bowel was edematous, and the fascia was unable to be approximated without tension. A postpyloric soft feeding tube was placed intraoperatively, and the temporary abdominal vacuum pack (VP) was reapplied before she was returned to the SICU. At this point, her hemodynamics had normalized; her UOP improved to 1 cc/kg/h, and lactate was 1 mmol/L and no longer acidotic. Over the next 48 hours, the patient was diuresed with furosemide to target 1.5 L net fluid negative per day, and enteral feeds were started at 10 cc/h. On POD 4, she underwent washout of her abdomen, sigmoid colostomy, and primary closure of her fascia and skin. She was then extu-bated and transferred to the surgical ward and had an uneventful recovery. Nine weeks later, she underwent colostomy takedown without incident.

DAMAGE CONTROL LAPAROTOMY

Damage control laparotomy (DCL) refers to a sequence of an abbreviated initial lapa-rotomy with the initial goals of controlling hemorrhage and contamination, a period of resuscitation, subsequent operations, and a definitive abdominal wall closure.[74] DCL was formalized 20 years ago by Rotondo and colleagues[75] as a method of reducing the morbidity and mortality associated with severe intra-abdominal injury. Over the past 15 years, there has been widespread adoption of DCL techniques, and the open abdomen has become commonplace in surgical ICUs. The open abdomen tech-nique has long been used to treat severe intra-abdominal infections.[76] Indications for DCL in severe IAI are similar to those in severe abdominal trauma: temperature less than 35°C, pH less than 7.20, a base deficit greater than 8, and laboratory or clinical evidence of coagulapathy.[77,78] Additionally, indications include massive volume resuscitation, ongoing contamination, inadequate source control, hemodynamic in-stability, need for second-look procedure, primary prevention of abdominal compart-ment syndrome (ACS), and development of multisystem organ failure.[74,79,80]

The sequence of damage control laparotomy as described for trauma is adapted to IAI with several modifications.[81] The initial resuscitation and evaluation period, termed ground zero, is generally longer, requiring several hours to restore adequate perfusion in the septic patient. The goals of this period are to replace circulating volume with crystalloids and to begin correcting the acidosis and coagulapathy associated with sepsis.

Once the patient has undergone a period of resuscitation, an exploratory laparotomy for source control is undertaken. The goals of this initial operation are to drain any intra-abdominal abscess and resect ischemic or necrotic tissue before the patient succumbs to physiologic fatigue. Most often this involves resecting a portion of hollow viscus and leaving the bowel in discontinuity.

After source control is obtained, the method of temporary abdominal closure (TAC) needs to be considered. The principles of TAC are containing the intra-abdominal contents, protection of the bowel, preservation of the fascia, and control of the peritoneal effluent. Numerous strategies for TAC have been described, ranging from skin-only closures with towel clips or running monofilament, absorbable or nonabsorbable mesh closure, VP, and vacuum-assisted wound management.[82,83] Primary skin closure and mesh placement have largely been replaced by vacuum dressings. They offer the advantage of easy placement and removal to facilitate multiple subsequent procedures, control and quantification of the peritoneal effluent, and preservation of the fascia. The VP, as described by Barker and colleagues,[84] has become the most widely used method of TAC and is the current standard of care.[79] Most commonly, the VP is constructed in 3 layers. A sterile polyvinyl sheet (1010 large bowel bag, 3M Health Care, St. Paul, Minnesota) is placed directly above the abdominal viscera and below the anterior abdominal wall. Either a moist towel or gauze is placed in the subfascial space, and 2 large silicone drains or nasogastric tubes are brought out through the superior portion of the wound. Finally, large adhesive drape (Ioban, 3M Health Care) is used to cover the entire defect, and the drains are connected to suction via a Y connector to provide continuous negative pressure.

A commercially available vacuum assisted closure device is available for TAC (VAC Abdominal Dressing System and AbThera, KCI San Antonio, Texas). It is constructed similar to the VP. A nonadherent plastic drape is placed below the abdominal wall; however, the towel is replaced by a porous polyurethane sponge. An adhesive drape and drain complete the dressing. Excellent rates of fascial reapproximation and low rates of enterocutanous fistula have been reported with vacuum-assisted closure devices.[85] At this point, no prospective comparison of VP dressings and vacuum-assisted closure devices has been undertaken.

After TAC has been performed, the patient returns to the ICU for a continued period of resuscitation. It is not uncommon for the patient to need aggressive resuscitation for 24 to 48 hours after the initial laparotomy for source control. The patient should be resuscitated based on the principles previously described. Within 24 to 48 hours, the patient should be taken back to the operating room for re-exploration and evaluation for closure. The TAC is removed, and the abdomen is re-explored, taking care to examine the site of the source of the intra-abdominal sepsis. Frequently, further debridement of necrotic tissue or drainage of accumulated purulent fluid is necessary. Extensive intra-abdominal lavage with sterile saline is undertaken to decrease the bacterial burden and remove any nonadherent hematoma or fibrous material. Existing staple lines and anastomoses should be gently examined for their integrity. Restoration of gastrointestinal continuity is delayed until the degree of peritonitis has decreased.[74] In some patients with intra-abdominal sepsis, creation of an end stoma may be preferable over primary anastomosis. Alternatively, a diverting loop ileostomy protecting a distal colonic primary anastomosis is a safe strategy.[65,66] If a prolonged period of an open abdomen is anticipated, stomas should be placed as far lateral as possible on the abdominal wall to provide maximal abdominal wall mobility during closure.[83] This can be done at the initial relaparotomy or delayed to a subsequent procedure.

At this point, an evaluation for closure is undertaken. If bowel edema has resolved, and the fascia can be brought together without undo tension, then primary closure should be attempted. Communication with the anesthesia team at this point is important; if the peak inspiratory pressures increase by more than 10 mm Hg during closure, then fascial closure should be abandoned. A rise in peak pressure can place the patient at risk for dehiscence or abdominal compartment syndrome.[86] Most patients undergoing DCL for IAI will have a significant amount of bowel and mesenteric edema precluding early closure.[83] At this point, the TAC should be reapplied and patient returned to the ICU.

It may take up to 7 to 10 days, during which the patient undergoes relaparotomy every 48 to 72 hours for the visceral edema and inflammatory response to subside enough to allow closure. However, during this time period, the fascia retracts laterally and becomes fused to the overlying fat; this makes primary closure impossible. Several methods may prevent the retraction of the myofascial unit, namely removable prostheses, dynamic retention sutures, and the VAC dressings.[82,87] Wittman developed a burr-like device consisting of 2 sheets of a Velcro-like material sutured to the fascia.[88] As in the VP, a plastic drape is placed under the abdominal wall, and the Wittman Patch (Starsurgical, Burlington, Wisconsin) is sewn in and the sheets compressed together and adhered. A dressing similar to the VP is placed above the patch to control the peritoneal effluent. At subsequent relaparotomies, the sheets are easily separated and trimmed and then reapproximated until the fascia can be closed. Several groups have reported success using this technique with closure rates of 75% to 100%.[89–92] Dynamic retention sutures can be used to maintain the myofascial unit and can be tightened at the bedside in the ICU.[93,94] The VAC dressing as described previously can provide excellent fascial reapproximation with success rates ranging from 65% to 100% in trauma patients.[85,95,96] Unfortunately, closure rates after sepsis are much lower overall.[97] This lower rate persists with the VAC dressing, as Wondberg reported a fascial closure rate of 33% in patients with IAI.[98]

If the abdominal fascia is not closed within 10 to 14 days using the previously described techniques, it is recognized that the fascia will not come together because of massive visceral edema, loss of domain, and the presence of a fixed visceral block. The open abdomen is then allowed to granulate in, and a split-thickness skin graft (STSG) is used to cover the wound.[99] Over the ensuring 6 to 12 months, the inflammatory response resolves, and the granulation tissue dissipates: at this time the skin can be elevated from the underlying viscera. The STSG is removed, and the fascial defect is closed, either with a primary closure, biologic mesh, or a component separation.[96]

REFERENCES

1. Levy MM, Fink MP, Marshall JC, et al. 2001 SCCM/ESICM/ACCP/ATS/SIS International Sepsis Definitions Conference. Intensive Care Med 2003;29(4):530–8.
2. Dellinger RP, Levy MM, Carlet JM, et al. Surviving Sepsis Campaign: international guidelines for management of severe sepsis and septic shock: 2008. Crit Care Med 2008;36(1):296–327.
3. Rivers E, Nguyen B, Havstad S, et al. Early goal-directed therapy in the treatment of severe sepsis and septic shock. N Engl J Med 2001;345(19):1368–77.
4. Parrillo JE. Pathogenetic mechanisms of septic shock. N Engl J Med 1993; 328(20):1471–7.
5. Sihler KC, Nathens AB. Management of severe sepsis in the surgical patient. Surg Clin North Am 2006;86(6):1457–81.

6. Human albumin administration in critically ill patients: systematic review of randomised controlled trials. Cochrane Injuries Group Albumin Reviewers. BMJ 1998; 317(7153):235–40.

7. Wilkes MM, Navickis RJ. Patient survival after human albumin administration. A meta-analysis of randomized, controlled trials. Ann Intern Med 2001;135(3):149–64.

8. Finfer S, Bellomo R, Boyce N, et al. A comparison of albumin and saline for fluid resuscitation in the intensive care unit. N Engl J Med 2004;350(22):2247–56.

9. LeDoux D, Astiz ME, Carpati CM, et al. Effects of perfusion pressure on tissue perfusion in septic shock. Crit Care Med 2000;28(8):2729–32.

10. Holmes CL, Walley KR. Bad medicine: low-dose dopamine in the ICU. Chest 2003;123(4):1266–75.

11. Sakr Y, Reinhart K, Vincent JL, et al. Does dopamine administration in shock influence outcome? Results of the Sepsis Occurrence in Acutely Ill Patients (SOAP) Study. Crit Care Med 2006;34(3):589–97.

12. De Backer D, Biston P, Devriendt J, et al. Comparison of dopamine and norepinephrine in the treatment of shock. N Engl J Med 2010;362(9):779–89.

13. De Backer D, Aldecoa C, Njimi H, et al. Dopamine versus norepinephrine in the treatment of septic shock: a meta-analysis*. Crit Care Med 2012;40(3):725–30.

14. Holmes CL, Patel BM, Russell JA, et al. Physiology of vasopressin relevant to management of septic shock. Chest 2001;120(3):989–1002.

15. Patel BM, Chittock DR, Russell JA, et al. Beneficial effects of short-term vasopressin infusion during severe septic shock. Anesthesiology 2002;96(3):576–82.

16. Russell JA, Walley KR, Singer J, et al. Vasopressin versus norepinephrine infusion in patients with septic shock. N Engl J Med 2008;358(9):877–87.

17. Russell JA. Bench-to-bedside review: vasopressin in the management of septic shock. Crit Care 2011;15(4):226.

18. da Silva Ramos FJ, Azevedo LC. Hemodynamic and perfusion end points for volemic resuscitation in sepsis. Shock 2010;34(Suppl 1):34–9.

19. Varpula M, Tallgren M, Saukkonen K, et al. Hemodynamic variables related to outcome in septic shock. Intensive Care Med 2005;31(8):1066–71.

20. Marik PE, Baram M, Vahid B. Does central venous pressure predict fluid responsiveness? A systematic review of the literature and the tale of seven mares. Chest 2008;134(1):172–8.

21. Michard F. Changes in arterial pressure during mechanical ventilation. Anesthesiology 2005;103(2):419–28 [quiz: 449–5].

22. Michard F, Boussat S, Chemla D, et al. Relation between respiratory changes in arterial pulse pressure and fluid responsiveness in septic patients with acute circulatory failure. Am J Respir Crit Care Med 2000;162(1):134–8.

23. Mayer J, Suttner S. Cardiac output derived from arterial pressure waveform. Curr Opin Anaesthesiol 2009;22(6):804–8.

24. Nguyen HB, Rivers EP, Knoblich BP, et al. Early lactate clearance is associated with improved outcome in severe sepsis and septic shock. Crit Care Med 2004;32(8):1637–42.

25. Jones AE, Shapiro NI, Trzeciak S, et al. Lactate clearance vs central venous oxygen saturation as goals of early sepsis therapy: a randomized clinical trial. JAMA 2010;303(8):739–46.

26. Zubert S, Funk DJ, Kumar A. Antibiotics in sepsis and septic shock: like everything else in life, timing is everything. Crit Care Med 2010;38(4):1211–2.

27. Kumar A, Roberts D, Wood KE, et al. Duration of hypotension before initiation of effective antimicrobial therapy is the critical determinant of survival in human septic shock. Crit Care Med 2006;34(6):1589–96.

28. Gaieski DF, Mikkelsen ME, Band RA, et al. Impact of time to antibiotics on survival in patients with severe sepsis or septic shock in whom early goal-directed therapy was initiated in the emergency department. Crit Care Med 2010;38(4):1045–53.

29. Brook I, Frazier EH. Aerobic and anaerobic microbiology in intra-abdominal infections associated with diverticulitis. J Med Microbiol 2000;49(9):827–30.

30. Solomkin JS, Mazuski JE, Bradley JS, et al. Diagnosis and management of complicated intra-abdominal infection in adults and children: guidelines by the Surgical Infection Society and the Infectious Diseases Society of America. Clin Infect Dis 2010;50(2):133–64.

31. Byrnes MC, Mazuski JE. Antimicrobial therapy for acute colonic diverticulitis. Surg Infect (Larchmt) 2009;10(2):143–54.

32. Weigelt JA. Empiric treatment options in the management of complicated intra-abdominal infections. Cleve Clin J Med 2007;74(Suppl 4):S29–37.

33. Jacobs DO. Clinical practice. Diverticulitis. N Engl J Med 2007;357(20):2057–66.

34. Marshall JC, Maier RV, Jimenez M, et al. Source control in the management of severe sepsis and septic shock: an evidence-based review. Crit Care Med 2004;32(Suppl 11):S513–26.

35. Wacha H, Hau T, Dittmer R, et al. Risk factors associated with intra-abdominal infections: a prospective multicenter study. Peritonitis Study Group. Langenbecks Arch Surg 1999;384(1):24–32.

36. Lopez N, Kobayashi L, Coimbra R. A Comprehensive review of abdominal infections. World J Emerg Surg 2011;6:7.

37. Annane D, Sebille V, Charpentier C, et al. Effect of treatment with low doses of hydrocortisone and fludrocortisone on mortality in patients with septic shock. JAMA 2002;288(7):862–71.

38. Sprung CL, Annane D, Keh D, et al. Hydrocortisone therapy for patients with septic shock. N Engl J Med 2008;358(2):111–24.

39. Bernard GR, Vincent JL, Laterre PF, et al. Efficacy and safety of recombinant human activated protein C for severe sepsis. N Engl J Med 2001;344(10):699–709.

40. Abraham E, Laterre PF, Garg R, et al. Drotrecogin alfa (activated) for adults with severe sepsis and a low risk of death. N Engl J Med 2005;353(13):1332–41.

41. Ely EW, Laterre PF, Angus DC, et al. Drotrecogin alfa (activated) administration across clinically important subgroups of patients with severe sepsis. Crit Care Med 2003;31(1):12–9.

42. Finfer S, Ranieri VM, Thompson BT, et al. Design, conduct, analysis and reporting of a multi-national placebo-controlled trial of activated protein C for persistent septic shock. Intensive Care Med 2008;34(11):1935–47.

43. Savel RH, Munro CL. Evidence-based backlash: the tale of drotrecogin alfa. Am J Crit Care 2012;21(2):81–3.

44. Rafferty J, Shellito P, Hyman NH, et al. Practice parameters for sigmoid diverticulitis. Dis Colon Rectum 2006;49(7):939–44.

45. Hulnick DH, Megibow AJ, Balthazar EJ, et al. Computed tomography in the evaluation of diverticulitis. Radiology 1984;152(2):491–5.

46. Werner A, Diehl SJ, Farag-Soliman M, et al. Multi-slice spiral CT in routine diagnosis of suspected acute left-sided colonic diverticulitis: a prospective study of 120 patients. Eur Radiol 2003;13(12):2596–603.

47. Hinchey EJ, Schaal PG, Richards GK. Treatment of perforated diverticular disease of the colon. Adv Surg 1978;12:85–109.

48. Kaiser AM, Jiang JK, Lake JP, et al. The management of complicated diverticulitis and the role of computed tomography. Am J Gastroenterol 2005;100(4):910–7.

49. Ambrosetti P, Grossholz M, Becker C, et al. Computed tomography in acute left colonic diverticulitis. Br J Surg 1997;84(4):532–4.
50. Mueller MH, Glatzle J, Kasparek MS, et al. Long-term outcome of conservative treatment in patients with diverticulitis of the sigmoid colon. Eur J Gastroenterol Hepatol 2005;17(6):649–54.
51. Brandt D, Gervaz P, Durmishi Y, et al. Percutaneous CT scan-guided drainage vs antibiotherapy alone for Hinchey II diverticulitis: a case–control study. Dis Colon Rectum 2006;49(10):1533–8.
52. Alvarez JA, Baldonedo RF, Bear IG, et al. Presentation, management and outcome of acute sigmoid diverticulitis requiring hospitalization. Dig Surg 2007; 24(6):471–6.
53. Shaikh S, Krukowski ZH. Outcome of a conservative policy for managing acute sigmoid diverticulitis. Br J Surg 2007;94(7):876–9.
54. Evans J, Kozol R, Frederick W, et al. Does a 48-hour rule predict outcomes in patients with acute sigmoid diverticulitis? J Gastrointest Surg 2008;12(3):577–82.
55. Sra HK, Shipman K, Virk HS. Does a 48-hour rule predict outcomes in patients with acute sigmoid diverticulitis? J Gastrointest Surg 2009;13(10):1892.
56. Rao PM, Rhea JT, Novelline RA, et al. Helical CT with only colonic contrast material for diagnosing diverticulitis: prospective evaluation of 150 patients. AJR Am J Roentgenol 1998;170(6):1445–9.
57. Ambrosetti P, Becker C, Terrier F. Colonic diverticulitis: impact of imaging on surgical management —a prospective study of 542 patients. Eur Radiol 2002; 12(5):1145–9.
58. Siewert B, Tye G, Kruskal J, et al. Impact of CT-guided drainage in the treatment of diverticular abscesses: size matters. AJR Am J Roentgenol 2006;186(3):680–6.
59. Ambrosetti P, Chautems R, Soravia C, et al. Long-term outcome of mesocolic and pelvic diverticular abscesses of the left colon: a prospective study of 73 cases. Dis Colon Rectum 2005;48(4):787–91.
60. Ferzoco LB, Raptopoulos V, Silen W. Acute diverticulitis. N Engl J Med 1998; 338(21):1521–6.
61. Salem L, Flum DR. Primary anastomosis or Hartmann's procedure for patients with diverticular peritonitis? A systematic review. Dis Colon Rectum 2004; 47(11):1953–64.
62. Maggard MA, Zingmond D, O'Connell JB, et al. What proportion of patients with an ostomy (for diverticulitis) get reversed? Am Surg 2004;70(10):928–31.
63. Nelson R, Singer M. Primary repair for penetrating colon injuries. Cochrane Database Syst Rev 2003;(3):CD002247.
64. Singer MA, Nelson RL. Primary repair of penetrating colon injuries: a systematic review. Dis Colon Rectum 2002;45(12):1579–87.
65. Constantinides VA, Heriot A, Remzi F, et al. Operative strategies for diverticular peritonitis: a decision analysis between primary resection and anastomosis versus Hartmann's procedures. Ann Surg 2007;245(1):94–103.
66. Schilling MK, Maurer CA, Kollmar O, et al. Primary vs. secondary anastomosis after sigmoid colon resection for perforated diverticulitis (Hinchey Stage III and IV): a prospective outcome and cost analysis. Dis Colon Rectum 2001;44(5): 699–703 [discussion: 703–5].
67. Breitenstein S, Kraus A, Hahnloser D, et al. Emergency left colon resection for acute perforation: primary anastomosis or Hartmann's procedure? A case-matched control study. World J Surg 2007;31(11):2117–24.
68. Bauer VP. Emergency management of diverticulitis. Clin Colon Rectal Surg 2009; 22(3):161–8.

69. O'Sullivan GC, Murphy D, O'Brien MG, et al. Laparoscopic management of generalized peritonitis due to perforated colonic diverticula. Am J Surg 1996; 171(4):432–4.

70. Favuzza J, Friel JC, Kelly JJ, et al. Benefits of laparoscopic peritoneal lavage for complicated sigmoid diverticulitis. Int J Colorectal Dis 2009;24(7):797–801.

71. Karoui M, Champault A, Pautrat K, et al. Laparoscopic peritoneal lavage or primary anastomosis with defunctioning stoma for Hinchey 3 complicated diverticulitis: results of a comparative study. Dis Colon Rectum 2009;52(4):609–15.

72. Myers E, Hurley M, O'Sullivan GC, et al. Laparoscopic peritoneal lavage for generalized peritonitis due to perforated diverticulitis. Br J Surg 2008;95(1): 97–101.

73. Taylor CJ, Layani L, Ghusn MA, et al. Perforated diverticulitis managed by laparoscopic lavage. ANZ J Surg 2006;76(11):962–5.

74. Waibel BH, Rotondo MF. Damage control in trauma and abdominal sepsis. Crit Care Med 2010;38(Suppl 9):S421–30.

75. Rotondo MF, Schwab CW, McGonigal MD, et al. 'Damage control': an approach for improved survival in exsanguinating penetrating abdominal injury. J Trauma 1993;35(3):375–82 [discussion: 382–3].

76. Ivatury RR, Nallathambi M, Rao PM, et al. Open management of the septic abdomen: therapeutic and prognostic considerations based on APACHE II. Crit Care Med 1989;17(6):511–7.

77. Asensio JA, McDuffie L, Petrone P, et al. Reliable variables in the exsanguinated patient which indicate damage control and predict outcome. Am J Surg 2001; 182(6):743–51.

78. Aoki N, Wall MJ, Demsar J, et al. Predictive model for survival at the conclusion of a damage control laparotomy. Am J Surg 2000;180(6):540–4 [discussion: 544–5].

79. Diaz JJ Jr, Cullinane DC, Dutton WD, et al. The management of the open abdomen in trauma and emergency general surgery: part 1-damage control. J Trauma 2010;68(6):1425–38.

80. Adkins AL, Robbins J, Villalba M, et al. Open abdomen management of intra-abdominal sepsis. Am Surg 2004;70(2):137–40 [discussion: 140].

81. Waibel BH, Rotondo MF. Damage control for intra-abdominal sepsis. Surg Clin North Am 2012;92(2):243–57.

82. Rutherford EJ, Skeete DA, Brasel KJ. Management of the patient with an open abdomen: techniques in temporary and definitive closure. Curr Probl Surg 2004;41(10):815–76.

83. Schecter WP, Ivatury RR, Rotondo MF, et al. Open abdomen after trauma and abdominal sepsis: a strategy for management. J Am Coll Surg 2006;203(3): 390–6.

84. Barker DE, Kaufman HJ, Smith LA, et al. Vacuum pack technique of temporary abdominal closure: a 7-year experience with 112 patients. J Trauma 2000; 48(2):201–6 [discussion: 206–7].

85. Garner GB, Ware DN, Cocanour CS, et al. Vacuum-assisted wound closure provides early fascial reapproximation in trauma patients with open abdomens. Am J Surg 2001;182(6):630–8.

86. Miller RS, Morris JA Jr, Diaz JJ Jr, et al. Complications after 344 damage-control open celiotomies. J Trauma 2005;59(6):1365–71 [discussion: 1371–4].

87. De Waele JJ, Leppaniemi AK. Temporary abdominal closure techniques. Am Surg 2011;77(Suppl 1):S46–50.

88. Wittmann DH, Aprahamian C, Bergstein JM. Etappen lavage: advanced diffuse peritonitis managed by planned multiple laparotomies utilizing zippers, slide

fastener, and Velcro analogue for temporary abdominal closure. World J Surg 1990;14(2):218–26.

89. Tieu BH, Cho SD, Luem N, et al. The use of the Wittmann Patch facilitates a high rate of fascial closure in severely injured trauma patients and critically ill emergency surgery patients. J Trauma 2008;65(4):865–70.

90. Weinberg JA, George RL, Griffin RL, et al. Closing the open abdomen: improved success with Wittmann Patch staged abdominal closure. J Trauma 2008;65(2): 345–8.

91. Fantus RJ, Mellett MM, Kirby JP. Use of controlled fascial tension and an adhesion-preventing barrier to achieve delayed primary fascial closure in patients managed with an open abdomen. Am J Surg 2006;192(2):243–7.

92. Cipolla J, Stawicki SP, Hoff WS, et al. A proposed algorithm for managing the open abdomen. Am Surg 2005;71(3):202–7.

93. Koniaris LG, Hendrickson RJ, Drugas G, et al. Dynamic retention: a technique for closure of the complex abdomen in critically ill patients. Arch Surg 2001;136(12): 1359–62 [discussion: 1363].

94. Verdam FJ, Dolmans DE, Loos MJ, et al. Delayed primary closure of the septic open abdomen with a dynamic closure system. World J Surg 2011;35(10): 2348–55.

95. Burlew CC, Moore EE, Biffl WL, et al. One hundred percent fascial approximation can be achieved in the postinjury open abdomen with a sequential closure protocol. J Trauma Acute Care Surg 2012;72(1):235–41.

96. Diaz JJ Jr, Dutton WD, Ott MM, et al. Eastern association for the surgery of trauma: a review of the management of the open abdomen–part 2 "Management of the open abdomen". J Trauma 2011;71(2):502–12.

97. Tsuei BJ, Skinner JC, Bernard AC, et al. The open peritoneal cavity: etiology correlates with the likelihood of fascial closure. Am Surg 2004;70(7):652–6.

98. Wondberg D, Larusson HJ, Metzger U, et al. Treatment of the open abdomen with the commercially available vacuum-assisted closure system in patients with abdominal sepsis: low primary closure rate. World J Surg 2008;32(12):2724–9.

99. Fabian TC, Croce MA, Pritchard FE, et al. Planned ventral hernia. Staged management for acute abdominal wall defects. Ann Surg 1994;219(6):643–50 [discussion: 651–3].

Two Case Studies of Cardiopulmonary Effects of Intra-abdominal Hypertension

Ram Nirula, MD

KEYWORDS

- Cardiopulmonary effect • Intra-abdominal hypertension • Pulmonary hypertension
- Abdominal compartment syndrome

KEY POINTS

- Intra-abdominal hypertension (IAH) falsely elevates the pulmonary artery occlusion pressure (PAOP). Volumetric pulmonary artery catheter monitoring may more accurately reflect preload in this clinical condition.
- Treatment of IAH and abdominal compartment syndrome (ACS) begins with medical interventions but requires a decompressive laparotomy for definitive management.
- Pulmonary hypertension effects cardiac function. Hypoxia may be improved with increased Fio_2, increased positive end-expiratory pressure (PEEP) and use of inotropic agents that simultaneously reduce pulmonary artery pressure.
- Ventricular dysfunction can be managed with reduction in preload by mechanical means when pharmacologic means fail.

CASE 1: ABDOMINAL COMPARTMENT SYNDROME

A 24-year-old woman had a liver transplant 2 days ago and required 15 L of fluid resuscitation. Her heart rate (HR) is 130 and blood pressure (BP) 80/50. She has a peak airway pressure of 45 with a tidal volume set at 400 mL at a rate of 14, Fio_2 100%, and PEEP of 10 cm H_2O and arterial blood gas (ABG) 7.1, Pco_2 52, Po_2 66, bicarbonate (HCO3) 16, and lactate 6. Her urine output has been 5 mL/h for the past 3 hours and her bladder pressure is 28 mm Hg. Her cardiac index (CI) is 2 L/min, pulmonary artery pressure (PAP) 52/26, and central venous pressure (CVP) 14.

This physiologic derangement is that of ACS. In general, normal adult intra-abdominal pressure (IAP) is considered 5 mm Hg to 7 mm Hg. IAH has been defined by the World Society of the Abdominal Compartment Syndrome (www.wsacs.org) as sustained increased IAP greater than or equal to 12 mm Hg and ACS as IAP greater than or equal to 20 mm Hg with new organ dysfunction or failure. IAP in excess of

---

Division of General Surgery, University of Utah School of Medicine, 30 North 1900 East, 3B 110, Salt Lake City, UT 84132, USA
E-mail address: r.nirula@hsc.utah.edu

Surg Clin N Am 92 (2012) 1679–1684
http://dx.doi.org/10.1016/j.suc.2012.08.017
0039-6109/12/$ – see front matter © 2012 Elsevier Inc. All rights reserved.

25 mm Hg, a level of IAH commonly associated with significant organ dysfunction, is generally accepted as suggesting the need for abdominal decompression.[1,2]

CARDIAC EFFECTS OF IAH

Even modest elevations of IAP can cause a reduction in inferior vena cava blood flow and cardiac preload due to reduced venous return, which results in a drop in cardiac output. Furthermore, elevation of the diaphragm and elevated intrathoracic pressures transmitted from the IAH cause compression of the lungs, which increase the pulmonary vascular resistance. This leads to overdistension of the right ventricle and right ventricular failure, which reduces left ventricular preload. The case (described previously) demonstrates the altered pulmonary artery catheter pressure measurements observed in the setting of ACS. The elevated PAPs may lead to an assumption that preload is adequate, or even excessive, but the actual intravascular volume may be inadequate due to the reduced compliance of the thoracic cavity from the IAH. Administration of fluids may provide a temporary benefit but, without decompression of the abdomen, excessive fluid leads to overdistension of the right ventricle, worsening cardiac output.[2]

Traditionally, PAOP and CVP are used as surrogates for left ventricular end-diastolic volume. Although likely valid in normal healthy individuals, the multiple assumptions necessary to use PAOP and CVP as estimates of left ventricular preload status and right ventricular preload status, respectively, are not necessarily true in critically ill patients with IAH/ACS. This inaccuracy exists because these pressures reflect the sum of the intrathoracic pressure and the intravascular pressure. Because the intrathoracic pressure is elevated, the correlation between PAOP and CVP to left ventricular end-diastolic volume is abolished. As a rule of thumb, a quick estimate of transmural (tm) filling pressures can be obtained by subtracting half the IAP from the measured filling pressure (PAOPtm = PAOP - IAP/2).[1–3]

Additionally, the compliance of the ventricle is affected by the underlying disease, causing increased ventricular edema as well as elevated intrathoracic pressures. In general, the presence of IAH causes a flattening and rightward shift of the ventricular compliance curve. Therefore, a given PAOP does not correlate with left ventricular end-diastolic volume.

Resuscitation to absolute PAOP and CVP in patients with IAH/ACS should be avoided because such a practice can lead to underresuscitation, inappropriate administration of diuretics, and inappropriate end-organ perfusion. Instead, volumetric monitoring with newer-generation pulmonary artery catheters that provide a measure of the right ventricular end-diastolic volume have shown a better correlation with preload recruitable increases in cardiac output. Right ventricular end-diastolic volume goal-directed fluid resuscitation leads to a reduction of hard clinical endpoints, such as multiple organ failure and death.[4] Many studies report that at high levels of PEEP, right ventricular end-diastolic volume consistently maintained a highly significant correlation with cardiac output, whereas PAOP and CVP frequently exhibited inverse correlations with cardiac output.[4]

IAH falsely elevates the PAOP. Volumetric pulmonary artery catheter monitoring is a better option for monitoring preload in this clinical condition.

PULMONARY EFFECTS OF IAH

On average, 50% of the increased IAP is transmitted to the intrathoracic compartment. IAH causes an increase in alveolar pressures, dead space, and shunt fraction. IAH causes a decrease in transpulmonary pressures, functional residual capacity, and static compliance of the chest wall. The combined effect of these changes is hypoxemia and hypercapnia. The elevated abdominal pressures are compromising pulmonary function in these patients, evidenced by the elevated peak airway pressures in the setting of small tidal volumes compromising ventilation. Furthermore, significant hypoxia is present despite modest PEEP and maximum inspired oxygen content.[2,3,5]

To reverse this process, the abdominal cavity needs to be decompressed immediately.[2–5] To improve perfusion while measures are taken to open the abdomen, a volume challenge may be warranted. Increasing the respiratory rate and tidal volume to improve minute ventilation reduces respiratory acidosis. This may require use of sedation and chemical paralysis, which is complicated by a patient's hypotension. Unfortunately, this intervention often elevates peak airway pressures even when sedation and chemical paralysis are used. The concern about elevated airway pressures producing barotrauma is not warranted in the setting of ACS because the transalveolar pressure is the important factor. In this setting, the elevated airway pressures are not a result of overdistension of alveoli from the ventilator but are due to elevated pressures from the ACS pushing against the lung. The transmural plateau pressure takes into account the IAP and is calculated by subtracting the half the IAP from the plateau pressure. This is the value that should be kept below 30 cm H_2O to 35 cm H_2O if lung-protective strategies are used.[3–5]

The acidotic pH affects cardiac function and the heart's ability to respond to pressors. Given the patient's poor cardiac function, the administration of HCO3 to elevate the pH may benefit cardiac function. Furthermore, on opening the abdomen, there is often a washout of lactate that further drops the pH, which could lead to further myocardial depression that may be fatal. The addition of epinephrine to improve cardiac contractility is necessary given the low cardiac output and hypotension. Dobutamine may contribute to reflex hypotension, which may be detrimental in this setting. Although it is tempting to use dobutamine, because of the elevated PAPs, the observed elevated pressure is not because of intrinsic pulmonary artery hypertension but is a reflection of elevated intrathoracic pressure. Dobutamine or milrinone can reduce intrinsic pulmonary vascular resistance but would have no effect on this patient's elevated intrathoracic pressure.

Treatment of IAH and the ACS begins with medical interevntions but requires a decompressive laparotomy for definitive management.

In summary, pressure-directed resuscitation and ventilator management must take into account the effect of transmitted IAH to the thoracic cavity. Volume-based monitoring should be used in terms of cardiac function and resuscitation because this approach correlates better with cardiac function. Treatment aims to improve tissue perfusion by improving cardiopulmonary function. When medical interventions fail, surgical intervention is immediate decompressive laparotomy.

CASE 2: PULMONARY HYPERTENSION

A 70-year-old man with a history of pulmonary hypertension was in a motor vehicle crash 24 hours ago. He is intubated for hypoxia and tachypnea with multiple rib fractures. His HR is 120, BP 90/60, and urine output is 10 15 mL/h to 15 mL/h. Chest radiograph shows bilateral patchy infiltrates, PAP is 68/40, CI 1.8 is L/min, and CVP is 18. Transesophageal echocardiogram shows a distended right ventricle with global hypokinesis worse in the right ventricle, indicative of cardiac contusion. His ventilator is set at a tidal volume of 600 mL, respiratory rate 16, FiO_2 60%, and PEEP 14 with an ABG pH 7.25, PcO_2 50, PO_2 90, HCO3 20, and lactate 3. He is started on ECMO and his lungs eventually recover, but when attempts are made to decannulate, his CI drops to 1.8 L/min, HR increases to 120 bpm, BP is 150/100, mixed venous oxygen saturation (Svo_2) drops to 50%, CVP is 5 cm H_2O, pulmonary wedge pressure increases to 24 cm H_2O, and systemic vascular resistance (SVR) is 4440 dyn*s/cm^5.

This case illustrates the complexities of managing patients with underlying cardiac disease—in this case pulmonary hypertension—complicated by pulmonary contusion and tissue hypoperfusion. The goals of management for this patient are to (1) improve tissue perfusion, (2) minimize further lung injury, and (3) minimize the difference between myocardial oxygen demands and contractility.

ACUTE MANAGEMENT OF PULMONARY HYPERTENSION

Patients who have evidence of pulmonary hypertension, defined as a pulmonary artery diastolic pressure greater than 15 mm Hg and a pulmonary systolic pressure greater than 25 mm Hg in the setting of chest trauma, pose unique challenges. To optimize perfusion without increasing the difference between myocardial oxygen demands and cardiac contractility, the right ventricular end-diastolic pressure must be reduced. Overdistension of the right ventricle must be avoided to optimize right ventricular function and minimize the effects of right ventricular distension on left ventricular function. These 2 goals are accomplished if pulmonary vascular resistance is reduced.

Minimizing hypoxia and acidosis helps reduce pulmonary vascular resistance, so Fio_2 may need to be increased to minimize pulmonary vasoconstriction that reflexively occurs with hypoxia. The net effect of high PEEP, however, may reduce tissue perfusion due to increasing pulmonary vascular resistance, which worsens right ventricular function. Therefore, accepting higher Fio_2 and minimizing PEEP if the elevated PEEP leads to a reduced CI may be necessary.

Ventilator strategies that minimize intrathoracic pressure are necessary to facilitate right ventricular function by minimizing pulmonary vascular resistance. Keeping intrathoracic pressures low also avoids barotrauma to the lung, reducing the inflammatory response within the lung. Reducing tidal volumes and accepting a higher Pco_2 (permissive hypercapnea) achieve this goal. Care must be taken that the acidosis does not diminish cardiac function. At times, the use of an HCO3 solution to combat the acidosis may be necessary during the acute resuscitation. Finally, pharmacologic reduction of the pulmonary pressures may be achieved with inotropes, such as dobutamine or milrinone, while simultaneously augmenting contractility.[6]

Inhaled nitric oxide (iNO) therapy also provides a pharmacologically rational approach in that it reduces ventilation-perfusion mismatch due to preferential vasodilation of the pulmonary capillaries that perfuse alveoli that are sufficiently distended to receive the inhaled nitric oxide. This improves oxygenation while reducing pulmonary vascular resistance and, hence, offloads the right ventricle. Dosing of iNO, according to the guidelines of the European Society of Cardiology, involves iNO at 10 ppm to 20 ppm for 5 minutes. They defined vasoreactivity as a reduction of mean PAP greater than or equal to 10 mm Hg to reach an absolute value of mean PAP of less than 40 mm Hg with an increased or unchanged cardiac output.[7] Despite these physiologic benefits, there are insufficient data to support the routine use of inhaled nitric oxide in this clinical setting because there are no large prospective studies showing that this affects mortality. Thereafter, oral agents, such as phosphodiesterase inhibitors (sildenafil), can be used for long-term management and should be overlapped with iNO.

Pulmonary hypertension affects cardiac function. Improving oxygenation with high Fio_2, keeping intrathoracic pressure low using low tidal volumes, and vasoactive drugs to lower pulmonary pressures are all treatment options.

EXTRACORPOREAL MEMBRANE OXYGENATION

The benefits of ECMO are 2-fold: ECMO provides the ability to oxygenate the blood in the setting of pulmonary damage and it reduces right ventricular preload, thereby reducing right ventricular end-diastolic volume and pressure. The latter effect is important for patients who have borderline right ventricular function at baseline, which cannot compensate for additional increases in pulmonary vascular resistance and volume resuscitation. If such conditions develop, as in the previously described case, and are temporary or reversible, then the use of ECMO may be warranted.[8] Several case series and a randomized trial describe the use of ECMO in patients with severe acute lung injury with improved survival.[8–10] The use of ECMO also reduces the amount of ventilator support required and, therefore, ventilator pressures can be reduced, which further augment right ventricular function.[9]

Previous randomized controlled trials of ECMO enrolled patients who had severe hypoxemia (P_{AO_2}:F_{IO_2} <0.2). Patients with bleeding disorders, recent cerebrovascular accident or gastrointestinal hemorrhage, evidence of traumatic brain injury, or severe underlying nonreversible systemic disease that greatly limits the likelihood of survival were excluded.[11,12] Typically, femoral-femoral or femoral-jugular cannulae are inserted for venovenous ECMO and heparinization is required to keep partial thromboplastin time between 45 seconds and 60 seconds.[13] In patients with left ventricular dysfunction, venoarterial ECMO is indicated.

Settings of mechanical ventilation for patients on venovenous ECMO should minimize ventilator-associated lung injury and permit higher degrees of protective lung ventilation. High PEEP levels (>10 cm H_2O) should be maintained to prevent further lung collapse after the institution of ECMO. Blood oxygenation and decarboxylation through the ECMO circuit also allow tidal volume reduction to limit plateau pressure (suggested plateau pressure <25 cm H_2O). F_{IO_2} on the ventilator should be reduced to the minimal value to keep arterial saturation greater than 85%.[13]

Weaning of venovenous ECMO should be considered when pulmonary function has improved, as indicated by higher lung compliance (increasing tidal volumes on pressure controlled ventilation), resolving lung infiltrates, and improvement in arterial P_{CO_2} and P_{O_2}. Mechanical ventilation should be set to lung-protective levels of support (eg, tidal volume 6 mL/kg, plateau pressure <30 cm H_2O, PEEP 8–12 cm H_2O, and F_{IO_2} <60%). Then the fresh gas flow to the oxygenator can be switched off while maintaining previous blood flow through the circuit. If a patient remains stable and adequately ventilated after a few hours of observation, and if echocardiography reveals no evidence of severe acute cor pulmonale, ECMO cannulae can be simply pulled out. Other methods of weaning include gradual decreasing of the level of ECMO support.[13]

ELEVATED SYSTEMIC VASCULAR RESISTANCE

In the case described, the patient is unable to come off ECMO, demonstrating signs of left ventricular overload with an elevated pulmonary wedge pressure. The management of left ventricular failure requires reduction in preload, a reduction in afterload, and an increase in contractility when preload and afterload manipulation have been optimized. Preload reduction with diuresis may facilitate ECMO discontinuation. Patients with diastolic heart failure are usually difficult to wean from the ventilator due to cardiogenic pulmonary edema because ventilator pressures are reduced, leading to increased flow to the left ventricle. The treatment of these patients aims at reducing pulmonary venous pressure and congestion, and such treatment usually requires diuretic therapy. Aggressive diuresis may result in serious hypotension in patients with diastolic heart failure because of the steepness of the curve of left ventricular diastolic pressure in relation to volume. Moreover, tachycardia may cause insufficient time for complete relaxation, resulting in an increase in diastolic pressure that compromises left ventricular filling, leading to elevated left-sided filling pressures. Therefore, afterload reduction should be used when possible to manage the elevated SVR. SVR is a calculated value ([MAP - CVP] $\times$ 80/CO), where *MAP* is mean arterial pressure and *CO* is cardiac output. Therefore, afterload elevation may not be the cause of the increased SVR but instead may be the result of a substantial drop in cardiac output. When SVR increases are due to the latter, contractility agents, such as epinephrine, are necessary. Agents, such as dobutamine or milrinone, have the added advantage of reducing afterload while simultaneously increasing contractility and should be used in the case described.

Ventricular dysfunction can be managed with reduction in preload by mechanical means when pharmacologic means fail.

REFERENCES

1. Malbrain ML, Ameloot K, Gillebert C, et al. Cardiopulmonary monitoring in intra-abdominal hypertension. Am Surg 2011;77(Suppl 1):S23–30.
2. Ameloot K, Gillebert C, Desie N, et al. Hypoperfusion, shock states, and abdominal compartment syndrome (ACS). Surg Clin North Am 2012;92(2):207–20.
3. Papavramidis TS, Marinis AD, Pliakos I, et al. Abdominal compartment syndrome—intra-abdominal hypertension: defining, diagnosing, and managing. J Emerg Trauma Shock 2011;4(2):279–91.
4. Chang MC, Miller PR, D'Agostino R Jr, et al. Effects of abdominal decompression on cardiopulmonary function and visceral perfusion in patients with intra-abdominal hypertension. J Trauma 1998;44(3):440–5.
5. Cheatham ML, Malbrain ML, Kirkpatrick A, et al. Results from the International Conference of Experts on Intra-abdominal Hypertension and Abdominal Compartment Syndrome. II. Recommendations. Intensive Care Med 2007;33(6):951–62.
6. Subramaniam K, Yared JP. Management of pulmonary hypertension in the operating room. Semin Cardiothorac Vasc Anesth 2007;11(2):119–36 Review.
7. Gruenig E, Michelakis E, Vachiéry JL, et al. Acute hemodynamic effects of single-dose sildenafil when added to established bosentan therapy in patients with pulmonary arterial hypertension: results of the COMPASS-1 study. J Clin Pharmacol 2009;49:1343–52.
8. Cordell-Smith JA, Roberts N, Peek GJ, et al. Traumatic lung injury treated by extracorporeal membrane oxygenation (ECMO). Injury 2006;37(1):29–32.
9. Madershahian N, Wittwer T, Strauch J, et al. Application of ECMO in multitrauma patients with ARDS as rescue therapy. J Card Surg 2007;22(3):180–4.
10. Peek GJ, Elbourne D, Mugford M, et al. Randomised controlled trial and parallel economic evaluation of conventional ventilatory support versus extracorporeal membrane oxygenation for severe adult respiratory failure (CESAR). Health Technol Assess 2010;14(35):1–46.
11. Morris AH, Wallace CJ, Menlove RL. Randomized clinical trial of pressure-controlled inverse ratio ventilation and extracorporeal CO2 removal for adult respiratory distress syndrome. Am J Respir Crit Care Med 1994;149(2 Pt 1):295–305.
12. Australia and New Zealand Extracorporeal Membrane Oxygenation (ANZ ECMO) Influenza Investigators, Davies A, Jones D, Bailey M, et al. Extracorporeal membrane oxygenation for 2009 influenza A(H1N1) acute respiratory distress syndrome. JAMA 2009;302(17):1888–95.
13. Combes A, Bacchetta M, Brodie D, et al. Extracorporeal membrane oxygenation for respiratory failure in adults. Curr Opin Crit Care 2012;18(1):99–104.

Index

Note: Page numbers of article titles are in **boldface** type.

A

Abdominal compartment pressure monitoring
    in ICU, 1397–1398
Abdominal compartment syndrome
    case study, 1679–1681
Acute hypertension
    in SICU
        treatment of, 1591–1595
Acute kidney injury (AKI), **1503–1511**
    biomarkers in, 1506–1507
    defined, 1503–1504
    diagnostic approach to, 1505–1506
    differential diagnosis of, 1507–1511
    imaging in, 1507
    medication review in, 1507
    RIFLE criteria for, 1504
Acute respiratory distress syndrome (ARDS)
    ventilator strategies for, 1467–1472
        corticosteroids, 1469
        ECMO, 1471–1472
        fluid management–related, 1468–1469
        HFOV, 1471
        inhaled vasodilators, 1469–1470
        low tidal volume ventilation, 1467–1468
        PEEP, 1468
        prone positioning in, 1470–1471
        recruitment maneuvers, 1468
        salvage therapies, 1469
Adenosine
    for ventricular arrhythmias in SICU, 1597
Advance directives
    critically ill patient–related, 1639
Airway pressure release ventilation (APRV), 1467
Airway swelling
    during weaning and extubation, 1480
AKI. *See* Acute kidney injury (AKI)
Aminoglycosides
    in SICU, 1604
Amiodarone
    for atrial fibrillation in SICU, 1596

Surg Clin N Am 92 (2012) 1685–1705
http://dx.doi.org/10.1016/S0039-6109(12)00219-8
0039-6109/12/$ – see front matter © 2012 Elsevier Inc. All rights reserved.

surgical.theclinics.com

Moving?

Make sure your subscription moves with you!

To notify us of your new address, find your **Clinics Account Number** (located on your mailing label above your name), and contact customer service at:

Email: journalscustomerservice-usa@elsevier.com

800-654-2452 (subscribers in the U.S. & Canada)
314-447-8871 (subscribers outside of the U.S. & Canada)

Fax number: 314-447-8029

Elsevier Health Sciences Division
Subscription Customer Service
3251 Riverport Lane
Maryland Heights, MO 63043

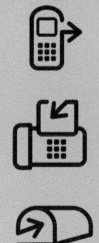

Moving?

Make sure your subscription moves with you!

To notify us of your new address, find your Clinics Account Number (located on your mailing label above your name), and contact customer service at:

Email: journalscustomerservice-usa@elsevier.com

800-654-2452 (subscribers in the U.S. & Canada)
314-447-8871 (subscribers outside of the U.S. & Canada)

Fax number: 314-447-8029

Elsevier Health Sciences Division
Subscription Customer Service
3251 Riverport Lane
Maryland Heights, MO 63043

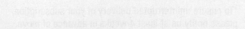

To ensure uninterrupted delivery of your subscription, please notify us at least 4 weeks in advance of move.

Printed and bound by CPI Group (UK) Ltd, Croydon, CR0 4YY

03/10/2024

01040431-0009